49.50

OSTEOARTHROMECHANICS

Editor

Dhanjoo N. Ghista, Ph.D.
McMaster University

⬤ Hemisphere Publishing Corporation
Washington New York London

McGraw-Hill Book Company
New York St. Louis San Francisco Auckland Bogotá
Guatemala Hamburg Johannesburg Lisbon London Madrid Mexico
Montreal New Delhi Panama Paris San Juan São Paulo
Singapore Sydney Tokyo Toronto

To Him, Lord Ananda Murtiji,
to my father, the late Dr. Noshir R. Ghista,
and to my mother, Khorshed N. Ghista

NOTICE

Medicine is an ever-changing science. As new research and clinical experience broaden our knowledge, changes in treatment and drug therapy are required. The editors and the publisher of this work have made every effort to ensure that the drug dosage schedules herein are accurate and in accord with the standards accepted at the time of publication. Readers are advised, however, to check the product information sheet included in the package of each drug they plan to administer to be certain that changes have not been made in the recommended dose or in the contraindications for administration. This recommendation is of particular importance in regard to new or infrequently used drugs.

This book was set in Press Roman by Hemisphere Publishing Corporation. The editors were Valerie M. Ziobro, Edward Millman, and J. Dereck Jeffers; the production supervisor was Miriam Gonzalez.
R. R. Donnelley & Sons Company was printer and binder.

OSTEOARTHROMECHANICS

1 2 3 4 5 6 7 8 9 0 D O D O 8 9 8 7 6 5 4 3 2 1

Library of Congress Cataloging in Publication Data
Main entry under title:

Osteoarthromechanics.

   Includes bibliographies and index.
   1. Orthopedia. 2. Bone. 3. Joints (Anatomy)
4. Human mechanics. I. Ghista, Dhanjoo N.
RD732.085   617'.3   81-6513
ISBN 0-07-023168-0   AACR2

CONTENTS

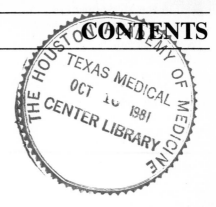

CONTRIBUTORS

THOMAS P. ANDRIACCHI, Ph.D.
Department of Orthopedic Surgery
Rush-Presbyterian—St. Luke's Medical
  Center
Chicago, Illinois

R. COLLINS, Ph.D.
Department of Medical Biophysics
Université Paul Sabatier
Toulouse Cedex, France

DHANJOO N. GHISTA, Ph.D.
Departments of Medicine
  and Biomedical Engineering
McMaster University
Hamilton, Ontario, Canada

STEVEN J. HAMPTON, Ph.D.
Department of Orthopedic Surgery
Rush-Presbyterian—St. Luke's Medical
  Center
Chicago, Illinois

RAE R. JACOBS, M.D.
Department of Orthopedic Surgery
University of Kansas Medical Center
Kansas City, Kansas

H. B. KINGSBURY, Ph.D.
Department of Mechanical and Aerospace
  Engineering
University of Delaware
Newark, Delaware

J. E. LONSTEIN, M.D.
Twin Cities Scoliosis Center
Minneapolis, Minnesota

J. L. NOWINSKI, Ph.D.
Department of Mechanical and Aerospace
  Engineering
University of Delaware
Newark, Delaware

JAMES PUGH, Ph.D.
Division of Bioengineering
Hospital for Joint Diseases
Orthopaedic Institute
New York, New York

GORDON C. ROBIN, M.D.
Orthopedics Department
Hadassah University Hospital
Jerusalem, Israel

SUBRATA SAHA, Ph.D.
Department of Orthopedics
Louisiana State University Medical Center
Shreveport, Louisiana

A. W. M. SCHIJVENS, Ph.D.
Department of Mechanical Engineering
Eindhoven University of Technology
Eindhoven, Holland

J. M. SEROO, Ph.D.
Department of Mechanical Engineering
Eindhoven University of Technology
Eindhoven, Holland

J. G. N. SNIJDER, Ph.D.
Department of Mechanical Engineering
Eindhoven University of Technology
Eindhoven, Holland

C. J. SNIJDERS, Ph.D.
Department of Mechanical Engineering
Eindhoven University of Technology
Eindhoven, Holland

LARS SONNERUP, Ph.D.
Department of Mechanical Engineering
Chalmers Institute of Technology
Goteborg, Sweden

PETER S. WALKER, Ph.D.
Orthopedics Division
Howmedica, Inc.
Rutherford, New Jersey

R. B. WINTER, M.D.
Twin Cities Scoliosis Center
Minneapolis, Minnesota

ZVI YOSIPOVITCH, M.D.
Orthopedics Department
Hadassah University Hospital
Jerusalem, Israel

PREFACE

Joint and spine disorders and failures constitute a major category of crippling problems, the understanding and treatment of which would benefit considerably from a biomechanical inquiry. Hence, it was decided to prepare a book on (1) a quantitative biomechanical elucidation of joint and spine functions and failures and (2) biomechanical design analyses of their correctional, fixation, and replacement devices.

This volume describes the mechanics of bone strength under physiologically representative dynamic loading, explaining how bone strength is impaired by holes and perforations induced by fixation devices. Joint lubrication and assessment of joints, including the mechanical factors in osteoarthritis, are discussed, along with the design criteria and analyses of artificial joints. Comprehensive coverage is given to the mechanical assessment of spinal function and disorders, as well as to the criteria, techniques, and devices used to correct spinal deformities and fractures.

The underlying theme of the book is to demonstrate how mechanics fundamentals and rigor can be invoked to provide quantitative analyses of joint and spine mechanisms, disorders, and prosthetic devices. The mechanics treatment of the material requires undergraduate level knowledge of structural mechanics, elasticity theory, lubrication theory, and finite element techniques. The book could serve as a major reference book for a biomechanics course, as well as a resource book for a biomechanical perspective of joint and spine mechanisms, disorders, and treatment.

ACKNOWLEDGMENTS

When primitive people first started realizing that physical force bowed down to psychic force, they began to wonder about the source from which they derived their psychic strength. That query marked a fundamental step in the true "evolution" of humankind. Thereafter, as people entered the "inner" world, they became increasingly obsessed with their internal imperfections, until they started pondering whether if by consolidating their psychic propensities they were to merge with that Supreme Power, would they not have permanent liberation from their imperfections? That was the second fundamental query of humankind.

Thus, from time immemorial, the noble aspects of the history of human existence have been sagas of struggle to attain macrocosmic statehood. Human evolution, as recognized in the conventional sense, merely constitutes manifestation of the physicopsychic changes that have accompanied this noble march—this inner march. It took thousands of years of evolution for this second fundamental query to occur to humans. But today's people do not have to struggle in quest of the answers to these fundamental queries. By the grace of Lord Ananda Murtiji, today's people are blessed to be afforded that realization and the means of moving toward their Supreme Desideratum.

Dhanjoo N. Ghista

CHAPTER ONE

THE DYNAMIC STRENGTH OF BONE
AND ITS RELEVANCE

Subrata Saha

Characterization of the tolerance limits of bone is important to safety engineers who are interested in the prevention of bone fracture. This chapter reviews the existing literature on the dynamic and impact properties of standardized bone specimens and whole bones. The tensile impact properties of bone and their relation to microstructure are discussed in detail. The fractographic analysis of bone fracture surfaces to determine the micromechanics of bone fracture is also described.

1 INTRODUCTION (NEED AND JUSTIFICATION)

The mechanical properties of bone have been more extensively investigated than those of any other biological tissue materials. Although our understanding of the mechanical properties and fracture behavior of bone is continuously improving, as yet it is far from complete. The area most lacking in information is the strength properties of bone in dynamic-loading situations—the subject of this chapter.

At present there is mounting concern for the improvement of safety and reduction of injury levels in accidents associated with high-speed transportation, industrial work, and recreational activities. Bone fracture is a common form of

This chapter was written during the time Dr. Saha was a faculty member of the Department of Engineering and Applied Science, Yale University, New Haven, Connecticut.

The author wishes to express his sincere appreciation to Prof. W. C. Hayes of Stanford University for his advice and encouragement during this investigation.

injury in such accidents. Therefore, engineers are interested in the tolerance limits of bones subjected to impact loads, for example, in an automobile accident, because such tolerance data are essential for the rational design of safety features to prevent bone fractures in the design of crashworthy vehicles. Basic information on the response and tolerance limits of human tissue must be obtained before the specifications for a safe design can even be formulated. Furthermore, if protective systems are to be optimally designed, it is important that tolerance data be obtained as accurately as possible. The tolerance limits of bone should also be established for a variety of design parameters such as velocity of impact and force duration, and for such biological factors as injury site, age, and sex.

The forces sustained by the human skeletal structure in vehicular and recreational accidents are characterized by abrupt onset, short duration, and high magnitude. However, the current state of knowledge concerning human impact tolerance is incomplete, and very few data are available on the tolerance limits of individual body components against localized impacts. Evans [1] observed that

> The chief conclusion to be drawn from a survey of the available literature is the need for more controlled studies of the impact tolerance of human bones in the intact body. This is especially important with respect to relatively low velocity impacts, as in the second collision in car and airplane crashes. Such data is badly needed by the safety engineer in many different fields.

The dynamic strength of bone is important because most bone fractures occur under dynamic-loading conditions. Moreover, all the bones in our bodies are constantly subjected to dynamic external loads, owing to our movements. Intrinsic muscle forces of changing magnitude also act constantly on the bones of our skeletal system. These dynamic forces affect the growth and remodeling activities of bone, as postulated by Wolff's law, and its electrical and chemical activities [2 to 4]. Thus the dynamic properties of bone are also of interest to orthopedic surgeons, anatomists, and many other biomedical scientists.

The dynamic properties of bone can be investigated at various levels of organization. One can investigate the forces acting on the whole body to determine their effect on the skeletal structure [5]. For instance, in studying the pilot-ejection problem, one can investigate the effects of rapid acceleration and deceleration on the spinal column [6]. At the next levels of organization, one can test whole bones and bone as a tissue material, using standardized test samples of bone. At a microstructural level, one can also test single osteons, as has been done by Ascenzi and his co-workers [7, 8]. For complete understanding of the dynamic behavior of bone, it is necessary to attack this problem at all these levels. Until now, the majority of the work has been in the testing of whole bones [9], with some work being done using standardized bone specimens [10]. No information is as yet available on the dynamic strength of bone at a microstructural level.

Because of the presence of submicroscopic channels and cavities in its structure (e.g., Haversian canals, resorption cavities, etc.), bone, like most other brittle materials, is weak in tension, as tensile stress tends to propagate these cracks, which are perpendicular to the axis of principal tensile stress. Rixford [11], on the basis of clinical experience, also pointed out the importance of tension in the fracture mechanisms of long bones. By using brittle coating methods, Evans and his colleagues [12, 13] demonstrated that most bone fractures occur in tension under both static and impact loads. Therefore, it is surprising to note that although the impact tolerance of whole bones and the dynamic strength of standardized bone specimens have been investigated in modes other than tension [14 to 18], no attempt has been made to determine the tensile impact strength of compact bone at high loading rates.

The objectives of the present investigation were therefore to provide data on the tensile impact strength and elastic properties of bone and to correlate these with microstructure and fracture-surface topography. Instrumented impact testing was used to record load-time histories throughout impact, which allowed the calculation of dynamic mechanical properties during failure. This has a significant advantage over conventional impact testing, which provides only the total energy to fracture.

The energy to fracture is a function of the force times the distance through which the force operates. Two materials may have properties that result in equal tensile impact energies from the same specimen geometry, arising in one from a large force associated with a small elongation and in the other from a small force associated with a large elongation. This investigation showed that bone samples having equivalent failure-energy readings could yield very different characteristic load-elongation or stress-strain curves. The use of a single number, the total energy to fracture, without consideration of how the energy is absorbed, may thus be misleading when the data are applied in a design.

It has been shown previously that the mechanical properties of bone are rate sensitive [17, 19, 20]. In this investigation, the static tensile strength of bone was compared with the tensile impact strength to explore the strain-rate sensitivity of compact bone. Some notched samples were also tested in tensile impact, to determine the effect of a notch on impact tolerance.

Because changes in bone microstructure can be expected to influence the mechanical properties of bone, attempts were made to correlate the dynamic strength properties of bone with its microstructure. To gain further insight into the influence of microstructure on fracture strength and to study the micromechanics of bone fracture, fractographic analysis of the tested specimens was also performed.

2   STRUCTURE OF BONE

To understand the micromechanics of bone fracture and the influence of bone microstructure on its mechanical properties, it is almost a prerequisite to study the biological structure of bone. The microstructure of bone is well documented in the medical literature [21 to 26].

The adult human skeleton is composed of 206 bones, which on the basis of shapes can be classified as long (humerus, radius, and ulna in the upper extremity, and femur, tibia, and fibula in the lower extremity), short (bones of the wrist and ankle, and sesamoid bones), flat (bones of the cranium, the scapula, and the ribs), or irregular (vertebrae). On the basis of gross structure, bone tissue is either compact (the hard, dense outside layer of all bones; also called cortical bone) or cancellous (like a sponge, containing many small cavities that are filled with marrow; also called spongy or trabecular bone).

2.1 Microstructure of Bone

Bone is an osseous form of connective tissue, distinguished by its hardness, which results from the deposition of a calcareous inorganic material in a complex crystalline form within a fine organic matrix of collagen fibers. The most characteristic feature of adult bone tissue is its lamellar structure, the collagen fibers and the calcified matrix being organized in thin layers of lamellae (4 to 12 μm thick) arranged in various ways. In most cases, the collagen fibers in each layer have a dominant direction that is different from those in adjacent layers, and the lamellation is a result of this differing orientation of the collagen fibrils in each of the superimposed lamellae [27].

In general, the central shaft (diaphysis) of a long bone consists of several layers of inner and outer circumferential lamellae enclosing a middle zone of longitudinally oriented osteons. An osteon can be defined as an irregular, branching, and anastomosing cylinder composed of a more or less centrally placed neurovascular canal (5 to 100 μm in diameter) surrounded by concentric, cell-permeated lamellae of bone matrix [28]. Osteons have often been described as the basic unit structure of compact bone [22, 25, 29, 30]. But this unit-structure idea is often overemphasized, and although much of the adult human compact bone is composed of osteons, contrary to popular belief, osteons are almost totally absent from the bones of many species, e.g., white rats [31]. Compact beef bone samples were also found to be predominantly nonsteonal in character [32].

As a part of the continuous remodeling activity in living bone, bone-destroying cells (osteoclasts) enlarge some of the existing vascular canals to form resorption cavities. Subsequently, bone-forming cells (osteoblasts) deposit concentric layers of bone matrix in the resorption cavity, replacing it with a new osteon, called a *secondary osteon* or *Haversian system*. This osteon is termed secondary because it replaces an existing form of bone. Figure 1 is a photomicrograph of a transverse section of a compact bone specimen showing secondary oesteons and a resorption cavity.

Compact bone has several anastomosing vessel systems that carry nutrients to the bone cells (osteocytes). The most important of these is the central canals (Haversian canals, Fig. 1) of osteons, which communicate with each other and with the marrow cavity through transverse Volkmann's canals. The osteocytes live within minute lenticular cavities, called lacunae, and receive their nutrients through a system of numerous interconnecting minute channels called canaliculi, some of which also extend up to the Haversian and Volkmann's canals.

2.2 Ultrastructure of Bone

The ultrastructure of bone is beyond the range of the optical microscope, and thus most ultrastructural study has been accomplished recently with the use of the

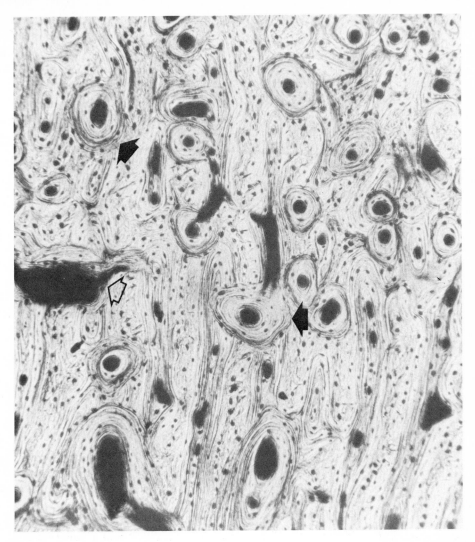

Figure 1 Microstructure of a compact beef bone specimen showing secondary osteons with Haversian canals at its centers (dark arrows) and a resorption cavity (open arrow).

electron microscope and with x-ray diffraction analysis. The dry weight of bone is composed of 60 to 75 percent inorganic hydroxyapatite (both crystals and amorphous) and 25 to 35 percent organic matrix. Collagen accounts for as much as 90 to 97 percent of the organic matrix, the remainder being amorphous ground substance, mainly mucopolysaccharides. Individual collagen fibers are about 500 to 2000 Å thick, several micrometers in length, and have cross striations at about 640-Å spacings. The hydroxyapatite crystals are deposited around the periphery of the collagen fibers, with their C axes parallel to the long axis of the collagen fibrils. The exact nature of the bonding between the collagen and the hydroxyapatite is now known. Controversy also exists about the size and shape of apatite crystals. It is generally believed that they are 200 to 400 Å long and 10 to 50 Å in width or in diameter, depending on whether the crystals are believed to be plates or needles.

It is important to note that marked variations are found in the microscopic structure of bone among different animals, among different bones of the same individual, and among different areas of the same bone. The characteristic microscopic appearance of constantly remodeling bone tissue reflects its response to both structural and biochemical demands and can be explained in terms of the growth process. It should also be noted that, although bone is created and maintained by living cells, bone is primarily a nonliving substance composed of collagen fibers and hydroxyapatite crystals.

3   THE PRESENT STATE OF KNOWLEDGE

The present state of knowledge of the mechanical properties of bone has been well reviewed by Evans [9, 10], Kraus [29], Swanson [33], Currey [34], and Herrmann and Liebowitz [35]. Because the subject of this chapter is the dynamic strength of bone in tension, this section reviews previous investigations of the static tensile and dynamic properties of bone. Reviews are presented of (1) the static tensile strength of bone; (2) the dynamic properties and fracture characteristics of bone; and (3) the impact tolerance of whole bones.

3.1   Tensile Strength of Bone

The first systematic studies of the mechanical properties of bone were conducted by Wertheim [36]. He tested strips of compact bone from femurs and fibulas of fresh cadavers aged 1 to 74 yr. He found no correlation between tensile strength and age but did find the average ultimate tensile strength (UTS) for males to be 13,200 lb/in², and for females 9540 lb/in². In 1876, Rauber [37] took fresh longitudinal samples of cortical bone from the middle diaphysis of the human humerus, femur, and tibia and found their average UTS to be 14,560 (8,880 to 18,670) lb/in², 17,640 (15,110 to 24,170) lb/in², and 12,850 (8,170 to 18,840) lb/in², respectively. A third investigation, by Hulsen [38], used dry human femurs and indicated an average UTS of 16,850 (14,260 to 21,720) lb/in².

More recently, Carothers [39] determined the ultimate tensile strength of samples from the femoral diaphysis of embalmed cadavers and found it to average 22,000 (16,600 to 31,500) lb/in². Evans and Lebow [12, 40] studied embalmed human cortical samples and found that the middle third of the shaft had not only the greatest ultimate tensile strength, modulus of elasticity, and hardness but also the greatest percentage elongation under tension. Wet samples (rehydrated) always showed a greater percentage elongation than did dry ones from the same region. Comparative studies show the tibia to have the greatest average tensile strength, and the fibula the greatest percentage elongation under tension.

Another study to determine ultimate tensile strength was performed by Dempster and Liddicoat [41]. Their samples, from femurs, tibiae, and humeri, gave values of $11,428 \pm 1,540$ lb/in^2 for wet bone and $17,090 \pm 3,940$ lb/in^2 for dry bone. Dempster and Coleman [42] obtained tensile strength data along and across the grain from museum specimens of the human tibia and mandible (dry and water soaked). The cross-grain UTS ranged from about 8 to 16 percent less than the parallel-to-grain strength.

Evans [43], in a comprehensive study of the tensile strength of human compact bone, tested 394 embalmed femoral and 192 tibial specimens under wet conditions and compared the results with tests of unembalmed and dry specimens. Some of his conclusions were: (1) embalmed wet- and dry-tested tibias are stronger than unembalmed specimens; (2) specimens from the middle third of the femoral diaphysis are stronger than those from the proximal shaft; (3) unembalmed dry-tested femurs are stronger than wet-tested femurs.

Sedlin [19] and Sedlin and Hirsch [44] performed a series of tests on human cortical bone to determine the effects of temperature, humidity, fixation method, and sample-size variation on the mechanical properties of bone. Currey [45] tested bovine specimens in tension and concluded that bone containing Haversian systems has less tensile strength than bone with no Haversian systems. Currey's work is discussed in more detail in the section on the influence of microstructure.

In a recent study, Sweeney et al. [46] obtained the mechanical properties of decalcified beef bone. The mean ultimate tensile strength was 18,660 (14,300 to 22,300) lb/in^2 in the longitudinal direction. In the transverse direction the UTS was only 8135 (6,840 to 10,500) lb/in^2. This difference in strength in different directions again emphasizes the anisotropic nature of bone. Their result also showed that bone is of lower strength than collagen fibers. This is similar to the difference between the strength of structural materials and that of single crystals.

Hirsch and Evans [47] are the only authors to report on the mechanical properties of infant compact bone. They tested standarized specimens from the femurs of infants (newborn to 6 mo of age) and from a 14-yr-old boy and obtained higher ultimate tensile stress and strain than those of fresh specimens from adult femurs. They also noted that the range of variation in the modulus of elasticity of specimens from infants was considerably less than that of similar specimens from adult bones.

Previous investigations of the mechanical properties of bone display a wide scatter in the data reported by different authors [29]. Wall et al. [48] dwelt on the origin of this scatter in bone strength tests and have listed a number of factors that may influence the results of such tests. The factors influencing the mechanical properties of bone are discussed in a later section. Table 1 lists bone ultimate tensile strengths as determined by different investigators and illustrates the wide range of values obtained.

The ultimate tensile stress of bone is an important mechanical property in any consideration of bone as a material. Traditionally, static tensile strength has been used as a criterion for judging the quality of metals. Similarly, the ultimate tensile stress of bone can be used as a parameter for judging the bone quality—for instance, to determine the effect of nutrition on bone strength. Static tensile strength also provides a baseline with which the ultimate stresses at various strain rates can be compared. As the maximum stress of bone generally increases with strain rate (see

Table 1 Bone ultimate tensile strengths

Index	Bone	Reference	Samples		Ultimate tensile strength (kg/mm²)		Specimen source, etc.
			No.	Condition	Average	Range	
A							
(a)	Femur (proximal)			Wet	7.91	4.91–10.09	Only cortical bone used–all spongy bone removed. Bone obtained from Caucasian males 47–81 yr of age.
				Dry	10.59	6.35–15.09	
(b)	Femur (middle)			Wet	8.48	6.92–10.89	
				Dry	11.35	6.55–15.11	
(c)	Femur (distal)			Wet	8.25	6.55–10.89	
				Dry	10.56	6.15–14.19	
(d)	Femur (anterior)	[12]		Wet	7.99	6.36–10.75	
				Dry	10.12	6.55–13.95	
(e)	Femur (posterior)			Wet	8.16	5.96–10.68	
				Dry	11.04	7.31–14.76	
(f)	Femur (medial)			Wet	8.20	4.91–9.91	
				Dry	11.21	6.76–15.11	
(g)	Femur (lateral)			Wet	8.51	7.18–10.00	
				Dry	11.32	8.67–14.67	
(h)	Femur (overall)		141	Wet	8.32	4.91–10.89	
			141	Dry	10.77	6.14–15.11	
B							
(a)	Tibia	[42]	10	Wet	9.2 ± 2.7		Rectangular test piece cut parallel to grain.
			20	Dry	14.01 ± 2.2		
(b)	Tibia	[42]	1	Wet	9.18		Circular test piece cut parallel to grain.
			6	Dry	13.45 ± 2.2		
(c)	Tibia	[42]	9	Wet	1.00 ± 0.29		Rectangular test piece cut across the grain.
			20	Dry	1.15 ± 0.33		Bones from an osteological collection–no details known.

	Bone	Ref	n	Wet/Dry	Value	Range	Notes
C							
(a)	Femur	[44]	16	Wet	9.9 ± 1.5		62-yr-old male.
(b)	Femur		10	Wet	8.3 ± 1.6		67-yr-old male.
(c)	Femur		8	Wet	8.0		34-yr-old male.
(d)	Femur		4	Wet	8.9		34-yr-old male.
(e)	Femur		9	Wet	8.3		69-yr-old male.
(f)	Femur		5	Wet	9.5		76-yr-old male.
D							
(a)	Femur (δ)	[126]	29	Dry	14.1 ± 0.2	12.2–16.1	
(b)	Humerus (δ)		27	Dry	14.9 ± 0.2	12.0–17.5	
(c)	Femur ($\circleddash$)		30	Dry	13.4 ± 0.3	8.5–16.7	
(d)	Humerus ($\circleddash$)		16	Dry	15.1 ± 0.5	11.9–15.1	
E							Bone from both sexes, white and black, none of whom had primary bone disease.
(a)	Femur	[108]	405	Wet	8.22		
(b)	Tibia		193	Wet	9.84		
(c)	Fibula		37	Wet	9.45		
F							
(a)	Femur (right)	[123]		Wet	11.39	9.35–13.0	39-yr-old female—worst result.
(b)	Femur (left)			Wet		10.4–12.8	
(c)	Femur (right)			Wet	15.19	15.0	57-yr-old female—best result.
(d)	Femur (left)			Wet		15.19–15.26	
(e)	Femur (right)			Wet	11.77	11.2–12.37	75-yr-old male—average result.
(f)	Femur (left)			Wet		11.8–12.16	
(g)	Femur		15	Wet	14.09 ± 0.36		All subjects under 60.
(h)	Femur		13	Wet	12.09 ± 0.32		All subjects over 60.
G	Single osteons of						Fully calcified osteons with longitudinal spiral course of fiber bundles.
(a)	Femur	[7]	20	Wet	11.29 ± 1.59		20-yr-old male.
(b)	Femur		10	Wet	11.00 ± 1.04		80-yr-old male.
H							
(a)	Femur	[47]	12	Wet	10.00	5.68–13.16	Newborn to 6 mo old.
(b)	Femur		4	Wet	17.625	14.70–22.44	14-yr-old boy.

Source: Wall et al. [48]. Reprinted with permission from *Medical and Biological Engineering*, vol. 8, J. C. Wall, S. Chatterjee, and J. W. Jeffery. On the Origin of Scatter in Results of Human Bone Strength Tests, Copyright 1970, Pergamon Press, Ltd.

next section), its static tensile strength might be considered as the lower limit of stress level, below which a bone sample is not expected to fail; thus, it can be used as a design criterion for appropriate cases.

3.2 Dynamic and Fracture Properties of Bone

Tsuda [49] conducted some Charpy impact tests of human femoral bone. The average impact energy absorbed per unit cross-sectional area was 13,700 N m/m^2 for wet specimens, and 11,800 N m/m^2 for dry specimens. Whether the specimens were notched was not reported. Further results of Charpy tests, using rectangular specimens with a V notch, were mentioned by Swanson [33] in his review article on the biomechanical characteristics of bone. Based on the results of 280 specimens from fresh human femurs, he concluded that: (1) the material is highly notch sensitive, although varying the notch root radius between 0.08 and 0.25 mm had no effect on the results; (2) longitudinal specimens are tougher than tangential specimens (impact ranges were 9.02 to 38.2 and 3.33 to 12.5 N mm, respectively); (3) there is no significant variation in impact strength, either along the length of one femur or with the quadrant of origin; and (4) the impact strength of the material seems to fall with age.

Hert et al. [15] tested cylindrical samples of bovine bone in a Charpy test in an attempt to correlate the impact bending strength with the degree of osteoniza- tion. They observed a large variability in their impact-test results (approximately 0.7 to 2.0 kg·cm), as compared with the compression-test results. Salkovitz [50] also commented on the large scatter of the results from impact tests of bone. He tested six samples from beef metatarsal in a pendulum-type impact bending tester and found the energy-absorption capacity to vary from 0.28 to 6.17 ft·lb.

Bird and Becker [51] and their associates (Bird et al. [18]) performed compressive impact tests on samples of fresh beef femur to seek a relationship between failure mode and impactor particle velocity. The modulus of elasticity decreased with stress rate, and the ultimate stress increased. One of their most interesting results was the considerably higher impact resistance of whole bones as compared with small specimens.

An important study on the dynamic properties of bone was reported by McElhaney and Byars [14] and McElhaney [20]. They performed constant-velocity compressive tests at strain rates of from 0.001 to 1500 s^{-1} on specimens from human (embalmed) and beef femurs and compared the results with those for engineering materials such as aluminum and nylon (Fig. 2a). For human bone, the ultimate compressive stress increased from 21.8 ksi at the lowest strain rate to 46.0 ksi at the highest, whereas the corresponding increase in the elastic modulus was from 2.2×10^6 to 5.9×10^6 lb/in^2. They indicated that a functional relationship of the form

$$\sigma_e = A \ln \dot{e} + B \tag{1}$$

could be used to represent the effect of strain rate $\dot{e}$ on the stress σ_e, where A and B are constants.

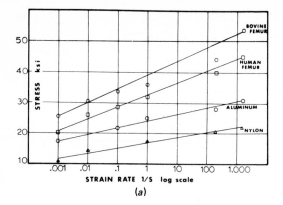

(a)

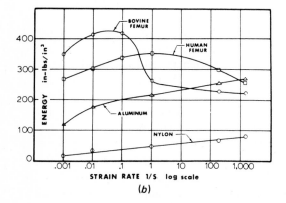

(b)

Figure 2 Changes in maximum stress and energy-absorption capacity as a function of strain rate. (a) Stress-strain rate curves; (b) energy-strain rate curves. (*After McElhaney [20]*.)

The energy-absorption capacity and maximum strain first increased to a maximum and then decreased with increasing strain rate (Fig. 2b). From this the authors postulated the existence of a *critical velocity*, which was in the neighborhood of s^{-1} for embalmed human bone and 0.05 s^{-1} for fresh beef bone. They found that at the lower rates of strain, shear failures occurred, but at the higher rates of strain the failures were accompanied by vertical splintering and multiple bone fragments.

The dynamic response of cranial bone was extensively studied by Wood [52, 53]. He tested 120 cranial bone specimens at various tensile strain rates ranging from 0.005 to 150 s^{-1}. Whereas the breaking stress and modulus of elasticity increased with strain rate, the breaking strain decreased, and the energy-absorption capacity remained strain-rate independent (Fig. 3). His results also showed that there was no detectable variation in the mechanical properties of cranial bone with changes in orientation tangent to the surface of the skull.

In a series of tests using both notched and unnotched beef bone specimens, Bonfield and Li [54] studied the temperature dependence of fracture of bone. The energy absorbed was greatest at about 0 to 25°C and was reduced at both lower and higher temperatures. With no notches, transverse specimens were much weaker than longitudinal specimens. The presence of a V notch of unspecified root radius

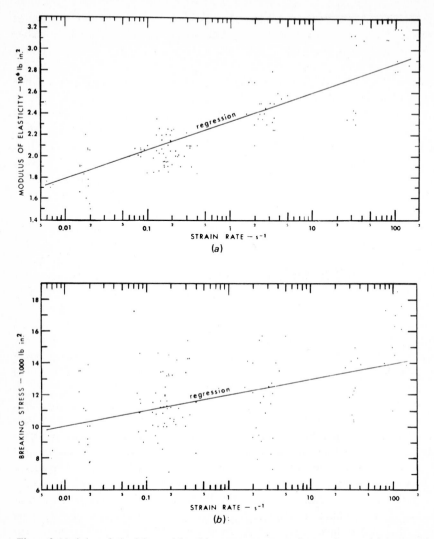

Figure 3 Modulus of elasticity and breaking stress versus strain rate for cranial compact bone. (*a*) Modulus of elasticity versus strain rate for cranial compact bone; regression line given by $E = (2.32 + 0.28 \log \dot{\epsilon}) \times 10^6$ lb/in^2. (*b*) Breaking stress versus strain rate for cranial compact bone; regression line given by $\sigma_B = 11.990 + 1000 \log \dot{\epsilon}$ lb/in^2. (*After Wood [53].*)

reduced the energy absorbed at 0°C to about one-eighth of the unnotched value for longitudinal specimens, and to about one-half that value for the transverse specimens.

By using notched beef bone specimens in three-point bending, Piekarski [55] measured the energy required to propagate a crack for high and low strain rates. At controlled crack propagation rates, bone displayed a high resistance to fracture, i.e., high fracture toughness, comparable even to some metallic materials. This was achieved by the pullout of Haversian systems and mineral components, thus creating a large amount of new fracture surface that absorbed large amounts of energy. At catastrophic crack propagation, brittle fracture occurred, with the crack extending through the cross section in substantially one plane. As a result, the fracture energy was drastically reduced.

Piekarski [55] also examined the bone fracture surface by optical and scanning electron microscopy and identified different mechanisms of fracture. The type of fracture had many similarities to that in fiber-reinforced composite materials. He also attempted to correlate the failure energy of bone to the failure energy of its constituent materials, mainly mineral and collagen. He concluded that Griffith's theory of fracture does not apply in the case of bone, as the actual critical crack length was much smaller than that required by Griffith's theory. It seems that critical crack length is one of many factors, including orientation and strain rate, and further work is necessary before a definite conclusion is reached.

Margel [56] also tested V-notched beef bone specimens in three-point bending at low to moderate (0.0002 to 2 in/min) cross-head speeds. She found that the strongest specimens were those with regular planar lamellae. Fracture strength was found to vary only slightly with strain rate (about 14 kg/mm^2 throughout the range of testing), but the work required to fracture the specimens changed appreciably (8.1 mm kg/mm^2 at 0.000176 to 0.00176 min^{-1}, and 4.5 mm kg/mm^2 at 0.0176 to 1.76 min^{-1}). Using Griffith's theory, she obtained a critical crack length of 0.25 mm and a fracture toughness of 21 ± 7 kg $mm^{1/2}/mm^2$ for beef bone. Although the load-deflection curves had shown plastic deformation in many cases, she assumed elastic behavior in calculating stresses at the crack tip. Thus, some of her conclusions seem questionable.

Pope and Outwater [30] also tested precracked long bones from dog, cow, rhesus monkey, and embalmed cadavers and determined the mean fracture toughness and fracture energy. Fresh anthropoid bone had a fracture energy of about 10.5 lb·in/in^2) in the transverse direction, and about 4 lb·in/in^2 in the longitudinal direction. These values decreased as a function of increased strain rate, aging, or preservation as cadavers, and the mode of failure also varied according to strain rate.

In a recent paper, Melvin and Evans [57] tested single-edge-notched beef specimens. They obtained a critical strain energy release rate of 7.9 to 14.6 in·lb/in^2 for longitudinal crack propagation, and 17.9 to 31.6 in·lb/in^2 for transverse crack propagation.

Black and Korostoff [58] recently reported a method that allows the dynamic elastic modulus of viable human cortical bone to be determined in tension in a near-physiological state. Elastic moduli of excised tibial specimens were found to vary between 6.35 and 10.0 × 10^9 N/m^2 at 35.4 Hz, increasing to a range of 12.1 to 14.9 × 10^9 N/m^2 at 353.6 Hz. They also found an interesting apparent relationship between modulus and percentage of bone mineral content. The modulus decreased with increasing inorganic content (and age) at 35.4 Hz, but increased with increasing inorganic content at 353.6 Hz. Their study also suggested that there may be a mechanical component in bone that has a characteristic mechanical time constant of $\frac{1}{200}$ s. This study indicates that if elastic modulus is used as a criterion for nondestructive measurement of bone mechanical properties, then a more precise determination of the frequency dependence of bone elastic properties is imperative.

It is clear from the previously mentioned studies on the dynamic and fracture properties of bone that our knowledge of even the basic dynamic mechanical properties of bone is incomplete. No data are available on the tensile impact strength of bone at high loading rates. Therefore, the objective of this investigation was to obtain data on the tensile impact tolerance of bone.

As discussed in the introduction to this chapter, the dynamic strength properties of bone are important because most bone fractures occur under dynamic conditions. Therefore, any design of safety equipment to prevent bone fractures should take into account the tolerance limits and fracture characteristics of bone, as described in this section. Although a safety engineer is interested mainly in the tolerance limits of whole bones, the advantage of testing standardized bone specimens is obvious from the fact that the dynamic strength properties of bone as a tissue can be obtained from such tests. Once the dynamic behavior of bone as a material is established for various modes of loading (tensile, compressive, bending, and shear) and for various strain rates, then the tolerance limits of whole bones can be calculated for any loading condition from a knowledge of the geometry and cross section of the individual whole bone. This would eliminate the necessity for extensive testing of whole bones at various strain rates and for different modes of loading.

3.3 Impact Testing of Whole Bones

The dynamic strength of whole bones has been investigated by many authors [9]. As the main emphasis of this chapter is on the dynamic strength of bone as a material, only a few of the previous investigations of the dynamic strength of whole bones will be reported here.

The subject of head injury due to impact is perhaps the most thoroughly investigated area of research on human tolerance levels. Various authors have discussed the mechanisms of injury to the brain and spinal cord, the levels of acceleration and force necessary to cause concussion and skull fracture, and the establishment of tolerance levels [59 to 62].

The impact response of intact cadaver heads was investigated by Evans et al. [63] using high-speed motion pictures (1000 frames/s) and accelerometers mounted on the cadaver. In this study, the available kinetic energy, the impact velocity, the peak impact acceleration, and impact duration were measured. Linear fractures were obtained with peak impact accelerations of 337, 555, 344, and 724 g with total time durations of 11.25, 9.03, 4.88, and 3.38 ms, respectively. Although the available kinetic energies for these tests were 471, 268, 561, and 581 ft·lb, respectively, the magnitude of the energy responsible for the fractures was probably 33 to 75 ft·lb, as most of the energy was expended in denting the impact surface, rather than in fracturing the skull.

These experiments clearly demonstrated that not only the magnitude of the available kinetic energy, but also its rate of absorption is important in the mechanics of skull fracture. Thus, the longer the time available for absorption of the energy, the greater the energy that can be tolerated without fracture. Other studies on skull fracture were conducted by Gurdjian et al. [64 to 67] and co-workers (Lissner et al. [68]).

Huelke et al. [69, 70] studied mandibular fractures due to impact using brittle-coating methods and high-speed motion pictures (up to 3000 frames/s). When the condyles were free to move, impacts to the chin area revealed that the mandible behaved like a pin-jointed arch. He showed that most of the fractures arose from failure of the bone caused by the tensile stresses produced by bending.

In a recent paper, Nahum et al. [71] experimentally obtained the forces necessary for fracture of the skull and facial bones under localized loading. The tolerances were relatively independent of impulse duration, in contrast with the tolerance of the brain to closed-skull injury. Significantly lower average strength was found for the female bone structure. Because acceleration rather than force was used in some earlier studies, the authors raised the question of correlation between force and acceleration, and which was a more accurate measurement for tolerance descriptions.

Injuries to the human vertebrae resulting from dynamic loading were investigated by Patrick [72] using instrumented cadavers. Human cadavers with strain gauges cemented to the body of the vertebrae were subjected to vertical acceleration, and the resultant forces on the vertebrae were calculated. Some of his results were: (1) forces to the human vertebrae are a linear function of caudocephalad acceleration up to the point where buckling or fracture takes place; (2) high rates of onset of acceleration produce high peaks of strain of short duration; (3) end-plate fractures occur in the lumber vertebrae at loads as low as 435 lb (muscle loads further reduce the external loads required to fracture the end plates); and (4) vertebral end-plate fractures are very difficult to find by x-ray examination.

The tolerance of the unembalmed adult human pelvis to impact, applied by a drop weight, was investigated by Fasola et al. [73]. A force of 830 lb was required to produce bilateral disjunction of the sacroiliac joint for the defleshed pelvis and femurs. They also tested some specimens with pelvic viscera, muscles, and ligaments intact, and, in this case, a force of 775 lb was required to produce the fracture disjunction of the sacroiliac joint. The authors also investigated rupture of the hip joint and the lateral wall of the acetabulum. They concluded that the combined strength of the femurs was greater than that of the weight-bearing arches of the pelvis. The effect of dynamic loading on the pelvis has also been studied by F. G. Evans' group (at the University of Michigan) by the brittle-coating method. They dropped specimens from a height that caused displacement of the acetabulum laterally and the pubic symphysis posteriorly, thus producing tensile-strain patterns in the iliopubic rami and acetabula.

Patrick et al. [74] conducted a recent study of the impact tolerance of the human knee-thigh-hip complex, an area that is often injured in car accidents. Ten human cadavers were tested by placing them in a car-crash simulator and applying impact forces to the patella. Fractures of the right hip were produced with loads of 1400, 1900, 2550, and 3850 lb. Some of these were severe multiple fractures. A load of 1600 lb caused fractures of the superior and inferior rami of the left pubis, and a load of 1950 lb caused severe multiple fractures.

Femoral fractures were produced at 950, 1650, 1850, and 2250 lb for supracondylar fractures, 1500 lb for a midshaft fracture, 1400 lb for an inter-trochanteric fracture, and 2650 lb for a dislocated trochanteric fracture. Fractures of the unpadded patella occurred at loads of 1550, 1800, 1950, 2000, 2100, and 2250 lb.

From their results, the authors concluded that it is impossible to predict with certainty whether fracture would occur first in the patella, the femur, or the pelvis. However, they suggested that the femur is the most vulnerable, because femoral fractures were most common and they occurred at a lower average load than fractures of the patella or the pelvis. They concluded that a load of 1740 lb is a reasonable tolerance limit, based on overall injury threshold level. In a later study using four unrestrained cadavers in simulated frontal collisions at 10 and 20 mi/h, no femoral fractures occurred up to axial loads of 1950 lb. It was thus suggested that the earlier injury threshold might be increased.

Evans, Pederson, and their colleagues [75, 76] studied brittle coated femurs in various orientations subjected to dynamic loading by dropping a 719-lb weight. They concluded that failure of the bone occurred owing to starting of fracture in tension.

Smith [77] also investigated the static and dynamic loads necessary to produce fractures in the proximal end of the human femur. As in previous studies, dynamic loading was applied by dropping a weight from various heights. An average of 250 ft·lb of energy was required for fractures of the ilium, dislocation of the hip joint, and intertrochanteric fractures of the femur. When the loading was applied to the greater trochanter from the side, it produced fractures of the iliac, acetabulum, and femoral shaft with an average energy of 306 ft·lb. Similarly, an average impact energy of 364 ft·lb applied to the neck of a horizontally placed femur produced subcapital, oblique, and transverse fractures of the femoral neck.

The effect of loading rates on the tolerance limits of bone is an important design consideration. This was studied by static and impact bending loading of 44 pairs of fresh adult femurs, reported by Mather [16]. In both tests, the femur was simply supported at the epiphyses, and a transverse load was applied at the central diaphysis. In the impact test, in which a striker fell on the femur with a velocity of 32 ft/s, the average energy required to fracture the femoral diaphysis was 31.3 ft·lb. The paired femurs tested under the static condition required a mean energy of 20.5 ft· lb to fracture. The ratio of two values calculated for each pair of femurs had a mean value of 1.66, but individual ratios ranged from 0.25 to 3.25. In this comparison, the kinetic energies transferred to the fractured elements were neglected. The author concluded that reliable tolerance estimates cannot be deduced from static tests of individual bones.

A similar comparison of the static and dynamic torsional loading of embalmed and fresh human tibiae was conducted by Burstein and Frankel [17]. The testing was conducted in a pendulum torsion machine, and the impact velocity was adjusted so that the loading duration was maintained at 0.1 s. A parallel series of tests was conducted at a loading duration of 1 min to obtain quasi-static strengths. The average energy absorbed for all specimens at low strain rates (0.00003 to

0.0003 s^{-1}) was 103 kg·cm, compared with an average of 229 kg·cm for all specimens at high loading rates (0.09 to 0.13 s^{-1}), an increase of 45 percent.

Similar increases were observed in a later paper utilizing paired canine long bones tested in torsion under static and dynamic conditions by the same authors and their co-workers [78]. In a recent investigation of mechanical properties of bone as a function of the rate of deformation, Panjabi et al. [79] tested rabbit femurs and ulnae in torsion at five loading rates ranging from 0.003 to 13.2 rad/s. The bones absorbed 67 percent more energy and had 33 percent more torque and torsional deflection and 5 percent more stiffness at the highest rate of deformation than at the lowest. They also showed the existence of a *critical strain rate* up to which the strength increased and beyond which it decreased.

Data on the impact testing of whole bones can be utilized to determine the maximum load levels to which these bones can be subjected without causing fracture. Such data are essential in the formulation of safety specifications, for instance, in the design of safe ski bindings. Similar data can also be used to determine how the shape and geometry of a whole bone affects its tolerance limits as calculated on the basis of bone-coupon tests.

3.4 Factors Affecting Mechanical Properties

Previous investigations of the mechanical properties of bone exhibit a large amount of scatter in the data. One of the main reasons for this is the fact that the mechanical properties of bone are strongly affected by many biological and mechanical factors. Thus, to specify the strength of a bone, it is necessary also to specify some of these important variables. The important factors affecting bone strength can be divided into two broad categories:

1. *Biological factors*:
    (*a*) physical conditions such as moisture content, embalmed or fresh, temperature;
    (*b*) species, age, sex, race; (*c*) variation within one bone and between bones, orientation; (*d*) microstructure; (*e*) degree of mineralization and collagen fiber orientation; (*f*) condition and length of storage; (*g*) pathological conditions such as influence of diet, effect of fluorosis, radiation, and other diseases.
2. *Mechanical factors*:
    (*a*) type of stress—tensile, compressive, or shear; (*b*) specimen dimensions and geometry; (*c*) strain rate; (*d*) presence of stress concentration, e.g., notches.

The details of previous investigations on the effects of these biological and mechanical factors will not be repeated here, as several excellent reviews have recently been published [9, 29, 33, 35, 44].

3.5 Mathematical Models

In recent years, numerous investigators have been engaged in the development of biodynamic models of the human skeletal system and its components, to study the dynamic responses of the body under impact or accelerative forces as encountered in the seat ejection of pilots or in automobile accidents. The need for such mathematical models is evident from the fact that human volunteers can be subjected to stress and acceleration levels only up to the threshold of injury, and cadavar experiments are difficult, expensive, and cannot always be extrapolated to simulate living conditions. Such mathematical representation is also essential to predict the injury probability in a new loading situation for which no test data may be available. Many such conceptual or mathematical simulations of various parts of the body have been discussed in a recent symposium on biodynamic models [80] and by other authors [81 to 86]. Owing to space limitations, these cannot be discussed here, and the reader is advised to consult individual references for further study. It is likely that as the models of body systems become more precise, they will contribute significantly to our understanding of the injury mechanisms resulting from dynamic forces. They will also make it possible to obtain the tolerance limits of the human body without going through extensive laboratory testing and without having to rely so heavily on extrapolation from animal research.

4 DYNAMIC PROPERTIES IN TENSILE IMPACT

4.1 Experimental Procedure and Resulting Data

Bovine and human femurs were utilized to prepare standardized compact bone specimens (Fig. 4) for the tensile impact testing. In the testing of biological specimens, the method of preparation and storage is important in preserving the *in vivo* strength properties. Thus the bone samples were machined under continuous water spray to minimize any possible thermal damage. They were stored frozen and were kept wet in Ringer's solution until the actual testing was done. The impact testing was conducted in an instrumented pendulum-type tensile impact tester (Fig. 5) with a striking velocity of 135 in/s, which corresponded to a 2-ft free fall of the pendulum head. A quartz load cell monitored the load, and the output of the load cell was recorded on an oscilloscope.

All the calculated mechanical properties were obtained from oscilloscope records of load-time curves. The dynamic stress-strain relations were obtained from the load-time curves. The dynamic stress-strain relations were obtained from the load-time curves using the following relations: During impact, the instantaneous velocity of the pendulum head at any time t is given by

$$V = V_0 - \frac{1}{m} \sum_{i=1}^{n} F_i \, \Delta t \qquad (2)$$

where V_0 = initial pendulum striking velocity
   m = pendulum mass (2.482 lb)
   n = number of increments Δt used in the integration
   F_i = force acting at time t_i

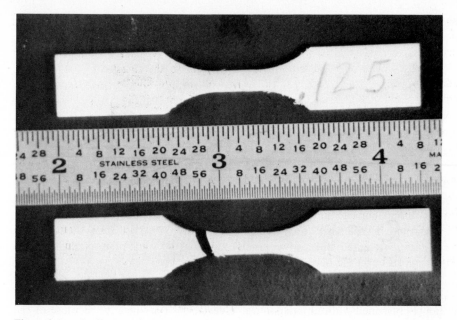

Figure 4 Longitudinal cortical bone specimens for tensile impact testing (0.065 in thick), before and after test.

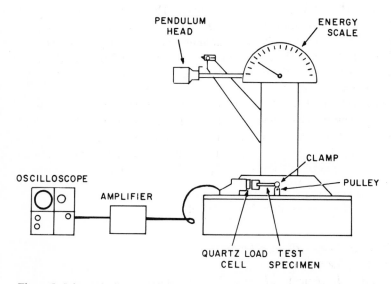

Figure 5 Schematic diagram of the test setup for tensile impact testing.

From the velocity-time curve, the displacement is obtained as a function of time, using the relation

$$x = \sum_{i=1}^{n} V_i \, \Delta t \qquad (3)$$

By combining the force-time and displacement-time curves, the curve of force versus displacement is obtained. This curve is proportional to the nominal stress-strain curve.

All the losses during impact reduced the velocity of the pendulum head by less than 4 percent, owing to the total energy loss in breaking the specimen and knocking the broken part away. Therefore, it was reasonable to assume a constant velocity during impact, and the displacement or total elongation of the specimen was calculated on the basis of an average velocity of 132.9 in/s. Thus, the load-time curves also represented the load-versus-elongation or dynamic stress-strain behavior of the samples in tensile impact.

Additional mechanical properties were calculated from the load-time curves in tensile impact (Fig. 6). The proportional limit σ_i was defined as the maximum stress the sample sustained without an appreciable deviation from linearity. Because of the irregular nature of the stress-strain curve, this limit was somewhat arbitrary. Most engineering structures are designed so that stresses do not exceed the proportional limit. But it has not been established yet whether the tolerance limit for bone should be based on this elastic limit, i.e., on the onset of plastic deformation or on the onset of catastrophic failure. Further information on the biological effects of plastic deformation in bone is required to answer this question.

The *modulus of elasticity* is a measure of the stiffness or rigidity of the material and is measured by the slope of the stress-strain curve. The initial secant modulus of elasticity E_i was calculated from the stress-strain data at the proportional limit. Similarly, a secant modulus of elasticity E_u was calculated from the stress-strain data at maximum stress, indicating the slope of the straight line joining the point of maximum stress to the origin. Thus, E_i equal to E_u indicated that the stress-strain curve was linear up to the point of maximum stress. If the stress-strain curve is assumed linear, as is commonly done in design, the secant modulus of elasticity is more meaningful than the tangent modulus of elasticity. Most previous

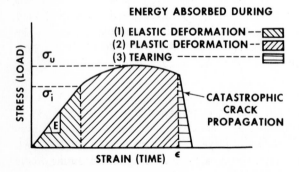

Figure 6 Idealized stress-strain (or load-time) curve in tensile impact showing the energy absorbed during elastic, plastic, and tearing phases.

investigators have reported the tangent modulus of elasticity, or have mentioned modulus of elasticity without specifying how it was calculated. The tangent modulus of elasticity E was calculated for fresh human bone samples to compare it with the reported value in the literature, obtained statically.

The *energy-absorption capacity* is defined as the energy required to fracture a specimen in an impact test and is a measure of toughness or impact strength. This was obtained by measuring the area under the load-time curve with a planimeter. As shown in Fig. 6, the use of an instrumented impact tester allowed the separation of the total energy to fracture into (1) energy absorbed during elastic deformation, (2) energy absorbed during plastic deformation, and (3) energy absorbed during tearing. The impact energy U was considered the sum of the energy absorbed during the elastic and plastic deformations. Separation of the total energy-absorption capacity in this way allows a more refined characterization of the fracture properties of bone. It also provides more design parameters based on various damage criteria. For instance, Bird et al. [18] showed that, after impact, some bone samples had undergone microcracks that were not noticeable by visual observation. It is likely that if the impact energy does not exceed the elastic energy-absorption capacity U_i, then the microcrack damage can be avoided. However, the total energy to produce failure is also important, because the inability of a bone to withstand the impact will cause fracture and consequently a much more severe injury.

Typical load-time curves for longitudinal compact bone samples are shown in Fig. 7. As shown in this figure, the dynamic stress-strain relations for compact bone in tensile impact are markedly nonlinear to the point of fracture. A majority of the specimens underwent plastic deformation as depicted in Fig. 7, c and d. The remainder exhibited elastic behavior (Fig. 7a) or strain-hardening effects (Fig. 7b). Other investigators also noted plastic deformation of bone in static tension [9, 88, 89], shear [89], bending [90], and dynamic compression [18, 20].

A comparison of the load-time curves made it clear that equal failure energies (characterized by the area under the load-time curve) could be obtained from specimens displaying markedly different dynamic stress-strain behavior. This shows the shortcomings of the conventional impact test, which provides only one-point data, the total energy to fracture. It further emphasizes that the characterization of the impact tolerance of bone with a single number, the total energy-absorption capacity, without consideration of how the energy is absorbed, can be misleading when such data are applied in design. Similar considerations also hold true in the selection of materials for prostheses and implants. Frankel and Burstein [91] have pointed out that "under static loading conditions the elastic limit may not be exceeded, but under dynamic conditions it may. Thus the amount of energy a material can absorb after it reaches its elastic limit becomes important."

Beef bone samples Table 2 shows the means and standard deviations (SD) for the tensile impact properties of 50 fresh beef bone specimens. The fact that E_u is less than E_i indicates that, on the average, beef bone samples underwent some plastic deformation, even though a few samples displayed strain-hardening effects (Fig. 7b). For samples exhibiting some plasticity, the impact energy U_i absorbed during elastic

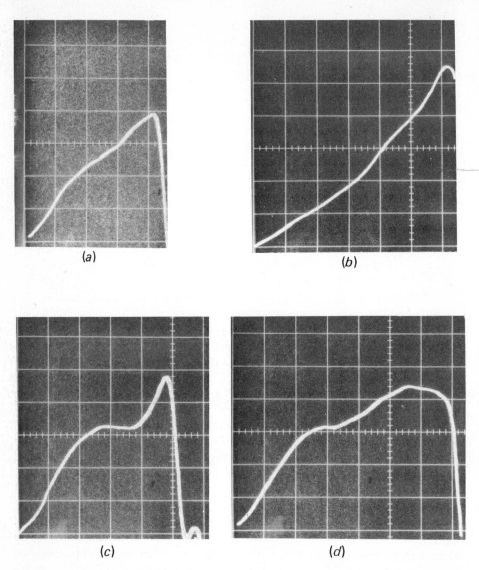

Figure 7 Typical examples of load-time or stress-strain curves of longitudinal compact beef bone samples in tensile impact. (*a*) Elastic failure; vertical scale, 25 lb or 3075 lb/in²; horizontal scale, 20 μs or 2658 μin/in. (*b*) Strain hardening; vertical scale, 25 lb or 3050 lb/in²; horizontal scale, 10 μs or 1329 μin/in. (*c*) and (*d*) Plastic deformation; vertical scale, 25 lb or 3100 lb/in²; horizontal scale, 20 μs or 2658 μin/in. (All scales are given per division.)

deformation was small compared with the total energy absorbed. For 39 such samples, the mean elastic energy U_i was 49.93 ± 18.33 in·lb/in², compared with 162 in·lb/in² for the total energy to rupture. If the impact tolerance of bone is based on the prevention of plastic deformation and microcracking, then this energy to produce yield may be an important design parameter.

Human bone samples Means and SD for the tensile impact properties of 42 embalmed and 49 fresh human compact bone samples are presented in Table 3. Table 3 shows that the tolerance limits for fresh human bone specimens are higher than those for embalmed specimens. This is probably because the embalmed bone specimens were from an older person (more than 60 yr of age) whereas the fresh specimens were from a 38-yr-old man.

Table 2 and 3 also show that the modulus of elasticity is the most consistent of the mechanical properties. Wood [53], in his study of the dynamic tensile behavior of cranial bone, also observed that the modulus of elasticity was the least variable of mechanical properties. The tangent modulus of elasticity for fresh human bone (Table 3) also agreed in general with the values reported in the literature.

Nineteen of 49 fresh human bone samples and 26 of 42 embalmed human bone samples underwent some plastic deformation prior to failure. The yield stress in tensile impact was 9.79 ± 2.72 ksi for the fresh human bone samples, and 8.45 ± 1.43 ksi for the embalmed bone samples. As for the beef bone specimens, the energy to produce yield was significantly smaller than the total impact-energy capacity.

Cancellous bone samples Eleven cancellous bone samples from the metaphyses of beef femurs were also tested in tensile impact. Owing to their low strength and fragility, it was difficult to manufacture and test standardized samples of cancellous bone. Stress-strain curves for these specimens in tensile impact were either elastic up to failure or were parabolic in nature (Fig. 8). These two types of stress-strain curves probably result from the different orientations of the bone samples. As shown in Fig. 8, the parabolic stress-strain relation was characterized by a smooth curve up to the point of total fracture, and thus did not exhibit any signs of catastrophic crack propagation. This may be related to the fact that, while some bony spicules in a specimen with irregular trabecular pattern reached their ultimate load-carrying capacity and underwent microcracking, the others still supported the load, preventing catastrophic failure.

An average ultimate tensile impact stress of 1.365 ksi was obtained for the 11 cancellous bone samples. The tensile impact strength was 2.12 ksi for the six specimens with linear stress-strain relation, and 0.457 ksi for the five specimens with parabolic stress-strain relation. The difference between these two groups is statistically significant. The six specimens that failed elastically had a mean secant modulus of elasticity of 0.168 (0.0742 to 0.3811) $\times 10^6$ lb/in^2, a mean impact-energy capacity of 14.09 (9.28 to 20.88) in·lb/in^2, and a mean ultimate strain of 1.29 (0.80 to 1.70 percent). The five specimens with parabolic stress-strain relations had a mean ultimate strain of 2.94 (2.67 to 4.0 percent).

The mechanical properties of cancellous bone are important, because it acts as a major shock-absorbing mechanism at the human articulating joints. Moreover, implanted prosthetic devices often rely on cancellous bone for their fixation, as in the case of a total hip replacement. Nevertheless, only a few studies of the mechanical behavior of cancellous bone have been reported in the literature, and most of these were concerned with its compressive or shearing properties [92 to

Table 2 Tensile impact properties of bone (mean ± 1 SD) for 50 longitudinal fresh bovine samples*

Stress [ksi (MPa)]		Maximum strain ϵ	Impact energy U [in·lb/in² (J/m²)]	Secant modulus of elasticity [10⁶ lb/in² (GPa)]	
Proportional limit σ_i	Ultimate σ_u			Initial E_i	Ultimate E_u
9.6 ± 4.1 (66.2 ± 28.2)	17.6 ± 5.3 (121.3 ± 36.5)	1.34 ± 0.54	142 ± 85 (24900 ± 18200)	1.83 ± 0.32 (12.6 ± 2.2)	1.50 ± 0.47 (10.3 ± 3.24)

*Values in SI units are shown in parentheses.
Source: Saha and Hayes [32].

Table 3 Means and SD of the mechanical properties of human bone specimens in tensile impact*

Condition	No. of samples	Ultimate stress σ_u [ksi (MN/m²)]	Maximum strain	Impact energy U [in·lb/in² (J/m²)]	Modulus of elasticity [10⁶ lb/in² (GN/m²)]	
					Tangent E	Secant E_i
Fresh	49	18.32 ± 4.80 (126.3 ± 33.1)	1.15 ± 0.30	107.3 ± 42 (18790 ± 7355)	2.11 ± 0.50 (14.5 ± 3.4)	1.80 ± 0.42 (12.4 ± 2.9)
Embalmed	42	14.3 ± 3.7 (98.6 ± 25.5)	0.982 ± 0.225	81.7 ± 31.5 (14308 ± 5517)		1.76 ± 0.23 (12.1 ± 1.6)

*Values in SI units are shown in parentheses.

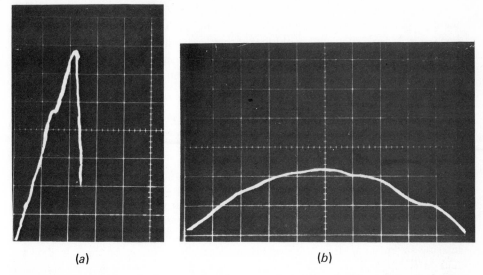

(a)   (b)

Figure 8 Characteristic load-time or stress-strain curves of cancellous beef bone in tensile impact. (a) Elastic failure; vertical scale, 5 lb or 334 lb/in²; horizontal scale, 50 μs or 6645 μin/in. (b) Parabolic nonlinear behavior; vertical scale, 10 lb or 600 lb/in²; horizontal scale, 20 μs or 2658 μin/in. (All scales are given per division.)

95]. As a result, our current knowledge of the dynamic response of cancellous bone is minimal, and the subject needs further attention.

Comparison of static and tensile impact properties It has already been pointed out that the mechanical properties of bone are strain-rate dependent. Thus some bone samples were also tested quasi-statically to compare static and impact strengths and to indicate the strain-rate sensitivity of compact bone in tensile impact. Data on the ultimate strength in static tension are presented and compared with those of other authors in Table 4. From Tables 2 and 4, we find the tensile impact strength σ_u of compact beef bone is 20 percent higher than the static value. Similarly, from Tables 3 and 4, it is evident that the tensile impact strength of fresh human bone samples was greater by 33.5 percent at the higher strain rate.

Table 4 Tensile strength of compact bone in static tension

Source	Condition	No. of samples	Yield stress σ_i (ksi)	Ultimate stress σ_u (ksi)	Ultimate stress σ_u from other references (ksi)
Human femur, male (38 yr)	Fresh, wet	13	11.13 ± 2.25	13.72 ± 1.47	13.85 (9.24–18.84) [37]
Beef femur	Fresh, wet	24		14.7 ± 2.8	13.3 ± 2.87 [123]

To ascertain if this increase in strength in tensile impact is affected by the number and location of sampling, the static tensile strength of each fresh human bone sample was compared with the impact strength of another sample from an adjacent region, i.e., from the same quadrant, same segment, and at the same radial distance from the center of the shaft. The percentage increase in strength was calculated for each pair using the formula

$$\text{Percentage increase} = \frac{\sigma_{u(\text{impact})} - \sigma_{u(\text{static})}}{\sigma_{u(\text{static})}} \times 100 \qquad (4)$$

Based on this, the percentage increase in ultimate stress was 26.4 percent for 13 fresh human compact bone specimens.

This comparison of static and dynamic strength in tensile impact showed that although there is a definite increase in tensile strength with increased strain rate, the percentage increase differs between beef and human bone. The increase is also somewhat affected by the source of the specimens. Wood [53, 54] also found an increase in breaking stress with increasing strain rate for cranial bone in dynamic tension (Fig. 3). In particular, he found an increase of approximately 40 percent in breaking stress between strain rates of 0.01 and 100 s^{-1}. The increase in maximum stress with increasing strain rate was also observed in bone in compression [14, 18] and torsion [78, 79].

The result showing an increased bone strength in tensile impact is in agreement with observations for engineering materials. Clark and Duwez [96] compared the static tensile strength and dynamic strength of steel at a strain rate of 190 s^{-1}. The increase in ultimate strength was of the order of 45 percent for carbon steel, about 30 percent for manganese steel, and about 30 percent for nickel-chromium steel, with some cases showing no change for a group of nickel-chromium specimens. In another paper, Clark and Wood [97] also showed that the ultimate strengths of some metals and alloys were greater under dynamic conditions than under static conditions, but at velocities above approximately 25 ft/s they did not seem to increase. They also observed that there was essentially no variation of tensile strength with change of gauge length. Similar observations, indicating an increase in ultimate stress with higher strain rates, have also been reported for other engineering materials [98, 99].

In static tension, Evans and Lebow [12, 40] obtained an energy-absorption capacity of 83.6 in·lb/in^3 for wet embalmed compact bone samples from the femur of a 78-yr-old male. Thus, the tensile impact energy of 81.7 obtained in this investigation (Table 3, expressed per unit volume) is in agreement with the value obtained by Evans and Lebow. These results do not exhibit the increase in energy-absorption capacity that was observed by Mather [16] and Burstein and Frankel [17] in their comparison of static and dynamic strengths. But the results of this investigation do agree with those of Wood [53, 54], who also did not find any increase in the energy-absorption capacity in his dynamic-tension test of cranial bone. McElhaney and Byars [14] reported the existence of a critical strain rate of 1 s^{-1} in bone, beyond which the energy-absorption capacity decreased even though it did increase with increasing strain rate up to that point. The applied strain rate of

$132 \ s^{-1}$ in this investigation was beyond this reported critical strain rate for bone, and thus it is not surprising that the energy-absorption capacity remained essentially constant.

On the basis of tests of 242 specimens from the human femur in static tension, Evans and Lebow [12] obtained percentage elongations from 1.15 to 1.27 percent, which is slightly higher than the 0.982 ± 0.225 percent obtained in tensile impact in this investigation (Table 3). This is expected, because with the higher strain rates, the material has less chance to deform plastically before failure, consequently reducing total elongation. Wood [53] also observed a decrease in breaking strain with increases in strain rate (Fig. 3). This decrease in ultimate strain with increasing strain rate is instrumental in the decrease in failure energy beyond a critical strain rate, even though the maximum stress increases. This also points out that in the design of safety equipment, to prevent bone fracture in high-speed collisions, the allowable strain must be appropriately reduced from the value obtained through testing at low strain rates.

A comparison of Tables 2 and 3 with Table 4 shows that the scatter in the tensile impact strengths of beef and fresh human bone samples was much larger under impact conditions than in the static case. This may be related to the fact that stress-concentration effects are much more critical at higher strain rates, as there is less chance to deform plastically to reduce the stress-concentration effect. Hert et al. [15] also observed a large variability in the impact bending strength of beef bone samples compared with the variation in static compression strength. Salkovitz [51] also commented on the large scatter in his data from impact tests of bone. This also suggests that, owing to the stress-concentration effect, a healing bone or a bone with a cavity is more susceptible to fracture in a dynamic-loading situation than in the static case.

4.2 Correlation between Elastic and Strength Properties

Pearson's product-moment correlation coefficients were used to determine correlations between elastic properties and bone strength. Such correlations are useful for the indirect determination of bone strength properties from its elastic coefficients, which can be measured nondestructively. The correlation matrix of tensile impact properties for 49 fresh human bone specimens is shown in Table 5. Similar correlation matrices were also obtained for the beef and embalmed human bone specimens [32, 100].

An extremely high correlation ($S = 0.001$) between impact energy-absorption capacity U and ultimate strain ϵ is noted for both human and beef bone samples. This indicates that the failure energy of bone in tensile impact can be estimated from its ultimate strain. Evans and Lebow [12, 40] also reported a strong correlation between maximum strain and energy absorption in the static tensile testing of human femoral specimens. In most cases, the correlation coefficient between U and ϵ is higher than the coefficient between U and ultimate stress σ_u. This raises the question of whether it may be more appropriate to base the

Table 5 Correlation matrix between elastic and strength properties for fresh human bone

	σ_u	U	E	ϵ	E_i	σ_i
Ultimate tensile stress σ_u	1.0000* (0) $S = 0.001$	0.6926 (49) $S = 0.001$	0.5303 (49) $S = 0.001$	0.1660 (49) $S = 0.127$	0.5458 (49) $S = 0.001$	0.4734 (19) $S = 0.020$
Impact energy U	0.6926 (49) $S = 0.001$	1.0000 (0) $S = 0.001$	−0.0549 (49) $S = 0.354$	0.7457 (49) $S = 0.001$	−0.0673 (49) $S = 0.323$	0.4142 (19) $S = 0.039$
Tangent modulus of elasticity E	0.5303 (49) $S = 0.001$	−0.0549 (49) $S = 0.354$	1.0000 (0) $S = 0.001$	−0.4144 (49) $S = 0.002$	0.8701 (50) $S = 0.001$	0.7589 (19) $S = 0.001$
Ultimate strain ϵ	0.1660 (49) $S = 0.127$	0.7457 (49) $S = 0.001$	−0.4144 (49) $S = 0.002$	1.0000 (0) $S = 0.001$	−0.4738 (49) $S = 0.001$	0.1568 (19) $S = 0.261$
Secant modulus of elasticity E_i	0.5458 (49) $S = 0.001$	−0.0673 (49) $S = 0.323$	0.8701 (50) $S = 0.001$	−0.4738 (49) $S = 0.001$	1.0000 (0) $S = 0.001$	0.7774 (19) $S = 0.001$
Yield stress σ_i	0.4734 (19) $S = 0.020$	0.4142 (19) $S = 0.039$	0.7589 (19) $S = 0.001$	0.1568 (19) $S = 0.261$	0.7774 (19) $S = 0.001$	1.0000 (0) $S = 0.001$

*Reading down, each set of data gives the correlation coefficient, cases (in parentheses), and significance.

tolerance limit of bone on *maximum strain* instead of maximum stress, as is customarily done.

Table 5 also shows that statistically significant correlations exist for (1) proportional limit σ_i and maximum stress σ_u with modulus of elasticity E and E_i, and (2) energy-absorption capacity U and maximum stress σ_u. Mather [101] also obtained significant correlations between breaking load and modulus of elasticity for human femurs in bending. Sedlin and Hirsch [44] obtained similar relationships between the modulus of elasticity of human bone and its ultimate breaking stress.

The highly significant correlation of initial modulus of elasticity E_i with proportional limit σ_i and maximum stress σ_u is important. The *in vivo* strength of living bone cannot be determined for human beings by any destructive test. However, methods are being developed whereby the modulus of elasticity may be measured *in vivo* by ultrasonic methods. Thus, it may be possible to develop noninvasive methods for determining bone strength. This is based on the fact that the velocity of ultrasonic wave propagation through an elastic medium is dependent on its modulus of elasticity and mass density and is given by

$$\text{Velocity} = \sqrt{\frac{\text{modulus of elasticity}}{\text{density}}} \qquad (5)$$

The density of bone is generally known or can be obtained *in vivo* by radiographic means, and if the velocity of ultrasound through it is measured, then the modulus may be calculated. Using normal and pathological human cortical bone specimens, Abendschein and Hyatt [102] found a high degree of correlation between the ultrasonic wave velocity and the elastic modulus and density of bone samples. Therefore, based on the previously mentioned correlations, it is possible to calculate bone strength from noninvasive measurements. Such methods are especially suitable for clinical evaluation of the strength of healing bone. Floriani et al. [103], Abendschein and Hyatt [104], and Brown and Mayor [105] have used such ultrasonic methods to determine the rate of fracture healing. Such correlations can also be used to calculate the bone strength of patients, by using small bone biopsy specimens that may be too small for mechanical testing, but whose elastic properties can be measured by ultrasonic or other means [59, 106, 107].

The elastic properties of bone have also been used as a criterion for judging the quality of bone and for measuring the effect of different diets on its load-carrying capacity. For instance, rachitogenic diets and diets rich in calcium produced changes in the elastic modulus and corresponding ultimate strength of bones of experimental animals. Thus nondestructive measurement of elastic modulus might also be utilized as a means for monitoring the effect of nutritional variables on the mechanical properties of bone.

4.3 Correlation between Microstructure and Dynamic Strength Properties

The microstructure of tested specimens was examined histologically in an attempt to determine if there is a structural basis for strength differences in specimens from a single bone, as well as specimens from different bones of different subjects. Photomicrographs showing the microstructure were taken successfully for 45 beef samples (Fig. 1) and for 55 fresh human bone samples, and were examined in a reflected-light optical microscope using metallographic techniques [100]. The percentage area of Haversian systems of secondary osteons and cavity areas (spaces occupied by Haversian canals, primary canals, resorption cavities, and Volkmann's canals), in each specimen was measured by a planimeter. A high correlation between some of the physical properties and histological elements was found.

Correlations between tensile impact strength, percentage of Haversian system, and cavity area Both beef and human bone specimens exhibited a strong negative correlation between ultimate tensile impact strength σ_u and the percentage of secondary osteon area. The relation for human bone specimens is shown graphically in Fig. 9. Currey [45], in testing 50 beef bone samples in static tension, obtained a high negative correlation ($S < 0.001$) between ultimate strength and the percentage of Haversian systems. Evans and Bang [108] also suggested a strong negative correlation between tensile strength and area of osteons.

As shown in Fig. 9, the general regression equation between tensile impact strength and area of secondary osteons in human bone is given by

$$\sigma_u = 28.05 - 0.236x \tag{6}$$

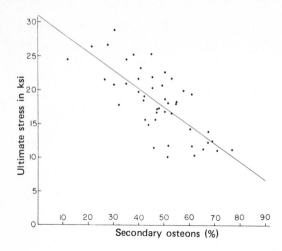

Figure 9 Relation between tensile impact strength and percentage area of secondary osteons in fresh human bone specimens.

where σ_u is given in ksi, and x is the percentage of Haversian systems in the specimens.

If cavity area is also considered as a dependent variable, then the tensile impact strength is given by

$$\sigma_u = 26.54 - 0.269x + 0.252y \tag{7}$$

where y is the percentage of cavity area in the test specimen. A positive coefficient for cavity area may seem surprising, but this is because of the significant positive correlation between cavity area and area of secondary osteons (correlation coefficient $= 0.311$, $s = 0.017$).

Similarly, from a linear regression analysis, the tensile impact strength for beef bone is given by

$$\sigma_u = 19.67 - 0.153x \tag{8}$$

This is similar to the linear regression equation

$$\sigma_u = 16.368 - 0.0565x \tag{9}$$

obtained by Currey [45] for the static tensile strength of beef bone.

Correlations betwen impact energy capacity, percentage of Haversian system, and cavity area The correlation coefficients also revealed a very high negative correlation (at the 0.001 significance level) between the impact-energy capacity U and the percentage of secondary osteon area x in the fresh human bone specimens. The relationship is shown graphically in Fig. 10. The linear regression equation describing the impact-energy capacity U is

$$U = 210.26 - 1.792x \tag{10}$$

where U is given in in·lb/in^2.

If the percentage of cavity area y is also considered, then the relationship is slightly modified to

$$U = 202.74 - 1.957x + 1.249y \qquad (11)$$

Unlike fresh human bone samples, test results from beef bone specimens did not show a statistically significant $(S = 0.05)$ correlation between the percentage of secondary osteon area and impact-energy capacity. The main reason for this may be that the range of secondary osteon area in beef bone samples is much smaller than that of the human bone samples, and that the beef bone samples were obtained from various subjects. Hert et al. [15] also tested cortical beef bone specimens in bending impact and did not find any correlation between the energy-absorption capacity and the percentage area of Haversian systems in the specimen.

There are two possible explanations for the negative correlations between the percentage area of Haversian bone and bone strength. These are the higher percentage of cavity area in Haversian bone and the fact that Haversian bone is less mineralized than primary bone. Currey [45] also expressed the opinion that both these causes may result in the weakness caused by the presence of Haversian systems. Another possible cause of the weakening effect of Haversian systems is the weak interface between the secondary osteons and the interstitial bone matrix [108]. This weak interface perhaps facilitates the propagation of the main crack front, causing an early failure. Evidence of this was found in the subsequent fractographic analysis of the bone fracture surfaces.

The dependence of the dynamic strength of human bone on its microstructure [109] leads to several implications that are of practical importance. First is the fact that the relationship enables us to predict the impact tolerance of bone from a knowledge of its microstructure. Lower ultimate strength and energy-absorption

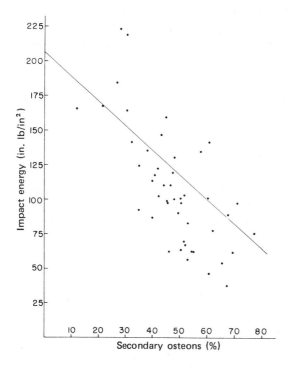

Figure 10 Relation between impact energy-absorption capacity and percentage area of secondary osteons in fresh human bone specimens.

capacity for bones with a larger percentage of Haversian systems may explain why the bones of older people having largely remodeled secondary bone are less pliable, and why geriatric fracture is quite common.

It has been shown previously that by using the correlations between the elastic and strength properties of bone, the maximum stress can be determined *in vivo* by ultrasonic and other means. Therefore, by using the relationships between the bone strength and its microstructure [e.g., Eqs. (6) and (8)], the microstructural features (e.g., the percentage area of secondary osteons) of a bone can also be estimated from *in vivo* measurements. These results are also helpful in developing mathematical models of bone as a composite material.

It is expected that further work in this direction will produce better insight into the ways in which different bone diseases affect the strength characteristics of bone by causing changes in its microstructure. This, in turn, may lead to new diagnostic or treatment methods.

Notched samples The presence of a discontinuity in the geometry or in a material property of a long bone can cause a stress concentration and thus seriously reduce its load-carrying capacity. Clinical evidence of such stress-concentration effects is found in cases where a fractured bone, which appeared completely healed in an x-ray examination, was refractured during the normal activity of the patient [110 to 112]. Such stress-concentration effects become more pronounced in a dynamic condition, as in a fall, increasing the likelihood of refracture.

To explore the notch sensitivity of bone in tensile impact, some single- and double-edge notched specimens were tested in the pendulum tester. These specimens required much less impact energy for fracture and showed reduced ultimate stress and strain. This suggests that bone is highly susceptible to the stress concentrations of surface defects and confirms that a large amount of impact energy is expended in crack initiation. The subsequent crack propagation requires a relatively small portion of the total failure energy. This behavior is evident from the steep slope of the tearing portion of the load-time curve (Figs. 6 and 7) and the small area under this portion of the curve.

The drastic reduction in both the ultimate stress and the energy-absorption capacity of notched bone specimens indicates that, by creating holes and notches for fixing implants as is often done in orthopedic surgery, we might significantly reduce the load-carrying capacity of the whole bone. This also suggests that, if possible, such defects should be confined to the portion of the bone that is predominantly in compression, as this reduces the likelihood of propagating the crack. Further research is necessary to determine the optimum sizes of drill holes and the spacings that would minimize the effect of stress concentration and thus the likelihood of fracture.

4.4 Fractography

Fractography is the systematic examination of fracture surfaces with an aim of analyzing fracture features to determine the causes and basic mechanisms of fracture. Material engineers have traditionally used fractographic methods as a valuable tool in the failure analysis of metals and composites [113, 114]. Such methods can also be profitably used in the study of the micromechanics of bone fracture [30, 56, 115, 116]. With this objective in mind, fractographic investigations of selected bone samples were conducted. The examination of fractured bone specimens involved several metallographic techniques, including reflected-light microscopy and scanning electron fractography [100, 117].

Most compact bone specimens failed without any significant change in their cross sections, indicating the brittle fracture behavior of mature bone (Fig. 4). Figure 11 is a scanning electron micrograph of three compact bone samples tested in tensile impact. As shown in this figure, macroscopically most fracture surfaces exhibited a fairly rough texture, and the majority of the failures could be characterized as a quasi-cleavage type of fracture (Fig. 11c).

Where signs of large plastic deformation were present, as in Fig. 11b, this was verified from the stress-strain record. The fracture surfaces sometimes contained a natural bone fault, such as a blood vessel, showing that the fracture might have originated there (Fig. 11b). On the other hand, when an advancing crack met a natural bone cavity, the crack was either stopped or it deviated, indicating that natural cavities in bone may also be helpful in containing the growth of the crack front.

Most bone specimens failed without any signs of osteon pullouts, unlike the fiber pullouts in the failure of composites. This is shown in Fig. 12, which also shows the concentric lamellar structure of an osteon. At controlled crack propagation rates, Piekarski [56] obtained osteon pullouts that also created large fracture surfaces. As the formation of a new fracture surface is the main mechanism by

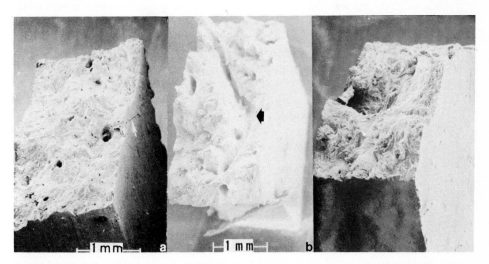

Figure 11 Scanning electron micrograph showing macroscopic views of tensile impact fracture surfaces of beef bone. (a) Brittle fracture, secondary crack shown by arrow, 25×; (b) ductile fracture, might have originated at the large blood vessel (arrow), 20×; (c) quasi-cleavage fracture, 25×.

which a material absorbs fracture energy, this explains why bone exhibits a high resistance to fracture when the crack is propagated at a controlled rate.

As shown in Figs. 11a and 13, secondary microcracks were often associated with the main fracture surface. The results indicate that, in the case of catastrophic failures, secondary microcracking—and not osteon pullout—was the main mechanism of plastic deformation. As the surface area of such secondary cracks is comparable to and sometimes larger than the main fracture surface, in applying linear elastic fracture mechanics to bone fracture, it is important to consider the surface energy required to produce such secondary microcracks. Owing to the increased fracture surface area, specimens with extensive secondary microcracks are likely to show a higher energy-absorption capacity than specimens in which they are absent. Thus the presence of such secondary cracks may explain some of the variations in the dynamic strength properties of the tensile impact specimens.

The results of this study showed that fractographic analysis of bone fracture surfaces can be very helpful in increasing our understanding of the micromechanics of bone fracture. The results also indicated that scanning electron microscopy can be utilized as a convenient means for studying bone microstructure and its relation to fracture properties.

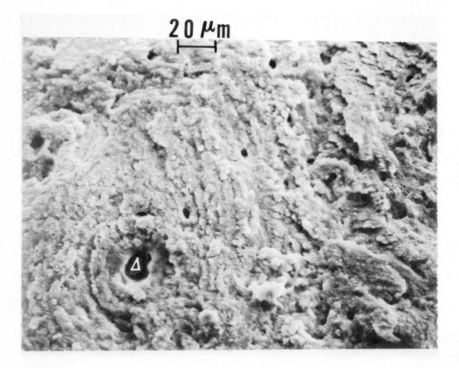

Figure 12 Scanning electron micrograph of the tensile impact fracture surface of a compact beef bone specimen showing the concentric lamellar structure of an osteon. Haversian canal at the center of the osteon (marked by Δ).

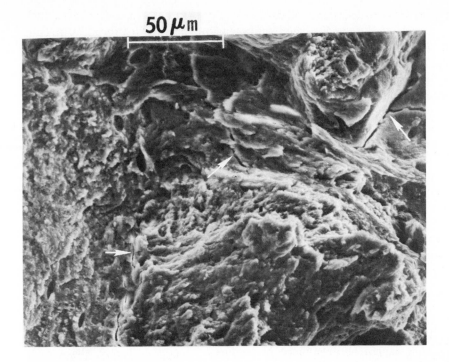

Figure 13 Scanning electron micrograph of the tensile impact fracture surface of a notched compact bone sample showing extensive secondary microcracking (marked by arrows).

5 CONCLUSIONS

Bone is a complex, anisotropic, nonhomogeneous material with time-dependent viscoelastic properties. Because of its strain-rate dependence, the maximum stress that bone can resist depends on a balance between the rate at which local displacements are imposed and the rate at which these displacements can be accommodated by elastic deformation and plastic flow. Thus we see that both an estimation of the local displacement rate and the resulting stresses are necessary to solve fracture problems in bone. Because of this rate dependence, static criteria for bone fracture are insufficient, and even a quasi-dynamic criterion may be inadequate. Unfortunately, much of the current design of safety equipment is based on the static tolerance of bone, rather than on its dynamic properties.

In static testing we generally characterize the strength of bone by the maximum stress that the specimen can withstand before failure. But until recently, it was difficult to measure the stress-strain behavior experimentally under high rates of loading. Therefore, in most previous impact studies, the dynamic or impact strength of bone was measured by the total energy required to fracture the specimen, which, for instance, in a pendulum testing machine, is given by the product of the weight of the pendulum and the difference between the initial and final heights. This investigation shows that bone samples with the same fracture energy might have very different stress-strain behavior. This emphasizes that the total work of fracture is not necessarily the most useful parameter that can be measured, because it masks such effects. This investigation demonstrates the utility of instrumented tensile impact tests in characterizing fracture behavior and in determining the impact tolerance of bone.

It should be noted that the method for the tensile impact testing of bone utilized in this investigation can easily be modified to test samples at different strain rates, by dropping the pendulum head from different heights. The simplicity of this test method and the ease of analyzing the results makes it suitable as a standard laboratory test for the determination of the dynamic strength of bone. This is especially true because, owing to the marked plastic yielding of bone in bending, ultimate stresses cannot be calculated accurately without a knowledge of the stress-strain relationships over the whole cross section [90]. Thus, transverse impact testing of bone, by Charpy or Izod methods, fails to provide data on ultimate stress, an important parameter in the calculation of tolerance limits.

5.1 Some Applications

Some applications of the tensile impact tolerance data obtained during this investigation are as follows. For obvious reasons, the *in vivo* strength of living human bone cannot be determined by loading a bone up to failure. One possible way to circumvent this difficulty is to estimate the dynamic strength of bone utilizing the correlations between bone strength and elastic properties obtained during this investigation. As discussed previously, *in vivo* nondestructive determination of elastic properties is possible using ultrasonic methods. This approach may find application in space flights where, due to calcium losses, bone strengths may be adversely affected. Additional applications may be found in determining the mechanical properties of healing fractures [103 to 105].

Study of the dynamic mechanical properties of bone is needed to develop quantitative specifications for substitute materials and to ensure effective mechanical compatibility of implants and prosthetic devices, which are often used to replace parts of defective or fractured bone. A mechanical mismatch because of greatly different elastic properties of the bone and the implant will produce a stress concentration that might lead to early failure. It might also introduce some spurious signals into some biological control loops, causing undesirable biological reactions. For instance, a rigid prosthesis that does not transmit any load to a bone might encourage osteoclastic action, resulting in bone resorption. Thus, the behavior of bone as a material and its static and dynamic load-carrying capacities are of direct importance in the design of bone plates, screws, nails, and other internal prostheses [118 to 120]. It is hoped that the data on the dynamic mechanical behavior of bone obtained during this investigation will be helpful in this regard.

Another important application of information concerning the dynamic response of human bone is in the development of model materials for anthropomorphic dummies to be used in crashworthiness experiments [121]. Once the ultimate impact strength of bone is known, suitable synthetic materials can be used in the skeletons of anthropomorphic dummies. These materials can then be expected to fail at the same tolerance limits as human bones.

5.2 Future Research Directions

Compared with structural materials, much remains to be learned about the dynamic and fracture behavior of bone. It is therefore difficult to select those directions that need immediate research attention.

It is clear that there is a need for the development of failure theories for bone along the lines used for structural materials. Existing failure theories for engineering materials, especially those for anisotropic materials, can be modified to apply to bone and should be checked with experimental observations. The main difficulty in developing an accurate failure theory for bone is the fact that no data are at present available on the mechanical behavior of bone under biaxial or multiaxial loading. Although, in practice, most bone fractures occur under a combined loading condition, most previous investigations have studied bone strength only for uniaxial stresses. Therefore, it is hoped that in future investigations more emphasis will be placed on testing bone under combined loading systems.

The formulation of constitutive laws for the rate sensitivity of bone will be of considerable importance in analyzing dynamic-loading problems. A common feature of such constitutive laws for engineering materials is the hypothesis of a reference static stress-strain relation. For multiaxial loading, this corresponds to a reference static yield surface, which grows in some prescribed manner with strain rate. Determination of such yield surfaces for various strain rates will be an important step forward in formulating a dynamic failure criterion for bone.

Additional future research directions relate to stress concentrators in bone. Bone contains a large number of natural cavities in the form of Haversian canals, Volkmann's canals, canaliculi, and resorption spaces, most of which are oriented longitudinally. These bear certain similarities to flaws in unidirectional composites. Thus stress concentration might play an important role in the initiation and propagation of cracks in bone. On the other hand, they might have a beneficial effect in arresting crack propagation. This happens when a sharp crack meets a natural cavity that blunts the crack tip, causing a reduction in stress concentration. Stress-concentration effects are especially important at high strain rates, as it has been shown that dynamic loading of a solid containing a crack may give rise to stress-intensity factors whose magnitudes exceed those generated by quasi-static loading [122]. The role of stress concentration (both static and dynamic) in bone is poorly understood and needs much further study to determine its effect on fracture strength.

It is evident from a review of the present literature on the mechanical properties of bone (see Sec. 3) that a wide gap exists between our understanding of the macroscopic and microscopic aspects of bone fracture. As aptly pointed out by Herrmann and Liebowitz [35], a correlation between observations on the microscopic and the macroscopic levels and their relationship to fracture needs to be systematically pursued. It appears that fractographic analysis of bone fracture surfaces can be a helpful tool in this pursuit and can contribute significantly to our understanding of the micromechanics of bone fracture [115, 116].

Fracture of bone depends simultaneously on many parameters, and a comprehensive understanding of the dynamic strength of bone requires knowledge of not only these separate effects but also of their interaction. Thus, studies on the influence of strain rate [18, 20, 53, 79], fatigue [13, 33], humidity [9, 19], temperature [89], age [12, 123], and microstructure [15, 45, 124, 125] must be related in a comprehensive failure theory. To synthesize these experimental results into a cohesive whole, fracture of bone needs to be explained in terms of its micromechanics, showing how these parameters affect the mechanisms causing fracture. Only then we will have a reasonably complete understanding of how bone behaves as a material.

APPENDIX: RELEVANT UNIT CONVERSION TABLE

1 pound force (lbf) = 4.448 Newton (N)
1 kilogram force (kgf) = 9.807 N
1 Joule (J) = 1 Newton meter (N m)
1 lb/in^2 (psi) = 6894.8 N/m^2
1 kip/in^2 (ksi) = 1000 lb/in^2
1 in lb/in^2 = 175.13 J/m^2
1 ft lbf = 1.3558 Joule
1 Pascal (Pa) = 1 N/m^2

REFERENCES

1. F. G. Evans, Impact Tolerance of Human Pelvic and Long Bones, in E. S. Gurdian, W. A. Lang, L. M. Patrick, and L. M. Thomas (eds.), "Impact Injury and Crash Protection," pp. 402–417, Thomas, Springfield, Ill., 1970.
2. J. Wolff, "Das Gesetz der Transformation der Knochen," Hirschwald, Berlin, 1892.
3. C. Bassett and R. O. Becker, Generation of Electric Potentials by Bone in Response to Mechanical Stress, *Science,* vol. 137, pp. 1063–1064, 1962.
4. J. D. Currey, The Adaptation of Bones to Stress, *J. Theor. Biol.,* vol. 20, pp. 91–106, 1968.
5. R. G. Snyder, "Impact. Bioastronautics Data Book," pp. 221–295, *NASA* SP-3006, 1973.
6. D. Orne and Y. K. Liu, A Mathematical Model of Spinal Response to Impact, *J. Biomech.,* vol. 4, pp. 49–71, 1971.
7. A. Ascenzi and E. Bonucci, The Tensile Properties of Single Osteons, *Anat. Rec.,* vol. 158, pp. 375–386, 1967.
8. A. Ascenzi, E. Bonucci, and A. Simkin, An Approach to the Mechanical Properties of Single Osteonic Lamellae, *J. Biomech.,* vol. 6, pp. 227–235, 1973.
9. F. G. Evans, "Stress and Strain in Bones," Thomas, Springfield, Ill., 1957.

10. F. G. Evans, "Mechanical Properties of Bone," Thomas, Springfield, Ill., 1973.
11. E. Rixford, The Mechanisms of Fracture, *J. Am. Med. Assoc.*, vol. 61, pp. 916–920, 1913.
12. F. G. Evans and M. Lebow, Regional Differences in Some of the Physical Properties of the Human Femur, *J. Appl. Physiol.*, vol. 3, pp. 563–572, 1951.
13. F. G. Evans and M. Lebow, Strength of Human Compact Bone under Repetitive Loading, *J. Appl. Physiol.*, vol. 10, p. 127, 1957.
14. J. H. McElhaney and E. F. Byars, Dynamic Response of Biological Materials, ASME paper 65-WA/HUF 9, 1965.
15. J. Hert, P. Kuchera, M. Vavra, and V. Volenik, Comparison of the Mechanical Properties of Both the Primary and Haversian Bone Tissue, *Acta Anat.*, vol. 61, pp. 412–423, 1965.
16. B. S. Mather, Observations on the Effects of Static and Impact Loading on the Human Femur, *J. Biomech.*, vol. 1, pp. 331–335, 1968.
17. A. H. Burstein and V. H. Frankel, The Viscoelastic Properties of Some Biological Materials, *Ann. N.Y. Acad. Sci.*, vol. 146, pp. 158–165, 1968.
18. F. Bird, H. Becker, J. Healer, and M. Messer, Experimental Determination of the Mechanical Properties of Bone, *Aerosp. Med.*, pp. 44–48, January, 1968.
19. E. D. Sedlin, A Rheological Model for Cortical Bone, *Acta Orthop. Scand. Suppl.*, vol. 83, pp. 5–77, 1965.
20. J. H. McElhaney, Dynamic Response of Bone and Muscle Tissue, *J. Appl. Physiol.*, vol. 21, pp. 1231–1236, 1966.
21. K. Rodahl, J. T. Nicholson, and E. M. Brown, "Bone as a Tissue," McGraw-Hill, New York, 1960.
22. A. W. Ham and T. S. Leeson, "Histology," Lippincott, Philadelphia, 1961.
23. H. M. Frost, "Bone Remodelling Dynamics," Thomas, Springfield, Ill., 1963.
24. H. M. Frost, "Bone Biodynamics," Little, Brown, Boston, 1964.
25. F. C. McLean and M. R. Urist, "Bone: Fundamentals of the Physiology of Skeletal Tissue," 3d ed., University of Chicago Press, Chicago, 1968.
26. G. H. Bourne, "The Biochemistry and Physiology of Bone," 2d ed., Academic, New York, 1971.
27. J. W. Smith, The Arrangement of Collagen Fibers in Human Secondary Osteons, *J. Bone J. Surg.*, vol. 42B, pp. 588–605, 1960.
28. R. R. Cooper, J. W. Milgram, and R. A. Robinson, Morphology of the Osteon, *J. Bone J. Surg.*, vol. 48A, pp. 1239–1271, 1966.
29. H. Kraus, On the Mechanical Properties and Behavior of Human Compact Bone, in S. N. Levine (ed.), "Advances in Biomedical Engineering and Medical Physics," vol. 2, pp. 169–204, Interscience, New York, 1968.
30. M. H. Pope and J. O. Outwater, The Fracture Characteristics of Bone Substance, *J. Biomech.*, vol. 5, pp. 457–465, 1972.
31. D. H. Enlow, "Principles of Bone Remodelling," Thomas, Springfield, Ill., 1963.
32. S. Saha and W. C. Hayes, Instrumented Tensile Impact Tests of Bone, *Exp. Mech.*, vol. 14, pp. 473–478, 1974.
33. S. A. V. Swanson, Biomechanical Characteristics of Bone, in R. M. Kenedi (ed.), "Advances in Biomedical Engineering," vol. 1, pp. 137–187, Academic, New York, 1971.
34. J. D. Currey, The Mechanical Properties of Bone, *Clin. Orthop. Relat. Res.*, no. 73, pp. 210–231, 1970.
35. George Herrmann and Harold Liebowitz, Mechanics of Bone Fracture, in H. Liebowitz (ed.), "Fracture: An Advanced Treatise," vol. VII, pp. 771–840, Academic, New York, 1972.
36. M. G. Wertheim, Memoire sur l'élasticité et la cohesion des principaux tissues du corps humain, *Ann. Chim. Phys.*, vol. 21, pp. 385–414, 1847.
37. A. A. Rauber, "Elasticitat und festigheit der Knochen," vol. IV, pp. 1–75, Engelmann, Leipzig, 1876.
38. K. K. Hulsen, Specific Gravity, Resilience and Strength of Bone, *Bull. Biol. Lab. St. Petersburg*, vol. 1, pp. 7–35, 1896 (in Russian).

39. C. O. Carothers, F. C. Smith, and P. Calabrisi, The Elasticity and Strength of Some Long Bones of the Human Body, *Nav. Med. Res. Inst. Rept.* NM 001 056.02.13, 1949.

40. F. G. Evans and M. Lebow, The Strength of Human Bone as Revealed by Engineering Techniques, *Am. J. Surg.,* vol. 83, p. 326, 1952.

41. W. T. Dempster and R. T. Liddicoat, Compact Bone as a Nonisotropic Material, *Am. J. Anat.,* vol. 91, pp. 331–362, 1952.

42. W. T. Dempster and R. F. Coleman, Tensile Strength of Bone along and across the Grain, *J. Appl. Physiol.,* vol. 16, pp. 355–360, 1961.

43. F. G. Evans, Significant Differences in the Tensile Strength of Adult Human Compact Bone, in H. J. J. Blackwood (ed.), "Proceedings of the First European Bone and Tooth Symposium," pp. 319–331, Pergamon, Oxford, 1964.

44. E. D. Sedlin and C. Hirsch, Factors Affecting the Determination of the Physical Properties of Femoral Cortical Bone, *Acta Orthop. Scand.,* vol. 37, pp. 29–48, 1966.

45. J. D. Currey, Differences in the Tensile Strength of Bone of Different Histological Type, *J. Anat. London,* vol. 93, pp. 87–95, 1959.

46. A. W. Sweeney, R. P. Kroon, and R. K. Byars, Mechanical Characteristics of Bone and Its Constituents, ASME paper 65-WA/HUF-7, 1965.

47. C. Hirsch and F. G. Evans, Studies on some Physical Properties of Infant Compact Bone, *Acta Orthop. Scand.,* vol. 35, pp. 300–313, 1965.

48. J. C. Wall, S. Chatterjee, and J. W. Jeffery, On the Origin of Scatter in Results of Human Bone Strength Tests, *Med. Biol. Eng.,* vol. 8, pp. 171–180, 1970.

49. K. Tsuda, Studies on the Bending Test and the Impulsive Bending Test on Human Compact Bone, *J. Kyoto Pref. Med. Univ.,* vol. 61, pp. 1001–1025, 1957.

50. E. Salkovitz, Structural Properties of Bone, in L. Stark and G. C. Agarwal (eds.), "Biomaterials," pp. 119–129, Plenum, New York, 1969.

51. F. Bird and H. Becker, Dynamic Experiments with Beef Femur, *Allied Research Associates Rept.* ARA322-2, Concord, Mass., 1966.

52. J. L. Wood, "Mechanical Properties of Human Cranial Bone in Tension," Ph.D. thesis, University of Michigan, Ann Arbor, Mich., 1969.

53. J. L. Wood, Dynamic Response of Human Cranial Bone, *J. Biomech.,* vol. 4, pp. 1–12, 1971.

54. W. Bonfield and C. H. Li, Deformation and Fracture of Bone, *J. Appl. Phys.,* vol. 37, pp. 869–875, 1966.

55. K. Piekarski, Fracture of Bone, *J. Appl. Phys.,* vol. 41, no. 1, pp. 215–223, 1970.

56. D. R. Margel-Robertson, "Studies of Fracture in Bone," Ph.D. thesis, Stanford University, Stanford, Calif., 1973.

57. J. W. Melvin and F. G. Evans, Crack Propagation in Bone, in Y. C. Fung and J. A. Brighton (eds.), "1973 Biomechanics Symposium,", pp. 87–88, ASME, New York, 1973.

58. J. Black and E. Korostoff, Dynamic Mechanical Properties of Viable Human Cortical Bone, *J. Biomech.,* vol. 6, pp. 435–438, 1973.

59. W. Goldsmith, Biomechanics of Head Injury, in Y. C. Fung, N. Perrone, and M. Anliker (eds.), "Biomechanics, Its Foundations and Objectives," pp. 585–634, Prentice-Hall, Englewood Cliffs, N.J., 1972.

60. A. E. Hirsch, A. K. Ommaya, and R. H. Mahone, Tolerance of Subhuman Primate Brain to Cerebral Concussion, in E. S. Gurdjian, W. A. Lange, L. M. Patrick, and L. M. Thomas (eds.), "Impact Injury and Crash Protection," pp. 352–369, Thomas, Springfield, Ill., 1970.

61. V. R. Hodgson, Physical Factors Related to Experimental Concussion, in E. S. Gurdjian, W. A. Lange, L. M. Patrick, and L. M. Thomas (eds.), "Impact Injury and Crash Protection," pp. 275–307, Thomas, Springfield, 1970.

62. F. J. Unterharnscheidt and E. A. Ripperger, Mechanics and Pathomorphology of Impact-related Closed Brain Injuries, in N. Perrone (ed.), "Dynamic Response of Biomechanical Systems," pp. 46–83, ASME, New York, 1970.

63. F. G. Evans, H. R. Lissner, and M. Lebow, The Relation of Energy, Velocity and Acceleration to Skull Fracture, *Surg. Gynecol. Obstet.,* vol. 111, pp. 329–338, 1958.

64. E. S. Gurdjian, J. E. Webster, and H. R. Lissner, The Mechanics of Production of Liner Skull Fracture, *Surg. Gynecol. Obstet.*, vol. 85, pp. 195-210, 1947.
65. E. S. Gurdjian, J. E. Webster, and H. R. Lissner, Studies on Skull Fracture with Particular Reference to Engineering Factors, *Am. J. Surg.*, vol. 78, pp. 736-742, 1949.
66. E. S. Gurdjian, J. E. Webster, and H. R. Lissner, The Mechanism of Skull Fracture, *J. Neurosurg.*, vol. 7, pp. 106-114, 1950.
67. E. S. Gurdjian, W. A. Lange, L. M. Patrick, and L. M. Thomas, "Impact Injury and Crash Protection," Thomas, Springfield, Ill., 1970.
68. H. R. Lissner, E. S. Gurdjian, and J. E. Webster, Mechanics of Skull Fracture, *Proc. Exp. Stress Anal.*, vol. 7, pp. 61-70, 1949.
69. D. F. Huelke, Deformation Studies of the Mandible under Impact, *Anat. Rec.*, vol. 136, p. 214, 1960.
70. D. F. Huelke, Mechanisms Involved in the Production of Mandibular Fractures: A Study with the "Stress Coat" Technique, *J. Dent. Res.*, vol. 40, pp. 1042-1056, 1961.
71. A. M. Nahum, J. D. Gatts, C. W. Gadd, and J. Danforth, Impact Tolerance of the Skull and Face, in "12th Stapp Car Crash Conference," pp. 302-316, New York, 1968.
72. L. M. Patrick, Caudo-Cephalad Static and Dynamic Injuries to the Vertebrae, in M. K. Cragun (ed.), "The Fifth Stapp Automotive Crash and Field Demonstration Conference," pp. 171-181, Center for Continuation Study, University of Minnesota, Minneapolis, Minn., 1962.
73. A. F. Fasola, R. C. Baker, and F. A. Hitchcock, Anatomical and Physiological Effects of Rapid Deceleration, *WADC Tech. Rept.*, pp. 54-218, Wright-Patterson Air Force Base, Ohio, 1955.
74. L. M. Patrick. C. K. Kroell, and H. J. Martz, Jr., Forces on the Human Body in Simulated Crashes, in M. K. Cragun (ed.), "Proceedings of the Ninth Stapp Car Crash Conference," pp. 237-259, University of Minnesota, Minneapolis, Minn., 1966.
75. H. E. Pedersen, F. G. Evans, and H. R. Lissner, Deformation Studies of the Femur under Various Loadings and Orientations, *Anat. Rec.*, vol. 103, pp. 159-185, 1949.
76. F. G. Evans, H. E. Pedersen, and H. R. Lissner, The Role of Tensile Stress in the Mechanism of Femoral Fractures, *J. Bone J. Surg.*, vol. 33A, no. 2, pp. 485-501, 1951.
77. L. D. Smith, Hip Fractures, *J. Bone J. Surg.*, vol. 35A, pp. 367-383, 1953.
78. G. J. Sammarco, A. H. Burstein, W. L. Davis, and V. H. Frankel, The Biomechanics of Torsional Fractures: The Effect of Loading on Ultimate Properties, *J. Biomech.*, vol. 4, pp. 113-117, 1971.
79. M. M. Panjabi, A. A. White, and W. O. Southwick, Mechanical Properties of Bone as a Function of Rate of Deformation, *J. Bone J. Surg.*, vol. 55A, pp. 322-330, 1973.
80. "Symposium on Biodynamic Models and Their Applications," *Aerospace Medical Research Laboratory Rept.* AMRL-TR-71-29, 1971.
81. Y. K. Liu and J. D. Murray, A Theoretical Study of the Effect of Impulse in the Human Torso, in Y. C. Fung (ed.), "Biomechanics," pp. 167-186, ASME, New York, 1966.
82. R. R. McHenry, Mathematical Models for Injury Prediction, in E. S. Gurdjian, W. A. Lange, L. M. Patrick, and L. M. Thomas (eds.), "Impact Injury and Crash Protection," pp. 214-233, Thomas, Springfield, Ill., 1970.
83. D. J. Segal, Computer Simulation of Body Kinematics Associated with Rapid Declerations, in N. Perrone (ed.), "Dynamic Response of Biomechanical Systems," pp. 23-45, ASME, New York, 1970.
84. A. P. Vulcan and A. I. King, Forces and Moments Sustained by Lower Vertebral Column of a Seated Human during Seat-to-Head Acceleration, in N. Perrone (ed.), "Dynamic Response of Biomechanical Systems," pp. 84-100, ASME, New York, 1970.
85. G. N. Bycroft, Mathematical Model of a Head Subjected to an Angular Acceleration, *J. Biomech.*, vol. 6, pp. 487-495, 1973.
86. V. H. Kenner and W. Goldsmith, Impact on a Simple Physical Model of the Head, *J. Biomech.*, vol. 6, pp. 1-11, 1973.
87. S. Saha and W. C. Hayes, Tensile Impact Properties of Bone, in Y. C. Fung and J. A. Brighton (ed.), "1973 Biomechanics Symposium," pp. 89-91, ASME, New York, 1973.

88. A. Ascenzi, E. Bonucci, and A. Checcucci, The Tensile Properties of Single Osteons Studied Using a Microwave Extensimeter, in F. G. Evans (ed.), "Studies on the Anatomy and Function of Bone and Joints," pp. 121–141, Springer-Verlag, Heidelberg, 1966.

89. W. Bonfield and C. H. Li, Anisotrophy of Nonelastic Flow in Bone, *J. Appl. Phys.*, vol. 38, no. 6, pp. 2450–2455, 1967.

90. A. H. Burstein, J. D. Currey, V. H. Frankel, and D. T. Reilly, The Ultimate Properties of Bone Tissue: The Effects of Yielding, *J. Biomech.*, vol. 5, pp. 35–44, 1972.

91. V. H. Frankel and A. H. Burstein, The Design of Orthopaedic Prostheses, in B. L. Segal and D. G. Kilpatrick (eds.), "Engineering in the Practice of Medicine," pp. 148–158, Williams and Wilkins, Baltimore, 1967.

92. F. G. Evans and A. I. King, Regional Differences in Some Physical Properties of Human Spongy Bone, in F. G. Evans (ed.), "Biomechanical Studies of the Musculo-Skeletal System, pp. 49–67, Thomas, Springfield, Ill., 1961.

93. J. W. Melvin, D. H. Robbins, and V. L. Roberts, The Mechanical Behavior of the Dipole Layer of the Human Skull in Compression, *Dev. Mech.*, vol. 5, pp. 811–818, 1969.

94. J. W. Pugh, R. M. Rose, and E. L. Radin, Elastic and Viscoelastic Properties of Trabecular Bone: Dependence on Structure, *J. Biomech.*, vol. 6, pp. 475–485, 1973.

95. C. M. Schoenfeld, E. P. Lautenschlager, and P. R. Meyer, Mechanical Properties of Human Cancellous Bone in the Femoral Head, *Med. Biol. Eng.*, vol. 12, pp. 313–317, 1974.

96. D. S. Clark and P. E. Duwez, The Influence of Strain Rate on Some Tensile Properties of Steel, *Proc. ASTM*, vol. 50, pp. 560–575, 1950.

97. D. S. Clark and D. S. Wood, The Influence of Specimen Dimension and Shape on the Results in Tension Impact Testing, *Proc. ASTM*, vol. 50, pp. 577–586, 1950.

98. H. C. Mann, The Relation between the Tension Static and Dynamic Tests, *Proc. ASTM*, vol. 35, pt. 2, pp. 323–340, 1935.

99. R. E. Ely, Review of a High Speed Tensile Testing Program for Thermoplastics, in A. G. H. Dietz and F. R. Eirich (eds.), "High Speed Testing," vol. 1, pp. 3–25, Interscience, New York, 1960.

100. S. Saha, "Tensile Impact Properties of Bone and Their Relation to Microstructure," Ph.D. thesis, Stanford University, Stanford, Calif., 1973.

101. B. S. Mather, Correlations between Strength and Other Properties of Long Bones, *J. Trauma*, vol. 7, no. 5, pp. 633–638, 1967.

102. W. Abendschein and G. W. Hyatt, Ultrasonics and Selected Physical Properties of Bone, *Clin. Orthop.*, no. 69, pp. 294–301, 1970.

103. L. P. Floriani, N. T. Debevoise, and G. W. Hyatt, Mechanical Properties of Healing Bone by the Use of Ultrasound, *Surg. Forum*, vol. 18, pp. 468–470, 1967.

104. W. Abendschein and G. W. Hyatt, Ultrasonics and Physical Properties of Healing Bone, *J. Trauma*, vol. 12, pp. 297–301, 1972.

105. S. A. Brown and M. B. Mayor, Some Ultrasonic Properties of Healing Fracture, *Proc. 2d New England Bioeng. Conf.*, pp. 377–385, Pergamon Press, New York, 1974.

106. S. B. Lang, Ultrasonic Method for Measuring Elastic Coefficients of Bone and Results on Fresh and Dried Bovine Bones, *IEEE Trans. BioMed. Eng.*, vol. BME-17, no. 2, pp. 101–105, 1970.

107. R. W. Smith and D. A. Keiper, Dynamic Measurement of Viscoelastic Properties of Bone, *Am. J. Med. Electron.*, pp. 156–160, October, 1965.

108. F. G. Evans and S. Bang, Differences and Relationships between the Physical Properties and the Microscopic Structure of Human Femoral, Tibial and Fibular Cortical Bone, *Am. J. Anat.*, vol. 120, pp. 79–88, 1967.

109. S. Saha, Dynamic Strength of Human Compact Bone as a Function of Its Microstructure, *Proc. 27th Ann. Conf. Eng. Med. Biol.*, vol. 16, p. 290, 1974.

110. L. P. Seimon, Re-fracture of the Shaft of the Femur, *J. Bone J. Surg.*, vol. 46B, pp. 32–39, 1964.

111. V. H. Frankel and A. H. Burstein, The Biomechanics of Refracture of Bone, *Clin. Orthop.*, vol. 60, pp. 221–225, 1968.

112. O. D. Chrisman and G. A. Snook, The Problem of Refracture of the Tibia, *Clin. Orthop.*, vol. 60, pp. 217-219, 1968.
113. R. E. Peterson, Interpretation of Service Fractures, in M. Hetenyi (ed.), "Handbook of Experimental Stress Analysis," pp. 593-635, Wiley, New York, 1950.
114. "Electron Fractography," *ASTM Tech. Pub.* 436, Philadelphia, 1968.
115. S. Saha, Application of Electron Fractography to Bone Fracture, *Proc. 2d New England Bioeng. Conf.*, pp. 349-354, Pergamon Press, New York, 1974.
116. S. Saha, Fractographic Analysis of Bone Fracture, *27th Ann. Conf. Eng. Med. Biol.*, vol. 16, p. 296, 1974.
117. S. Saha, Behavior of Human Compact Bone in Tensile Impact and Its Relation to Microstructure, *Proc. 2d New England Bioeng. Conf.*, pp. 339-347, Pergamon Press, New York, 1974.
118. G. Schmeisser, Jr., Progress in Metallic Surgical Implants, *J. Mater.*, vol. 3, pp. 951-976, 1968.
119. E. Korostoff and E. I. Salkovitz, Biomaterials, vol. II, "Future Goals of Engineering in Biology and Medicine," J. F. Dickson III and J. H. U. Brown (eds.), Academic, New York, 1969.
120. D. J. Lyman and W. J. Seare, Biomedical Materials in Surgery, in R. A. Huggins, R. H. Bube, and R. W. Roberts (eds.), "Annual Review of Materials Science," vol. 4, pp. 415-433, Annual Reviews, Palo Alto, Calif., 1974.
121. J. W. Melvin, P. M. Fuller, R. P. Daniel, and G. M. Pavliscak, Human Head and Knee Tolerance to Localized Impacts, *SAE paper* 690477, Midyear Meeting, Chicago, 1969.
122. J. D. Achenbach, Dynamic Effects in Brittle Fracture, in S. Nemat-Nasser (ed.), "Mechanics Today," vol. 1, pp. 1-57, Pergamon, New York, 1974.
123. R. A. Melick and D. R. Miller, Variations of Tensile Strength of Human Cortical Bone with Age, *Clin. Sci.*, vol. 30, pp. 243-248, 1966.
124. F. G. Evans and R. Vincentelli, Relation of Collagen Fiber Orientation to Some Mechanical Properties of Human Cortical Bone, *J. Biomech.*, vol. 2, pp. 63-71, 1969.
125. F. G. Evans and R. Vincentelli, Relations of the Compressive Properties of Human Cortical Bone to Histological Structure and Calcification, *J. Biomech.*, vol. 7, pp. 1-10, 1974.
126. O. Lindahl and A. G. H. Lindgren, Cortical Bone in Man. II. Variation in Tensile Strength with Age and Sex, *Acta Orthop. Scand.*, vol. 38, pp. 141-147, 1967.

TWO

EFFECTS OF HOLES AND PERFORATIONS ON THE STRENGTH AND STRESS DISTRIBUTION IN BONE ELEMENTS

J. L. Nowinski

Clinical situations are discussed in which cracks or failures of tubular bones occur caused by holes made intentionally by the orthopedic surgeon, or caused by perforations resulting from diseases or tumors. The influence of such apertures on the stress fields in bones is examined by modeling the osseous tissue as a poroelastic or viscoelastic material. Two illustrations are given. The first illustration emphasizes the risks involved in torsion of perforated or fractured bone; it concerns a tubular bone with an aperture subjected to torsional loading, modeled by a viscoelastic material. The problem, solved in the context of linear elastostatics with the aid of the self-equilibrated stress system, is transferred into the viscoelastic Kelvin-Voigt range by means of the correspondence principle. The second illustration deals with the stress concentrations around various shapes of apertures caused by longitudinal and bending loads. Solutions are provided for two-dimensional problems of apertures of arbitrary form in a poroelastic material, subjected to an arbitrary loading. Complex-variable techniques and conformal mapping are employed in these solutions. The two-dimensional results need to be rectified by a correction factor, for evaluating the stress concentration in a tubular bone; this factor is a function of the aperture size, tube radius, and wall thickness. Tables list possible stress peaks around openings of various shapes under various loading conditions.

1 INTRODUCTION AND CLINICAL SITUATIONS

The reader, noticing the abundance of mathematical formulas in this chapter, may wonder if it is necessary to wade through the mathematics to appreciate the practical utility of the chapter. It is our obligation to provide a brief answer to this question, in the same breath advising the reader not to be dismayed by the mathematics, which is almost entirely relegated to appendixes and which need not be read.

Before we start, we have to accept the obvious fact that, from an objective point of view, the musculoskeletal system constitutes a mechanical structure as good as (or rather better than) any other inert structure, such as an automobile, an airplane, and other complex machines. Perhaps the only fundamental difference between the two is that the former is self-propelled and enormously complex.

If we agree to this fact, then our second thought is that one may apply to living machines the abundance of knowledge gained during centuries of dealing with inanimate machines. In other words, it is reasonable to start analyzing the mechanical properties of the musculoskeletal system by applying the well-known and reliable methods of structural analysis of inert systems. Such an idea is not new. Long ago Galileo advocated the soundness of such an approach. Simple structural analyses of bones were also made more than a hundred years ago by Wertheim, then by Rauber, and at the beginning of this century, by an American anatomist, Koch, in his brilliant classical paper [1] on the laws of bone architecture. Since then, a sizable number of anatomists and biomechanicists (such as McElhaney [1a] and Frankel and Burstein [2]) have built a comprehensive experimental and ideological foundation for our concept of the human as an animate machine. The usefulness of this work was always appreciated by people who, in their daily practice, deal with difficult clinical problems, in particular with regard to prosthetics and orthotics. Thus, the internal effects produced by the actions of externally applied forces are of immediate clinical interest to the orthopedic surgeon, who reduces and fixes a dislocation, plates a fracture, or implants a device. Specifically, this matter is of importance when, in performing an operation, the surgeon alters and disturbs, more or less drastically, the natural equilibrium that exists in every part of a living organism, and is able to evaluate only intuitively the future performance of the operated part. The situation seems the more surprising if one makes the comparison with our knowledge of the action of inert systems. We know with considerable accuracy the effects of loads to which inanimate systems are subjected in actual service. Such systems are correspondingly designed quite accurately, and in the rare instances in which our information on their structural resistance is limited, we are able at least to work within the so-called coefficients of safety. On the other hand, with regard to living organisms the operating surgeon, or the orthopedist in postoperative or conservative therapy, is often able to do no more than use traditional rules or make a best guess.

1.1 Clinical Situations

A few examples taken from the work of two eminent orthopedists [2] may serve to illustrate the seriousness of the problem.

Figure 1 displays a fracture of the neck of a femur fixed with multiple threaded pins. The holes made by the pins are locations of high stress concentration, increased by the close proximity of the holes and the resulting superposition of effects. Because there was insufficient information on the magnitude of the forces acting on the joint and the strength of the pins, the center pin has failed in

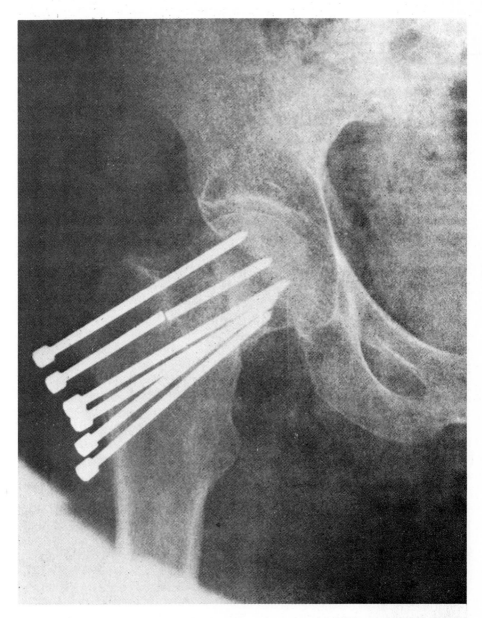

Figure 1 Femoral neck fixed with pins (one pin underwent a shear failure). (*After Frankel and Burstein [2].*)

shear. The removal of all but one of the pins is a routine procedure, but the extraction of the broken-off portion of the center pin requires special surgery, which could have been avoided if, prior to the original surgery, a better mechanical analysis had been available.

A similar situation is shown in Fig. 2, in which a femoral neck is fixed with a nail plate. Because the surgeon was insufficiently acquainted with the mechanics of the operation, the screws were not aligned strictly parallel to the holes in the nail plate, and a couple of screw heads broke. This necessitated additional (and rather superfluous) surgery involving the removal of the broken shafts of the screws.

Another mechanically hazardous situation is shown on the roentgenogram in Fig. 3, in which a femoral neck is strengthened by a common fixation device. The femur is here pierced by a number of pin holes, and its upper part is considerably weakened by insertion of a heavy bolt. It is still an open question whether the number (seven) of pins fixing the plate is right, because in similar cases five and even four pins are used; further, in experiments on commercial riveting, the fifth rivet placed in a row was always found useless.

A dangerous problem of a different kind results from insufficient acquaintance with the detrimental effects of holes on the strength of structures. Figure 4 displays such a case, involving a tibia. Here a fracture has originated from a long groove made for graft purposes. For this to occur it was sufficient for the patient merely to pivot on the foot. In another case (not shown here), a fracture in a tibia was found to spread from a small square hole with rather sharp corners. Again, this happened as the result of an imposed twisting moment. We can well understand that these fractures, propagating from the grooves or holes, are brought about by local stress concentrations and by the reduced resistance to twist of the open cross sections (relative to the closed section).

The foregoing are but examples of many clinical accidents that prove, beyond any reasonable doubt, the need for a more thorough analysis of the effects of external forces on the mechanical behavior of bones. To achieve this knowledge, however, one has to pay a price—exactly the same price as is paid every day in the structural analysis of inanimate systems. This price consists of considerable mathematical preparation and labor before final synthetic conclusions are reached. There is nothing unusual in this, as no scientific study provides royal roads to success. Likewise, there is no easy road to the structural analysis of bones, and this conclusion may serve as an answer to the question posed at the beginning of this introduction.

1.2 Scope of the Chapter

We have selected, for detailed analysis, a single problem that, with the background of the few accidents described above, may be considered particularly relevant in a clinical sense. This problem concerns the effects of holes in bones. In the first part of our investigation (Sec. 3) we analyze the influence of a perforation or hole on the resistance of a long bone to the action of torsional loading. The pertinent analysis has a clear connection with the failure illustrated in Fig. 4 and verifies the

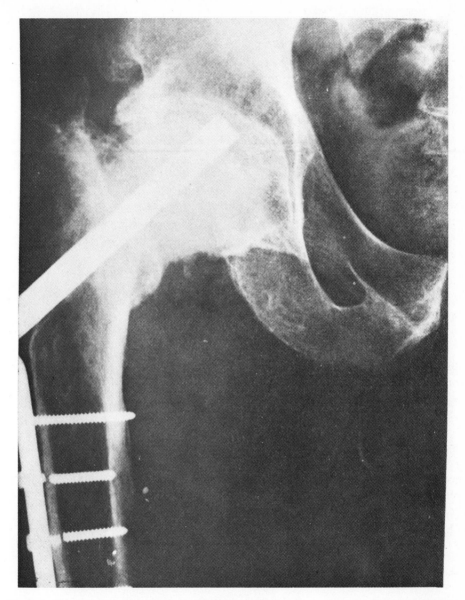

Figure 2 Femoral neck fixed with a nail plate (breakage of two screws). (*After Frankel and Burstein [2]*.)

clinical experience that holes reduce by many times the resistance of bones to torsional loading.

The concentration of stresses around holes, which—as mentioned above—may lead to hazardous situations of cracking or fracturing, constitutes the second part of our study (Sec. 4). This part confirms the clinical findings of high, and often

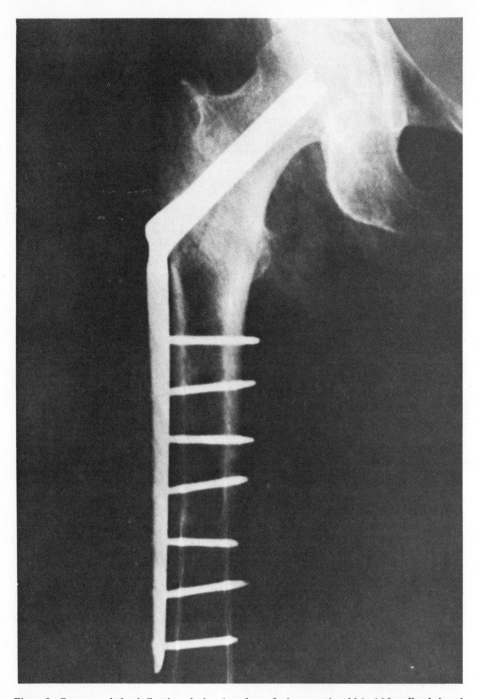

Figure 3 Common skeletal fixation device (number of pins questionable). (*After Frankel and Burstein [2].*)

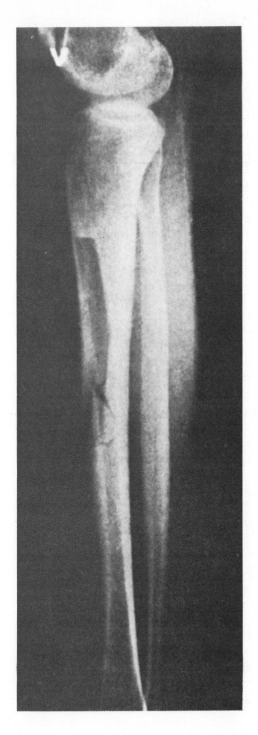

Figure 4 Fracture through a tibial donor site. (*After Frankel and Burstein [2].*)

dangerous, stress concentrations around openings, mostly in the vicinity of sharp corners.

It should be clearly and unequivocally stated that all conclusions derived from the structural analysis of such complicated bodies as bones must be accepted with great caution until a sufficiently large mass of theoretical-experimental evidence is accumulated. It is true that most properties of bone have been studied experimentally, and correlations developed that to some extent predict their gross behavior. However, it is equally true that the structure of the real bone *in vivo* is so intricate and individual, the actual situations in the living organism—especially if impaired by a disease or disrupted by a surgical intervention—so complex, that any model, however theoretically perfect, must be considered no more than a plausible conjecture. Nonetheless, the conclusions reached in the present state of the theory give at least some indications about the mechanical processes that develop in the human skeleton under the action of external forces. It seems justified to believe that in the absence of any theories or models at all, these processes would be totally obscure.

2 CONSTITUTIVE REPRESENTATIONS OF BONE ADOPTED IN THE ANALYSES

According to the experimental appraisal of the mechanical properties of bone, its structure is so complex and so variable that a characterization even of a single specimen requires an inordinate effort. In fact, the mechanical properties are found to be functions of numerous factors, such as the grain orientation of the specimen, preserving treatment (dry, wet, or embalmed), temperature, age and specific physical characteristics of the individual, location and orientation of the sample in the skeletal system, and rate of load application. Despite such difficulties, some facts related to bone structure are nowadays almost universally accepted. These are, for instance, that the osseous tissue is a viscoelastic material, that it it anisotropic (i.e., different in different directions), and that most often it must be treated as a nonhomogeneous substance, mainly on account of the irregular porosity. Furthermore (as with most biological materials), the solid phase of the bone—which is the osseous latticework—is most likely governed by nonlinear constitutive relations between the stress and deformation, and its liquid phase—which in the form of blood, marrow, nerve tissue, synovial and interstitial fluids, and others fills the cavities in the solid latticework—behaves like a strongly non-Newtonian fluid, that is, a fluid of complex viscosity.

With regard to the anisotropy of the bone, its material symmetries correspond to the crystallographic structures of the rhombic and hexagonal types. In other words, bone substance seems to have either three mutually orthogonal planes of material symmetry or a single axis of symmetry of an infinite order. It behaves, therefore, like an orthotropic or transversely isotropic body.[1] The effects of

---

[1] The reader interested in anisotropic materials may consult the book by Hearmon [3].

orientation reported by various researchers seem to indicate that the mechanical properties measured parallel to the grain exceed considerably those measured across the grain. According to some sources, the Young's modulus E_l parallel to the grain is, in a wet bone, about 2.33 times greater than the modulus E_r in the radial direction. On the other hand, this ratio with respect to the azimuthal direction is $E_l:E_t = 2.08$. In other words, if E_r is supposed equal to 1, then $E_l:E_t:E_r = 2.33:1.12:1$. In some vibration tests reported by Laird and Kingsbury [4], these ratios appear to be somewhat different, namely $1.6:1.3:1$. This is, however, relatively close to the above-mentioned results if one considers the strong non-uniformity of the material.

The prevailing opinion is that the viscoelastic properties of bone may adequately be described by the so-called standard linear viscoelastic body, which includes a spring connected in series with a Kelvin-Voigt element (the latter constituting a spring with a parallel dashpot) as in Fig. 5. This model—which, by the way, gives a scheme whose behavior, at least qualitatively, reproduces the response of many real bodies under load—seems to exhibit all three characteristic traits of bone material: instantaneous elastic response, bounded creep under load, and incomplete relaxation. Furthermore, the standard model has been thoroughly analyzed and is relatively simple to examine. A study of the rheological response of bone to external loading was performed by Sedlin [5] in his fundamental dissertation and a following paper. Some of the experimental results were confirmed by experiments made at the University of Delaware. Sedlin's extensive experimental research proved that under loads well below the fracture load the actual behavior of bone is well characterized by the standard linear viscoelastic model. Figures 6 and 7, reproduced from Sedlin's study, distinctly display the above-mentioned features of the standard model of Fig. 5. In Fig. 6 the instantaneous elasticity OA of the spring

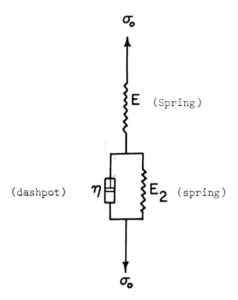

Figure 5 Linear standard model adopted according to experiments by Sedlin [5].

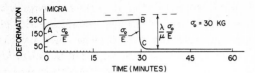

Figure 6 Change of deformation under constant load versus time according to experiments by Sedlin. (*After Sedlin [5].*)

E, exhibited under a constant load σ_0, is followed by the period of creep AB, which probably tends to the asymptotic value $(\lambda/\mu)(\sigma_0/E)$, where $\lambda = (E + E_2)/\eta$ and $\mu = E_2/\eta$. This is in accordance with the theoretical equation governing the standard model,

$$\dot{\sigma} + \lambda\sigma = E(\dot{e} + \lambda e) \tag{1}$$

in which a superposed dot denotes a time derivative, and e means a unit elongation associated with the tensile stress σ. Removal of the load at time $t = 30$ min causes the deformation to display the reversible elastic component BC, and then a gradual decay with time. The second basic feature of the bone is exhibited in Figs. 7 and 8, in which the relaxation AB of the specimens, under a deformation applied fairly suddenly (region OA) and then kept constant, is clearly visible. An opinion similar to that expressed by Sedlin is shared by practicing orthopedic surgeons Frankel and Burstein [2], although Zarek and Edwards [6] recommend a simplified model similar to a single Kelvin-Voigt two-element system (a spring in parallel with a viscous dashpot). On the other hand, Laird and Kingsbury [4] conclude from their dynamic experiments that the bone cannot be modeled with full accuracy by the standard model in the range of frequencies between 1 and 16 kHz. These authors do not suggest a model that would permit observed responses to be accounted for analytically. It should be noted, however, that even the standard model involves considerable mathematical difficulties when applied to concrete problems involving three-dimensional anisotropic viscoelastic bodies.

If the creep and relaxation curves of the standard model—which theoretically represent exponential functions—do not satisfactorily approximate experimental curves such as those in Figs. 6 to 8, it is always possible (at the cost of additional computational labor) to correct the imperfections of the model by adding combinations of higher-order derivatives of σ and e to both sides of the governing equation (1). It may also become possible to apply a representation in terms of suitable hereditary integrals, for which a great choice of kernels of exponentials, Abel's and

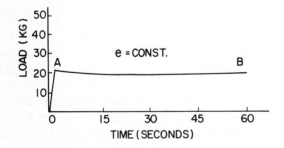

Figure 7 Relaxation of cortical bone under constant deformation according to experiments by Sedlin. (*After Sedlin [5].*)

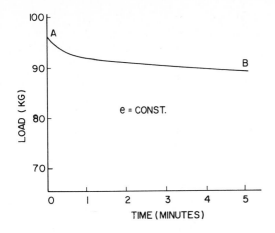

Figure 8 Relaxation of bovine bone under constant deformation, after experiments in Delaware [4].

other types, is available (consult, e.g., Robotnov [7]). Leaving, of necessity, the final judgment on the most perfect model of bone to posterity, we have to recognize that, whatever the actual constitution of the bone may be, to determine the stress and deformation fields in the skeletal elements on a more scientifice basis there seem to exist, among others, two possibilities. The first, given the porous structure of the bone, is to adopt any known theory of the mechanical behavior of poroelastic media. So far as can be determined, there exist three such theories: those of Biot [8], Heinrich and Desoyer [9], and Lubinski [9a], all applied to the consolidation theory of soil mechanics. A comprehensive review of these theories—in particular of Biot's approach—is given by Paria [10]. It must be admitted, however, that, despite the fact that the poroelastic model exhibits all the qualitative features mentioned above as pertaining to bone, such an approach to bone mechanics may be contested on the ground that the distinct features of this model make it perhaps less adaptable to the behavior of real bone, especially bone *in vivo*.

The other alternative is to treat bone as any other viscoelastic anisotropic material by employing the well-established methods of the conventional theory of viscoelasticity. Of the two illustrative studies that follow, the first applies the theory of linear viscoelasticity; the second is based on the theory of poroelastic bodies set forth by Biot.

To facilitate the calculations—already sufficiently laborious—we make some natural simplifications. We first assume that the distribution and concentration of pores in the bone are uniform, so that the bulk material may be regarded as quasi-homogeneous. As a result of this assumption the porosity, defined as the percentage of pores in a unit of bulk volume, is constant. Furthermore, in the poroelastic approach we assume that in the two-phase (solid skeleton, pore fluid) system, the solid skeleton is linearly and perfectly elastic and its deformations are small. Thus, the mechanical behavior of the solid component of the bone is governed by the linear Hooke's law. We consider the liquid phase as a Newtonian viscous fluid, and the flow of fluid produced by the deformation of the bone as governed by the linear Darcy's law. With regard to the internal forces, it is postulated that the stress in the bulk material is smoothly divided between, and uniformly distributed over, the solid phase; in the fluid phase the internal forces appear as hydrostatic pressures.

In the viscoelastic approach we adopt—as already mentioned—the apparatus of the linear theory of viscoelasticity with all its hypotheses and conclusions (consult, e.g., Flugge [11]). For the convenience of the reader, in each illustrative study the mathematical calculations are almost entirely confined to the associated appendix, and the main results and conclusions are discussed first. The meanings of the symbols used are explained in the notations section at the beginning of each appendix.

3 SIMULATION OF STRENGTH AND STRESS DISTRIBUTION IN A FRACTURED OR PERFORATED TUBULAR BONE RESULTING FROM TORSIONAL LOADING

As noted in the introduction to this chapter, this study simulates the clinical situation in which a fracture occurs or a hole is drilled in a long tubular bone, such as the femur or tibia, or a perforation is present as a result of bone disease. Because—according to the experimental evidence—the hazards of such situations lie especially in the weakness of the given bone elements to withstand torsional loadings, we analyze here the influence of a hole on the torsional strength of a tubular bone with an aperture bounded by two radial and two transverse cross

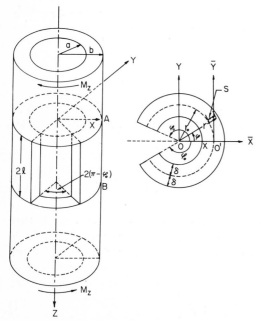

Figure 9 Geometry of the problem.

sections. The osseous tissue is simulated by a viscoelastic material of the standard linear type (Fig. 5) and is considered transverse isotropic with regard to its texture. The tube is subjected to sudden action of twisting couples M_z whose magnitude remains unchanged in time. Let us assume that the tubular bone has the form of a long circular cylinder in which an opening has been made that is bounded by two radial and two transverse cross sections, as shown in Fig. 9. The z axis of a Cartesian rectangular coordinate system x, y, z coincides with the axis of the cylinder, and the x axis lies in the axial plane of symmetry of the opening, whose length is $2l$ and whose width is $2(\pi - \phi_0)$.

The material of the tube is transverse isotropic, with the planes of isotropy perpendicular to the z axis. The cylinder is subjected to the twisting action of the couples M_z. If the cylinder had no opening, then determining the stress distribution would be a trivial problem of the theory of torsion of Saint-Venant. On the other hand, if the opening extended over the entire length of the cylinder ($l = \infty$), then the problem would degenerate into one concerning torsion in a bar with the cross section in the form of an annular sector. The problem under consideration constitutes, of course, a combination of these two cases, and requires first of all an analysis of the second case, torsion in an open annular cylinder.

3.1 The Stress State Resulting from a Perforation along a Portion of the Tube

It is well known that, whatever the cross section of a twisted bar, the axial displacement w, or warping, of the bar is given by the formula $w = \theta \Phi(x, y)$, where θ is the unit angle of twist, and $\Phi(x, y)$ is the so-called warping function. With the aid of this function we find that the only identically nonvanishing stress components according to the Saint-Venant theory of torsion and bending are

$$\tau_{zx} = G_z\theta \left(\frac{\partial \Phi}{\partial \bar{x}} - \bar{y}\right) \qquad \tau_{zy} = G_z\theta \left(\frac{\partial \Phi}{\partial \bar{y}} + \bar{x}\right) \tag{2}$$

where G_z is the shear modulus in planes parallel to the z axis, and $\bar{x}$ and $\bar{y}$ are axes of any reference frame, say, the one with the origin O' at the point $r = r_0$ and $\phi = 0$. In polar coordinates Eqs. (2) take the form

$$\tau_{zr} = G_z\theta \left(\frac{\partial \Phi}{\partial r} - r_0 \sin \phi\right) \qquad \tau_{z\phi} = G_z\theta \left(\frac{\partial \Phi}{\partial \phi}\frac{1}{r} + r - r_0 \cos \phi\right) \tag{3}$$

Except over a small range near the open ends, the shear lines in the annular sector may be considered circles. Thus, it is possible to adopt, instead of the above solution, the simplified solution given by Prescott [12] and Huber [13] (denoted by the superscript 0)

$$\tau_{zr}^0 = 0 \qquad \tau_{z\phi}^0 = G_z\theta \left(r - \frac{K}{r}\right) \tag{4}$$

where $K = (b^2 - a^2)/2(\ln b - \ln a)$. Although approximate, this solution seems sufficiently accurate for the present purposes. A comparison of equations (3) and (4) shows that, according to Prescott's solution, the warping $w^0 = w^0(r, \phi)$ of the cross sections of the open tube is represented by the formula

$$w^0 = \theta (r_0 r \sin \phi - K\phi) \tag{5}$$

so that the warping function becomes $\Phi^0 = r_0 r \sin \phi - K\phi$. The correctness of this conclusion is easily verified by inserting $\Phi^0 = w_0/\theta$ into Eq. (3), which then becomes identical with Prescott's Eq. (4). This formula would, of course, be valid if the open tube were free. In the present case, however, the terminal cross sections of the open segment AB of the tube (Fig. 9) are pieced together with the adjacent complete tubular portions, so that the warping of the cross sections is restrained and not free. This restraint is rather stringent because, as is well known, the cross sections of a twisted circular tube remain plane, and thus the terminal cross sections A and B of the open segment AB also have to remain undistorted.

To satisfy this requirement, it is necessary to superpose on the stress system Eq. (4), which accounts for the applied twisting couples, an auxiliary system of self-equilibrating stresses, which accounts for the fact that the open part of the tube is not free but attached to closed portions of the tube. As such a system we take the auxiliary system denoted by an asterisk in App. A and derived by Nowinski [14]. It is given by Eqs. (A1) and satisfies all necessary equilibrium and boundary conditions. The warping associated with this auxiliary stress sytem is denoted by w^*. For the open segment to form an interrupted hole with the adjacent portion, we require that

$$\int_{(A)} (w^0 - w^*)^2 \, dA = \text{minimum} \tag{6}$$

where A is the cross-sectional area of the annular segment. This condition, in combination with the Castigliano variational principle (equivalent to fulfillment of compatibility of deformations) leads to explicit expressions for the stress components of the auxiliary system. These stresses, on being added to the basic stresses given by Eqs. (4), yield the actual stresses appearing in the perforated tube. This completes the elastic part of the solution.

To determine the stress system in a tube of viscoelastic material, we apply the correspondence principle relating the viscoelastic and elastic stresses as explained in App. A. Furthermore, we assume that the viscoelastic material is of the standard type illustrated in Fig. 5. After a lengthy computation whose main steps are given in App. A, we find the resultant viscoelastic stresses at the moment directly after the application of the twisting moment M_z (that is, at time $t = +0$), and after a long period of time (denoted by $t = \infty$). We are mostly interested in the longitudinal stresses $\tau_{zz}^{*\text{visc}}$ and shear stresses $\tau_{z\phi}^{*\text{visc}}$, where, again, the asterisk denotes the auxiliary stress system, and the superscript visc the viscoelasticity of material. The stresses resulting from a very thin longitudinal slit in a thin tube, representing the

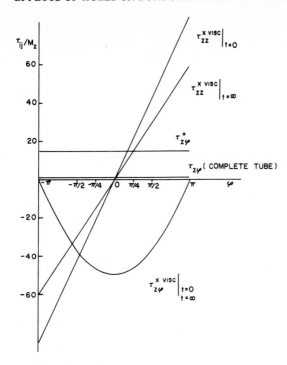

Figure 10 Stresses at the outer edge versus azimuthal angle ϕ: $\tau_{ij}^{*\text{visc}}$ = auxiliary stress; $\tau_{z\phi}^{0}$ = stress in fractured tube; total shear stress = $\tau_{z\phi}^{0} + \tau_{z\phi}^{*}$.

proximal part of the tibia, are calculated in the numerical example in App. A. The tube has an inner to outer radius ratio of 0.9:1.1. The stresses at the interface of the perforated and end portions, along the outer edge of the tube, are displayed in Fig. 10. Note the high concentration of shear stresses, at $\phi = 0$, diametrically opposite the slit. It is also seen that at the interface large normal stresses are generated, which would of course be absent in the free open tube. We shall return to this figure later.

3.2 Change in the Moment-Carrying Capacity Resulting from the Perforation

The relation between the twisting moment M_z and the unit angle of twist θ is given in the theory of elasticity as

$$M_z = G_z \theta \pi \frac{b^4 - a^4}{2} \tag{7}$$

where G_z is the shear modulus. If the thickness of the tube 2δ is small compared with the mean radius r_0, then with sufficient accuracy we can assert that

$$M_z = 4\pi G_z \theta r_0^3 \delta \tag{8}$$

On the other hand, if the tube has a thin slit all along its length, then on integrating the second of Eqs. (4) over the (open) cross section of the tube and equating the result to the twisting moment denoted now by M_z', we find the relation

$$M_z' = 4\pi G_z \theta r_0 \delta^3 \tag{9}$$

The ratio of the moments

$$\frac{M_z'}{M_z} = \frac{\delta^2}{r_0^2} \tag{10}$$

is independent of elastic constants and, therefore, in view of the elastic-viscoelastic correspondence principle, holds for viscoelastic materials. It is seen that for a thin tube for which, for example, $\alpha = \delta/r_0 = 0.1$, a corresponding open tube may bear no more than 0.01 of the moment carried by a complete tube. For a thick tube [for which the accuracy of Eq. (10) diminishes considerably] the ratio M_z'/M_z would, nonetheless, be of order $\frac{1}{16}$, which is still small. We observe here the fact—recorded in the introduction as a clinical fact—that an aperture (here in the form of a slit) in a tubular bone reduces its resistance to torsion in almost alarming proportion.

It is apparent that for relatively short and narrow apertures, the presence of portions of a complete tube at both ends of the open part of the tube must strengthen its resistance to the action of torsional loads. To find the restraining influence of such an arrangement it is necessary to find the strain energy of the middle portion of the tube [represented by the expression that comes after the variation sign δ on the left side of Eq. (A11)]. Putting this energy equal to the work done by the torque M_z on the total angle of twist $\psi = \theta l$ we find, after some calculations (here omitted), that

$$\psi = \frac{M_z}{4G_z \phi_0 r_0 \delta^3} \left(l + \frac{E_z}{2G_z} \sqrt{\gamma^*} \, \phi_0^2 r_0 \Lambda \right) \tag{11}$$

where

$$\Lambda = S_3 - \frac{E_z}{6G_z} \gamma^* S_2' + \frac{E_z}{15G} (\gamma^*)^2 \phi_0^2 \alpha^2 F_1 + \frac{E_z}{30G_z} \gamma^* \phi_0^2 S_2'' \tag{12}$$

[The symbols in Eq. (12) are defined at the beginning of App. A.] In the factor preceding the parentheses in Eq. (11), which we denote by θ_0, we recognize the angle of unit twist given by Eq. (9) for a tube opened along a generator along its full length (so that $\phi_0 = \pi$). Thus the second term in parenthesis in Eq. (11) exhibits the beneficial action of adjacent portions of a closed tube in reducing the twist of the open portion. For the ratio $\alpha = \delta/r_0 = 0.1$ and the values of the geometric and material coefficients in the numerical example in App. A, we find that the total angle of twist is

$$\psi = \theta_0 l \left(1 - 3.2 \frac{r_0}{l} \right) \tag{13}$$

It is seen that the effect of the constraint on the total angle of twist is small if the mean radius of the tube r_0 is small in comparison with the length of the aperture l. Because the Saint-Venant theory of torsion holds rigorously for slender bars, the accuracy of Eq. (13) decreases if the ratio r_0/l increases. However, for $r_0/l = \frac{1}{10}$, say, we may roughly estimate that the total angle of twist decreases by 30 percent.

This means that the transmitted moment M_z' given by Eq. (9) increases in the same proportion (for a fixed angle of twist), and that consequently the ratio of the moments in Eq. (10) increases slightly. This increase is, however, moderate, and only slightly alleviates the hazard of the situation.

3.3 Change in the Strength of the Tube Resulting from the Perforation

The strength of the tube with an aperture, viewed from the standpoint of the magnitude of the stresses, decreases in the presence of the end constraints. Before we verify this statement, let us note that to find the location of the most intense stresses in the cross sections $z = 0$ and $z = 2l$ (where the influence of the auxiliary stresses of restraint is greatest) would be a very complicated task. Let us, therefore, examine the stresses at the outer face of the tube, where the angle ϕ is $\pm\pi/2$. By consulting the graphs in Fig. 10, we find that at these places, say, immediately after the application of the load, the corresponding stresses are

$$\frac{\tau_{zz}^{*\text{visc}}}{M_z} \approx 42 \qquad \frac{\tau_{z\phi}^{*\text{visc}}}{M_z} \approx -36 \qquad \frac{\tau_{z\phi}^{0}}{M_z} \approx 15 \qquad (14)$$

To predict the combination of stress that produces failure of the tube under the action of the twisting moments M_z, it is necessary to use the so-called strength hypothesis. Unfortunately, for viscoelastic materials, whose mechanical properties depend on time, and in particular for osseous tissue, there exists no definite theory of strength. To find, at least, an estimate of the possible situation, let us examine the predictions obtained on the basis of the popular energy hypothesis of Huber-Mises-Hencky.[2] According to this hypothesis the stress at the moment of failure of the material is measured, in the present case, by the representative stress

$$\tau_{\text{repr}} = \sqrt{(\tau_{zz}^{*\text{visc}})^2 + (\tau_{z\phi}^{*\text{visc}} + \tau_{z\phi}^{0})^2} \qquad (15)$$

with the stresses under the radical associated with the faces of the tube. Introducing the values of Eqs. (14) into the last equation we find that, in the presence of the end restraints, $\tau_{\text{repr}}/M_z \approx 47$. On the other hand, if the restraining ends of the tube are absent, $\tau_{\text{repr}}/M_z = \tau_{z\phi}^{0}/M_z \approx 15$. This result indicates that, while the stiffness of the tube with a slit increases in the presence of restraints exerted by the terminal portions of the tube, its strength measured in terms of this representative stress decreases considerably. This result confirms our earlier conclusion on the hazards accompanying openings and perforations existing in tubular members subjected to the action of torsional moments.

---

[2] A comparison of the results of this hypothesis, universally accepted for elastoplastic materials, with the results of two other leading hypotheses, for a class of viscoelastic materials, may be found in [15].

4 SIMULATION OF THE STRESS DISTRIBUTION
AROUND HOLES IN BONE ELEMENTS

As noted in the introduction, apertures, whether resulting from perforations caused by bone disease or made intentionally at donor sites or by means of pins, nails, screws, and shafts, represent places that require special clinical attention. First, they reduce the strength of the bone elements by diminishing their working area and often strikingly changing their resistance patterns. This was discussed in detail in Sec. 3.

Other hazardous peculiarities of apertures are associated with their sharp corners and thin notches, which often become sites for the inception and propagation of cracks. In fact, according to the theory of Griffith [15a], if the energy necessary to lengthen an existing tiny cleft can be supplied by a reduction of the strain energy stored in the material, the crack extends spontaneously without the consumption of the total energy. This often leads to a complete breakdown of the structure.

Finally, any aperture constitutes a discontinuity in the relatively smooth geometry of a sound bone, and as such ordinarily becomes a stress raiser of considerable intensity. The resulting stress concentrations are of great clinical importance, because the actual stress close to the aperture may exceed by many times the average stress existing in the bone under given conditions and taken into account by the orthopedist.

In what follows we intend to discuss the stress distributions around holes in some detail from the point of view of the stress concentration. For definiteness and to facilitate the discussion, we assume, for the time being, that the dimensions of the hole are small compared with the dimensions of the bone. In such a case the effect of the hole is strictly local. The stress distribution in the vicinity of the hole is drastically changed, but in view of the Saint-Venant principle this change is small or even negligible at distances larger than the dimensions of the hole. Such a strictly localized character of the stress distribution around holes is often accepted as the justification for the approximate assumption that elements of finite width with small holes as compared with their width may be treated as very large plates with holes. We accept this approximate viewpoint in the first part of the discussion that follows. Later, we shall analyze the accuracy of such an approach.

4.1 Elliptic Hole in a Poroelastic
Material Plate under Tension

As a first step let us investigate the effect of an elliptic hole in a poroelastic material, applying the theory of Biot [8]. It is assumed that the bone member is subjected to a uniform tension P and that the insert in the hole exerts uniform pressure σ_0 on the fluid, and q_0 on the solid material.

Let σ_{ij} denote the stress acting on the solid phase, and σ the pressure in the fluid, both per unit area of the bulk material. In a cylindrical coordinate system r, θ, z, the major axis $2a$ of the ellipse is directed along the line $\theta = 0$, which also

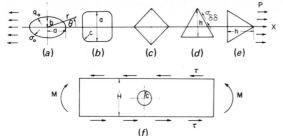

Figure 11 Various contours of holes.

points in the direction of the tension P (see Fig. 11a). Assuming that the strain is planar, we find the constitutive equations (stress-strain relations) of the poroelastic isotropic material, according to Biot's theory [8], as

$$\sigma_{rr} = 2Ne_{rr} + Ae + Q\epsilon$$

$$\sigma_{\theta\theta} = 2Ne_{\theta\theta} + Ae + Q\epsilon$$

$$\sigma_{zz} = Ae + Q\epsilon \qquad (16)$$

$$\sigma_{r\theta} = 2Ne_{r\theta}$$

$$\sigma = Qe + M\epsilon$$

Here[3] e_{ij} is the classical strain tensor associated with the solid phase; e and ϵ denote the dilatation of the solid and liquid phases, respectively; and uppercase letters represent material constants. If we treat the problem in the customary way as quasi-static (that is, if we neglect the influence of inertia), then the equilibrium equations are satisfied on introduction of the stress function $F(r, \theta, t)$ defined by

$$\sigma_{rr} + \sigma = \frac{1}{r}\frac{\partial F}{\partial r} + \frac{1}{r^2}\frac{\partial^2 F}{\partial \theta^2} \qquad \sigma_{\theta\theta} + \sigma = \frac{\partial^2 F}{\partial r^2}$$

$$\sigma_{r\theta} = \frac{1}{r^2}\frac{\partial F}{\partial \theta} - \frac{1}{r}\frac{\partial^2 F}{\partial r\, \partial \theta} \qquad (17)$$

where t denotes time. It remains now to satisfy the equation of compatibility of deformations. It was shown by Biot that this equation is satisfied if

$$\kappa\, \nabla^4 F = \nabla^2 \sigma \qquad (18)$$

where $\nabla^2 = \partial^2/\partial r^2 + \partial^2/r\, \partial r + \partial^2/r^2\, \partial^2\theta$ is the Laplace operator and we have used the notation $\kappa = [(A + 2N)M - Q^2]/2N(Q + M)$.

Another equation that must be satisfied and that regulates the flow of fluid through the pores is given by Darcy's law:

$$\nabla^2(Qe + M) = b\, \frac{\partial}{\partial t}(\epsilon - e) \qquad (19)$$

---

[3] See also the definitions at the beginning of App. B.

where b is the coefficient of permeability of the material. Manipulation of the last two equations leads to the following final form for the two governing equations:

$$K \nabla^6 F = b \frac{\partial}{\partial t} \nabla^4 F$$

$$K \nabla^4 \sigma = b \frac{\partial}{\partial t} \nabla^2 \sigma \tag{20}$$

each fortunately involving a single unknown function F or σ. In these equations the material coefficient $K = [(A + 2N)M - Q^2]/[A + M + 2(N + Q)]$.

An expedient solution procedure for these equations consists in suppressing the time variable t by means of the Laplace transformation, represented by

$$f^*(r, \theta; \xi) = \int_0^\infty f(r, \theta; t) e^{-\xi t} \, dt \tag{21}$$

with the asterisk denoting the transform of the function $f(r, \theta; t)$ and the Laplace parameter ξ replacing the time t. Then the transforms $F^*(r, \theta; \xi)$ and $\sigma^*(r, \theta; \xi)$ of the functions F and σ are represented by the relations

$$F^* = F_1^* + \frac{r_0^2}{K} \Sigma^* \qquad \sigma^* = \Sigma^* \tag{22}$$

where F_1^* is a biharmonic function satisfying the equation

$$\nabla^4 F_1^* = 0 \tag{23}$$

and Σ^* is a solution of the Helmholtz equation

$$r_0^2 \nabla^2 \Sigma^* - \Sigma^* = 0 \tag{24}$$

In these equations r_0^2 denotes the ratio $K/b\xi$, and the Σ^* terms in Eqs. (22) are chosen so as to satisfy automatically the condition (18) between the stress function F and the fluid pressure σ.

As the problem is formulated, it may be solved by using the technique of conformal mapping. In the present case, that of an elliptic aperture, this technique consists in mapping the exterior of the ellipse into the exterior of a unit circle in the plane of complex variables. The calculations are lengthy and cumbersome, and the main steps are relegated to App. B.[4] The final form of the stress components is given by Eqs. (B37) to (B39) in App. B, where, at the contour of the aperture, $\sigma_{\rho\rho}$ denotes the stress perpendicular to the contour, $\sigma_{\delta\delta}$ the tangential stress parallel to the contour, and $\sigma_{\rho\delta}$ the shear stress.

It is easily shown that the most informative stress, because it is the most intense, is the tangential stress $\sigma_{\delta\delta}$, which is representative of the stress concentration around the hole. It is displayed in Fig. 12 at time $t = +0$ (directly after

---

[4] More details of the mathematical analysis may be found in [16].

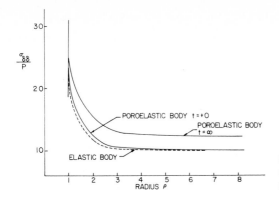

Figure 12 Azimuthal stress $\sigma_{\delta\delta}/P$ versus distance ρ along section $\delta = \pi/2$ for the elliptic hole.

the application of load) and at time $t = \infty$ (long after the application of load), along the cross section through the minor axis of the ellipse, where it reaches its maximum. It is also compared with the purely elastic case. The tensile load P is made equal to 1000 lb/in^2, whereas on the contour of the aperture the load on the elastic skeleton q_0 and the fluid pressure σ_0 are both taken as 100 lb/in^2. Furthermore, the material constant κ in Eq. (18) is assumed to be 0.30, and the eccentricity of the ellipse 0.20, which means that the ratio of the semiaxes is $a/b = 1.5$. On the boundary $\rho = 1$, the values of $\sigma_{\delta\delta}/P$ at time $t = +0$ and at time $t = \infty$ are comparable, equaling 2.33 and 2.54, respectively, but they diverge with increasing distance ρ to uniform distributions equal to $\sigma_{\delta\delta}/P = 1$ and 1.2, respectively. Clearly, the factor k of stress concentration around the aperture, measured as the ratio of the maximum stress at the aperture and the applied stress P, reaches the value 2.33 at time $t = +0$ and the value 2.1 at time $t = \infty$. Close to the boundary of the aperture there is little difference between the tangential stresses at $t = +0$ and at $t = \infty$, but at distances of a few aperture dimensions the stress $\sigma_{\delta\delta}$ at $t = +0$ is about 20 percent greater than that at $t = \infty$. Because the tangential stress calculated for the purely elastic material almost coincides with the viscoelastic stress at $t = +0$ and differs relatively little (by about 20 percent) from the elastic stress after a long period of time, it is reasonable to conjecture that, as a rough approximation, the elastic stress may serve as an estimate of the viscoelastic stress whatever the time of observation of the latter.

A plot of the variation of the tangential stress around the contour (that is, at $\rho = 1$) with changing angle δ is shown in Fig. 13. The stress $\sigma_{\delta\delta}$ reaches its maximum at the ends of the minor axis of the ellipse and is smallest at the ends of the major axis (directed along the external tensile forces).

Figures 12 and 13 both indicate that the stress increases with elapsing time. This makes plausible the conclusion that the overall state of stress intensifies with time and, in turn, builds up the deformation and sets the body—at least partially—into a state of creep. Such a finding implies that the present model of the poroelastic body displays a pattern followed by the standard linear three-parameter rheological model (elastic spring in series with a Kelvin-Voigt element) in Fig. 5. Its behavior seems, therefore, to be in agreement with the model proposed by Sedlin on the basis of comprehensive experimental observations.

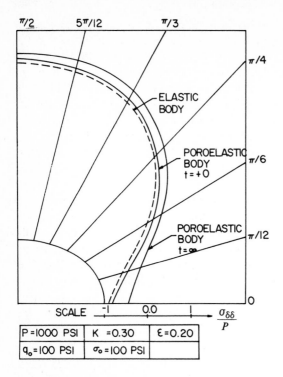

| P =1000 PSI | K =0.30 | ε=0.20 |
| q₀=100 PSI | σ₀ =100 PSI | |

Figure 13 Variation of the azimuthal stress $\sigma_{\delta\delta}/P$ around the contour ($\rho = 1$).

The calculations presented here for an elliptic contour may be similarly performed for any other aperture shape, but concrete results are still lacking. However, in view of the many unaccountable factors occurring in clinical situations, and our conclusion indicating a practically acceptable difference between elastic and viscoelastic materials, we hereafter concentrate solely on available theoretical data obtained for an elastic material.

4.2 Stress Concentrations in Bone Simulated by Elastic Plates with Small Apertures

We assume first that the dimensions of the aperture are small compared with the width of the bone element, and consider the hole as existing in a large plate. If not stated otherwise, the material is treated as isotropic. Three types of apertures are discussed: elliptic (with a circle and a slit as the limit cases), square, and equilateral triangular. Numerical data are listed according to Savin [17, 18].

Elliptic aperture—one-directional tension or compression The semiaxes of the ellipse are a and b (Fig. 11a). The external tension P per unit area of cross secton is directed along the semiaxis a. A general formula for the stress concentration factor k is

$$k = \frac{\sigma_{\delta\delta \, \max}}{P} = 1 + 2\frac{b}{a} \tag{25}$$

This checks with the value $k = 2.33$ for the elliptic hole discussed in App. B, for which $a/b = 1.5$. If $a = b$, the ellipse transforms into a circle and we get $k = 3$, which is the well-known classical result (see p. 80 of [19]). If the ratio a/b tends to zero, in other words if the ellipse becomes a narrow fissure perpendicular to the direction of tension, the concentration coefficient increases without limit. This means that at the tips of a slit perpendicular to the direction of the forces, the resistance of the material breaks down; the material becomes plastically deformed or cracks if it is brittle. On the other hand, if the slit is aligned with the external tension, when the ratio b/a tends to zero and the slit becomes a very narrow fissure, the stress concentration vanishes entirely.

Square aperture—one-directional tension or compression The side of the aperture is equal to a. It is found that the largest concentration of stress is near the corners of the square and depends considerably on the magnitude of the radius c of the rounded corners of the square. The coefficient k increases with decreasing ratio c/a. For instance, if the external tension is parallel to a side of the square as in Fig. 11b, the following values are obtained for the coefficient k at the corners:

$$\frac{c}{a} = \frac{1}{9} \qquad \frac{1}{20} \qquad \frac{1}{40}$$
$$k = 3.0 \qquad 4.6 \qquad 7.0$$

(26)

The alignment of the external tension with respect to the aperture is also of importance. For instance, if the tensile forces act parallel to a side (Fig. 11b), then we have

$$\frac{c}{a} = \frac{3}{50} \qquad \frac{1}{41}$$
$$k = 3.86 \qquad 4.46$$

(27a)

but if these forces are parallel to a diagonal (Fig. 11c), then

$$\frac{c}{a} = \frac{3}{50} \qquad \frac{1}{41}$$
$$k = 7.80 \qquad 11.52$$

(27b)

The form of Eq. (25) exhibits clearly the dependence of the coefficient k on the location of the aperture with regard to the external tension. This fact is confirmed with regard to the rectangular aperture. For instance, if the side of the rectangle of length a is located parallel to the direction of tension, we find the following maximum concentration coefficients at the corners of the rectangle:

$$\frac{a}{b} = \frac{1}{5} \qquad \frac{1}{3} \qquad \frac{1}{1} \qquad \frac{3}{1} \qquad \frac{5}{1}$$
$$k = 8.0 \qquad 6.2 \qquad 3.0 \qquad 3.2 \qquad 3.0$$

(28)

Elongation
perpendicular
to tension

Elongation
parallel to
tension

Equilateral triangular aperture—one-dimensional tension or compression The altitude of the triangle is h. Depending on the ratio c/h of the radius of the rounded vertices to the altitude, we have, for tensile forces acting parallel to a side (Fig. 11d),

$$k = 11.00 \text{ to } 17.60 \tag{29a}$$

and for forces acting perpendicular to a side (Fig. 11e),

$$k = 8.00 \text{ to } 12.80 \tag{29b}$$

the lower value corresponding to a larger ratio c/h (actually equal to $\frac{1}{14}$).

Elliptic, square, or triangular equilateral aperture—bending by a moment M Let the moment of inertia of the cross section of the strip in Fig. 11f be J. We find the concentration coefficient with the ratio $\sigma_{\delta\delta}/(MR/J)$, where for an ellipse $R = (a+b)/2$, for a square $R = 3a/50$ (a = length of a side), and for a triangle $R = 3H/2$ (H = width of the strip). Then we have

Circle, $k = 2.16$
Ellipse, $k = 0.67$
Square (sides parallel to sides of strip), $k = 1.67$ $\tag{30}$
Square (diagonal parallel to sides of strip), $k = 5.33$
Triangle (altitude parallel to length of strip), $k = 5.68$

In the above list the semiaxis a of the ellipse is directed along the length of the strip. If the semiaxis $b = 0$ and the semiaxis $a \neq 0$, then we have a slit of length $2a$ and there is no concentration of stress (the slit being located along the neutral line of the strip). If, on the other hand, $b \neq 0$ but $a = 0$, then at the ends of the slit the stress becomes unbounded. This leads to permanent plastic deformations or cracks.

4.3 Stress Concentrations Resulting from Holes in Plates of Finite Width

Heretofore our discussion involved apertures that are small compared with the width of the bone, which enabled us to treat the stress distribution as originating in a large plate. It hardly need be noted that such situations are rarely encountered in clinical practice, as in most cases the dimensions of plane surfaces are limited. The question arises, therefore, whether it is legitimate to apply data obtained for apertures in large plates, to plates of relatively small dimensions. Unfortunately, because of the considerable mathematical difficulties, the answer to this question is known for only a very few cases. We give some samples of known solutions.

If a strip of width H with a circular hole of radius c (Fig. 11f) is subjected to a longitudinal tension P (per unit area of cross section), the value of the stress concentration coefficient $k = \sigma_{\delta\delta}/P$ depends on the ratio $\lambda = 2c/H$ as follows ($\lambda = 0$ corresponds to a hole in a plate of infinite width):

$\lambda = 0$	0.1	0.2	0.3	0.4	0.5	
$k = 3.00$	3.03	3.14	3.36	3.74	4.32	(31)

It follows clearly from Eq. (31) that in the most hazardous case, when the hole covers half the width of the strip ($\lambda = 0.5$), the concentration coefficient is 1.44 (=4.32/3.00) times greater than the same coefficient evaluated for a large plate [compare formula (25) for $b = a$].

If the strip, instead of being extended, becomes sheared by external stresses τ applied along the long sides of the strip (Fig. 11f), then the concentration coefficient k, measured by the ratio $\tau_{r\delta}/\tau$, takes the following values:

$$\lambda = 0 \quad 0.1 \quad 0.2 \quad 0.3 \quad 0.4 \quad 0.5$$
$$k = 1 \quad 1.35 \quad 1.46 \quad 1.71 \quad 2.05 \quad 2.58$$

(32)

In this case, therefore, the increase in the coefficient k amounts to about 100 percent.

4.4 Influence of Tubularity on Stress Concentrations Resulting from Holes

In most clinically important cases the problem of stress distributions around holes involves tubular bones such as femurs or tibiae. In these cases it is important to know what errors are committed if we apply the results derived for plane plates to plates rolled up into close tubes. This complicated problem presents considerable difficulty, and its solution yielded numerical results in only a very few cases. But even worse, it was investigated only for thin tubes, known as shells, whereas in clinical situations the thickness of the tubular bones is most often significant. According to an approximate analysis of Lurie [20], the concentration coefficient k obtained for a plane plate must be multiplied by a coefficient k_1 to account for the curvature $1/a$ of the tube under longitudinal tension (a is the radius of its cross section). This coefficient is

$$k_1 = 1 + 0.43 \frac{c^2}{ah}$$

(33)

where c is the radius of the circular aperture, and h is the thickness of the tube (a being its radius). And so, for instance, in the proximal part of the tibia, say for $h/a = \frac{1}{5}$ and $c = h$, we find the magnification coefficient k_1 equal to about 1.09, by which one has, therefore, to multiply the coefficient $k = 3$ pertinent to a large plane plate [see formula (25) for $a = b$].

For a circular tube with a small equilateral triangular hole, subjected to twist by external shear stresses τh acting along the circular contours of the terminal cross sections of the tube (h is the thickness of the shell), Guz [21] evaluated the coefficient of stress concentration k defined as the ratio $\sigma_{\delta\delta}/\tau$, where $\sigma_{\delta\delta}$ is the tangential stress at the triangular contour (Fig. 11d) as follows: For the altitude of the triangle parallel to the generators of the tube (Fig. 11e),

$$k = \frac{\sigma_{\delta\delta}}{\tau} = +6.72$$

(34a)

and for the side of the triangle parallel to the generators of the tube (Fig. 11d),

$$k = \frac{\sigma_{\delta\delta}}{\tau} = -6.72 \qquad (34b)$$

APPENDIX A: MAJOR CALCULATIONS
FOR ANALYSIS IN SEC. 3

A1 NOTATION

a, b	inner and outer radii of tube
l	length of aperture
r_0	radius of middle surface of tube
r, ϕ, z	cylindrical coordinates
s	equal to $r - r_0$
h_1	equal to $1 + E_0/E_1$
h_3, h_{12}, h_{13}	defined by Eq. (A32) and characterizing response of three-dimensional standard model
w	longitudinal displacement (warping)
A, C, D	constants in Eqs. (A2)
α, A^*, C^*, D^*	parameters defined by Eq. (A10)
E_0, E_1, η_1	characteristics of Kelvin-Voigt model
E_z, E	Young's moduli parallel and perpendicular to the grain along z axis
E_z^*	defined by Eq. (A21)
$F_1, F_2, F_3, F_4,$	
$\beta, \lambda_{33}, \lambda_{312}$	defined by Eqs. (A22) to (A28)
G_z	shear modulus in planes parallel to z axis
K	equal to $(b^2 - a^2)/2(\ln b - \ln a)$
M_z	twisting moment
S_1, S_2, S_3	defined by Eqs. (A14) and (A15)
α^*	defined by Eq. (A18)
2δ	thickness of tube
$2(\pi - \phi_0)$	angle of opening of aperture
γ	parameter of stress decay
γ^*	equal to $\gamma^2 r_0^2$
$\gamma_0^*, \gamma_\infty^*$	defined by Eqs. (A42a) and (A43a)
τ_1	retardation time η_1/E_1
$\tau_3, \tau_{12}, \tau_{13}$	retardation times of three-dimensional standard model
$\tau_{zz}, \tau_{zr}, \tau_{z\phi}, \tau_{r\phi}$	stress components (longitudinal normal; shear in radial plane; shear in azimuthal plane; shear in cross section)
$x, y, z, \bar{x}, \bar{y}, z$	rectangular coordinates
Φ	warping function

θ, ψ unit and total angles of twist

overbar   denotes Laplace transform

*   denotes stress system (A1)

A2 THE ELASTIC STRESS FIELD

With the origin O of coordinate z located at the upper terminal cross section of the opening (Fig. 9), we take the auxiliary stress system in the following form:

$$\tau_{zz}^* = \frac{E_z\theta}{4}\, \gamma f_1 e^{-\gamma z}$$

$$\tau_{zr}^* = -\frac{E_z\theta}{8}\, \gamma^2 f_2 e^{-\gamma z}$$

$$\tau_{z\phi}^* = \frac{E_z\theta}{8}\, \gamma^2 f_3 e^{-\gamma z} \tag{A1}$$

$$\tau_{r\phi}^* = \frac{E_z\theta}{16}\, \gamma^3 f_4 e^{-\gamma z}$$

in which

$$f_1 = 4r(As\phi + Cr^2 s\phi^3 + Ds^3\phi) - [6A(\delta^2 - s^2)\phi$$
$$\quad + 10Cr^2(\delta^2 - s^2)\phi^3 + 3D(\delta^4 - s^4)\phi]$$

$$f_2 = r[2A(\delta^2 - s^2)\phi + 2Cr^2(\delta^2 - s^2)\phi^3 + D(\delta^4 - s^4)\phi] \tag{A2}$$

$$f_3 = r\{2[2A(\delta^2 - s^2)(\phi_0^2 - \phi^2) + \tfrac{3}{2}Cr^2(\delta^2 - s^2)(\phi_0^4 - \phi^4)$$
$$\quad + D(\delta^4 - s^4)(\phi_0^2 - \phi^2)] - r[2As(\phi_0^2 - \phi^2)$$
$$\quad + Cr^2 s(\phi_0^4 - \phi^4) + 2Ds^3(\phi_0^2 - \phi^2)]\}$$

$$f_4 = r^2[2A(\delta^2 - s^2)(\phi_0^2 - \phi^2) + Cr^2(\delta^2 - s^2)(\phi_0^4 - \phi^4)$$
$$\quad + D(\delta^4 - s^4)(\phi_0^2 - \phi^2)]$$

where E_z is Young's modulus in the z direction, and A, C, D, and γ are constants to be determined from additional conditions. If the radius $r_0 \to \infty$ and the angle of aperture $\phi_0 \to 0$ with $r_0\phi_0$ remaining constant, then Eqs. (A1) degenerate into those introduced by Nowinski [14] for constrained torsion of bars with rectangular cross section. The exponential terms in the stress system (A1) exhibit the strictly local character of this system, which, according to the principle of Saint-Venant, should have effect only in the region close to the existing discontinuity of the cross sections of the tube.

From the first equation of the system, with $\tau_{zz}^* = E_z\, \partial w^*/\partial z$, the warping of the cross sections associated with this system is derived as

$$w^* = -\theta\{A\theta[rs - \tfrac{3}{2}(\delta^2 - s^2)] + C\phi^3 r^2[rs - \tfrac{5}{2}(\delta^2 - s^2)]$$
$$\quad + D\phi[rs^3 - \tfrac{3}{4}(\delta^4 - s^4)]\}e^{-\gamma z} \tag{A3}$$

It is also straightforward to verify that the auxiliary stress system satisfies all the required equations of equilibrium in the differential form

$$\frac{1}{r}\frac{\partial \tau^*_{r\phi}}{\partial \phi} + \frac{\partial \tau^*_{rz}}{\partial z} = 0$$

$$\frac{\partial \tau^*_{r\phi}}{\partial r} + 2\frac{\tau^*_{r\phi}}{r} + \frac{\partial \tau^*_{\phi z}}{\partial z} = 0 \tag{A4}$$

$$\frac{\partial \tau^*_{rz}}{\partial r} + \frac{\tau^*_{rz}}{r} + \frac{1}{r}\frac{\partial \tau^*_{\phi z}}{\partial \phi} + \frac{\partial \tau^*_{zz}}{\partial z} = 0$$

as well as those in the integral form

$$\int_{(A)} \tau^*_{zz} \, dA = 0$$

$$\int_{(A)} \tau^*_{zx} \, dA = 0$$

$$\int_{(A)} \tau^*_{zy} \, dA = 0$$

$$\int_{(A)} \tau^*_{zz} y \, dA = 0 \tag{A5}$$

$$\int_{(A)} \tau^*_{zz} x \, dA = 0$$

$$\int_{(A)} \tau^*_{z\phi} r^2 \, dr \, d\phi = 0$$

where (A) denotes the annular cross section of the bar. The fulfillment of the homogeneous equations (A4) and (A5) shows that the system (A1) is in fact a self-equilibrating stress system, as asserted earlier. System (A1) also satisfies the prescribed boundary conditions

$$\tau^*_{zr} = 0 \qquad \text{at } s = \pm\delta$$

$$\tau^*_{z\phi} = 0 \qquad \text{at } \phi = \pm\phi_0 \tag{A6}$$

$$\tau^*_{r\phi} = 0 \qquad \text{at } s = \pm\delta \quad \text{and} \quad \phi = \pm\phi_0$$

A2.1 Matching the Open Segment with the Adjacent Tubular Portions

For the open segment of the tube to form one uninterrupted whole with the adjacent tubular portions, it is mandatory that the warping of portions coming into contact be identical. It seems almost impossible to satisfy this requirement pointwise. Instead, we content ourselves with an approximate fulfillment of this condition by demanding that the mean square disparity of the warping of the contacting sections be minimal:

$$\int_{(A)} (w^0 - w^*)^2 \, dA = \text{minimum} \tag{A7}$$

Because the above functional depends on three parameters A, C, and D, the following system of linear equations follows from condition (A7):

$$2a_{11}A + a_{12}C + a_{13}D = a_1$$
$$a_{12}A + 2a_{22}C + a_{23}D = a_2 \tag{A8}$$
$$a_{13}A + a_{23}C + 2a_{33}D = a_3$$

where we have used the following abbreviated notation:

$$a_1 = \tfrac{8}{9}K\phi_0^3 r_0 \delta^3$$
$$a_2 = \tfrac{8}{5}K\phi_0^5 r_0 \delta^3(\tfrac{1}{3}r_0^2 + \tfrac{1}{5}\delta^2)$$
$$a_3 = \tfrac{8}{15}K\phi_0^3 r_0 \delta^5$$
$$a_{11} = \tfrac{4}{3}\phi_0^3 r_0 \delta^3(\tfrac{1}{3}r_0^2 + \delta^2)$$
$$a_{12} = \tfrac{8}{5}\phi_0^5 r_0 \delta^3(\tfrac{1}{3}r_0^4 + \tfrac{28}{15}r_0^2\delta^2 + \tfrac{23}{35}\delta^4) \tag{A9}$$
$$a_{13} = \tfrac{8}{15}r_0 \delta^5(r_0^2 + \tfrac{23}{7}\delta^2)$$
$$a_{22} = \tfrac{4}{7}\phi_0^7 r_0 \delta^3(\tfrac{1}{3}r_0^6 + \tfrac{53}{15}r_0^4\delta^2 + \tfrac{85}{21}r_0^2\delta^4 + \tfrac{13}{21}\delta^6)$$
$$a_{23} = \tfrac{8}{5}\phi_0^5 r_0 \delta^5(\tfrac{1}{5}r_0^4 + \tfrac{10}{7}r_0^2\delta^2 + \tfrac{57}{105}\delta^4)$$
$$a_{33} = \tfrac{4}{3}\phi_0^3 r_0 \delta^7(\tfrac{1}{7}r_0^2 + \tfrac{7}{15}\delta^2)$$

At this juncture, it is convenient to introduce the symbols

$$\alpha = \frac{\delta}{r_0} \qquad A^* = \frac{r_0^2}{K}A \qquad C^* = \frac{r_0^4}{K}C \qquad D^* = \frac{r_0^4}{K}D \tag{A10}$$

Because it may be verified that the value of C^*, via the value of C, depends on the angle of aperture, we introduce an additional symbol $C^{**} = \phi_0^2 C^*$. A lengthy but trivial calculation leads to Table 1, which lists the values of A^*, C^{**}, and D^* versus the ratio α in the segment $[\tfrac{1}{10}, \tfrac{1}{3}]$.

We now turn to the determination of the still unknown parameter γ appearing

Table 1 Values of A^*, C^{**}, and D^*

α	$\frac{1}{10}$	$\frac{1}{7}$	$\frac{1}{6}$	$\frac{1}{5}$	$\frac{1}{4}$	$\frac{1}{3}$
A^*	1.064151	1.094976	1.104061	1.105206	1.082753	0.997359
C^{**}	−0.137242	−0.226104	−0.269428	−0.318957	−0.367676	−0.391988
D^*	−1.474485	−0.826771	−0.500041	−0.113189	0.301756	0.629779

in Eqs. (A1). Let us recall that the selection of the stress system (A1) rests on the fact that this system satisfies the static requirements of the problem, namely, the equations of equilibrium and the boundary conditions. The difficulty now is in making the system (A1) comply with the compatibility equations, say, in the form of Beltrami-Michell. However, in view of the fact that there is only a single parameter γ left at our disposal, we must apply, instead of the Beltrami-Michell equations, the Castigliano variational principle, which, as is well known, may be regarded as an equivalent of the compatibility equations. Taking the variation of the elastic strain energy, expressed in terms of the internal stresses, we obtain the equation

$$\delta \int_{-\delta}^{\delta} \int_{-\phi_0}^{\phi_0} \int_0^l \left[\frac{\tau_{zz}^2}{E_z} + \frac{1}{G_z} (\tau_{zr}^2 + \tau_{z\phi}^2) + \frac{\tau_{r\phi}^2}{G} \right] r \, dr \, d\phi \, dz = 0 \quad \text{(A11)}$$

where G is the shear modulus in the planes of isotropy, and it is agreed to minimize the strain energy over one-half the length of the open segment AB of the tube.[5]

Clearly, the stresses τ_{zz}, τ_{zr}, and $\tau_{r\phi}$ in Eq. (A11) have to be replaced with the corresponding expressions given by the first, second, and fourth of Eqs. (A1). The stress $\tau_{z\phi}$ is replaced by the sum of the third of Eqs. (A1) and the second of Eqs. (4).

In evaluating the integral (A11) we adopt the approximate relations[6]

$$\int_0^l e^{-\beta z} \, dz \approx \frac{1}{\beta} \qquad \int_0^l z e^{-\beta z} \, dz \approx \frac{1}{\beta^2} \quad \text{(A12)}$$

and after lengthy calculations obtain the following quadratic equation determining the value of the parameter $\gamma^* = \gamma^2 r_0^2$:

[5] In view of the symmetry of the problem with regard to the plane $z = l$, halving the full length of the tube, it is sufficient to consider one-half the tube only.

[6] It is shown below [see Eq. (A45)] that, for the values $\alpha = \frac{1}{10}$ and $\phi_0 = \pi$, the smallest value of $\gamma^* > 2$. Assuming the nondimensional length l of the donor site equal to 5 and (for simplicity and as a more hazardous situation) complete perforation of the bone wall, we find that $\gamma = (\gamma^*)^{1/2}/r_0 > 1.4$. Thus, $\gamma l \approx 7$, and consequently $e^{-\gamma l} \approx 0.001$. Thus, the disregarded terms in Eqs. (A12) are of order 10^{-3} as compared with 1. In view of this fact, the mutual interference of the self-equilibrated stress systems arising in the cross sections A and B of Fig. 9 may be ignored.

$$\frac{2}{3}\frac{E_z}{G}\,\alpha^2\phi_0^2 S_1(\gamma^*)^2 + \frac{E_z}{G_z}\,S_2\gamma^* + 2S_3 = 0 \tag{A13}$$

where

$$S_1 = \tfrac{1}{3}(A^*)^2(\tfrac{1}{5} + \tfrac{2}{7}\alpha^2 + \tfrac{1}{21}\alpha^4) + \tfrac{1}{3}(C^{**})^2(\tfrac{1}{15} + \tfrac{12}{35}\alpha^2 + \tfrac{2}{5}\alpha^4 + \tfrac{4}{33}\alpha^6 + \tfrac{1}{143}\alpha^8)$$

$$+ \tfrac{1}{3}(D^*)^2\alpha^4(\tfrac{1}{15} + \tfrac{10}{77}\alpha^2 + \tfrac{1}{39}\alpha^4) + \tfrac{8}{7}A^*C^{**}(\tfrac{1}{15} + \tfrac{1}{5}\alpha^2 + \tfrac{1}{9}\alpha^4 + \tfrac{2}{99}\alpha^6)$$

$$+ \tfrac{8}{3}A^*D^*\alpha^2(\tfrac{1}{35} + \tfrac{1}{21}\alpha^2 + \tfrac{1}{231}\alpha^4) + \tfrac{16}{21}C^{**}D^*\alpha^2(\tfrac{2}{35} + \tfrac{1}{5}\alpha^2 + \tfrac{4}{33}\alpha^4 + \tfrac{5}{429}\alpha^6) \tag{A14}$$

$$S_2 = S_2' + \phi_0^2 S_2'' \tag{A14a}$$

$$S_2' = \tfrac{1}{5}(A^*)^2\alpha^2(\tfrac{1}{3} + \tfrac{1}{7}\alpha^2) + \tfrac{3}{7}(C^{**})^2\alpha^2(\tfrac{1}{15} + \tfrac{1}{5}\alpha^2 + \tfrac{1}{9}\alpha^4 + \tfrac{1}{99}\alpha^6)$$

$$+ (D^*)^2\alpha^6(\tfrac{1}{45} + \tfrac{1}{77}\alpha^2) + \tfrac{2}{5}A^*C^{**}\alpha^2(\tfrac{1}{5} + \tfrac{2}{7}\alpha^2 + \tfrac{1}{21}\alpha^4)$$

$$+ \tfrac{4}{105}A^*D^*\alpha^4(2 + \alpha^2) + \tfrac{8}{35}C^*D^*\alpha^4(\tfrac{1}{5} + \tfrac{1}{3}\alpha^2 + \tfrac{1}{33}\alpha^4) \tag{A14b}$$

$$5S_2'' = (A^*)^2(\tfrac{1}{3} + 2\alpha^2 + \tfrac{5}{7}\alpha^4) + \tfrac{1}{3}(C^{**})^2(\tfrac{1}{3} + \tfrac{28}{5}\alpha^2 + \tfrac{66}{5}\alpha^4 + \tfrac{20}{3}\alpha^6 + \tfrac{38}{33}\alpha^8)$$

$$+ (D^*)^2\alpha^4(\tfrac{1}{7} + \tfrac{10}{9}\alpha^2 + \tfrac{5}{11}\alpha^4) + \tfrac{8}{21}A^*C^{**}(1 + \tfrac{51}{5}\alpha^2 + \tfrac{81}{7}\alpha^4 + \tfrac{37}{21}\alpha^6)$$

$$+ 2A^*D^*\alpha^2(\tfrac{1}{5} + \tfrac{10}{7}\alpha^2 + \tfrac{5}{9}\alpha^4) + \tfrac{8}{7}C^{**}D^*\alpha^2(\tfrac{1}{5} + \tfrac{121}{35}\alpha^2 + \tfrac{205}{63}\alpha^4 + \tfrac{55}{231}\alpha^6) \tag{A14c}$$

$$S_3 = \tfrac{1}{3}(A^*)^2(\tfrac{1}{3} + \alpha^2) + \tfrac{1}{21}(C^{**})^2(1 + \tfrac{53}{5}\alpha^2 + \tfrac{85}{7}\alpha^4 + \tfrac{13}{7}\alpha^6)$$

$$+ \tfrac{1}{3}(D^*)^2\alpha^4(\tfrac{1}{7} + \tfrac{7}{15}\alpha^2) + \tfrac{2}{3}A^*C^{**}(\tfrac{1}{3} + \tfrac{28}{15}\alpha^2 + \tfrac{23}{35}\alpha^4)$$

$$+ \tfrac{2}{15}A^*D^*\alpha^2(1 + \tfrac{23}{7}\alpha^2) + \tfrac{2}{5}C^{**}D^*\alpha^2(\tfrac{1}{5} + \tfrac{10}{7}\alpha^2 + \tfrac{19}{35}\alpha^4)$$

$$- \tfrac{4}{5}C^{**}(\tfrac{1}{3} + \tfrac{1}{5}\alpha^2) - \tfrac{4}{15}D^*\alpha^2 - \tfrac{4}{9}A^* \tag{A15}$$

The numerical values of the parameters S_1, S_2', S_2'', and S_3 appearing in the foregoing equations are given in Table 2.

It is clear that the discriminant of Eq. (A13),

$$\left(\frac{E_z}{G_z}S_2\right)^2 - \frac{16}{3}\frac{E_z}{G}\,\alpha^2\phi_0^2 S_1 S_3 \tag{A16}$$

is always positive in the range of values of α considered, because $S_3 < 0$ and $S_1 > 0$ in this range. Thus, the only physically admissible root of Eq. (A13) is

Table 2 Values of S_1, S_2', S_2'', and S_3

α	$\frac{1}{10}$	$\frac{1}{7}$	$\frac{1}{6}$	$\frac{1}{5}$	$\frac{1}{4}$	$\frac{1}{3}$
S_1	0.064644	0.062259	0.060733	0.058377	0.054389	0.047083
S_2'	0.000667	0.001236	0.001631	0.002249	0.003213	0.004816
S_2''	0.067026	0.067005	0.066858	0.066328	0.065057	0.062516
S_3	−0.324158	−0.315849	−0.310465	−0.302184	−0.288409	−0.262836

$$\gamma = \frac{1}{r_0} \left\{ \frac{-E_z S_2/G_z + \{(E_z S_2/G_z)^2 - 16 E_z \alpha^2 \phi_0^2 S_1 S_3/3G]^{1/2}}{4 E_z \alpha^2 \phi_0^2 S_1/3G} \right\}^{1/2} \tag{A17}$$

where the fraction inside the braces represents the parameter γ^*.

Introducing the notation

$$\alpha^* = \frac{2\alpha}{\ln\left[(1+\alpha)/(1-\alpha)\right]} \tag{A18}$$

we find $K = \alpha^* r_0^2$ in view of the earlier definition of the coefficient K following Eqs. (4). Note that in Eqs. (4) the symbol θ denotes the unit angle of twist of a tube of open cross section. Thus, if such a tube is acted on by a twisting moment M_z, then the unit angle of twist is

$$\theta = \frac{M_z}{4 G_z \phi_0 r_0^4 \alpha (1 + \alpha^2 - \alpha^*)} \tag{A19}$$

Its value is found by integrating the second of Eqs. (4) over the open cross section within the limits $a \leqslant r \leqslant b$, $-\phi_0 \leqslant \phi \leqslant +\phi_0$, and equating the result to the twisting moment M_z.

Equations (A1) can now be cast in the more elegant form

$$\tau_{zz}^* = E_z^* F_1(\alpha, r, \phi) \tag{A20a}$$

$$\tau_{zr}^* = -\frac{(\gamma^*)^{1/2}}{2} E_z^* F_2(\alpha, r, \phi) \tag{A20b}$$

$$\tau_{z\phi}^* = \frac{(\gamma^*)^{1/2}}{2} E_z^* F_3(\alpha, r, \phi) \tag{A20c}$$

$$\tau_{r\phi}^* = \frac{\gamma^*}{8} E_z^* F_4(\alpha, r, \phi) \tag{A20d}$$

where we have introduced the notation

$$E_z^* = \lambda_{33} \sqrt{\gamma^*} \exp\left(-\sqrt{\gamma^*}\,\frac{z}{r_0}\right) \tag{A21}$$

and

$$F_1(\alpha, r, \phi) = \beta \left\{ 2\,\frac{r}{r_0}\left(\frac{r}{r_0} - 1\right)\left[A^* + C^{**}\left(\frac{r}{r_0}\right)^2 \left(\frac{\phi}{\phi_0}\right)^2 + D^*\left(\frac{r}{r_0} - 1\right)^2 \right] \right.$$
$$\left. - \alpha^2 \left(1 - \frac{s^2}{\delta^2}\right)\left[3A^* + 5C^{**}\left(\frac{r}{r_0}\right)^2 \left(\frac{\phi}{\phi_0}\right)^2 + \frac{3}{2}D^*\alpha^2\left(1 + \frac{s^2}{\delta^2}\right) \right] \right\} \phi \tag{A22}$$

$$F_2(\alpha, r, \phi) = -\frac{\beta}{2}\,\frac{r}{r_0}\,\alpha^2 \left[A^* + C^{**}\left(\frac{r}{r_0}\right)^2 \left(\frac{\phi}{\phi_0}\right)^2 \right.$$
$$\left. + \frac{1}{2}D^*\alpha^2\left(1 + \frac{s^2}{\delta^2}\right) \right]\left(1 - \frac{s^2}{\delta^2}\right)\phi \tag{A23}$$

$$F_3(\alpha, r, \phi) = \frac{\beta}{2}\frac{r}{r_0}\left\{\alpha^2\left(1 - \frac{s^2}{\delta^2}\right)\left[2A^* + \frac{3}{2}C^{**}\left(\frac{r}{r_0}\right)^2\left(1 + \frac{\phi^2}{\phi_0^2}\right)\right.\right.$$

$$\left.+ D^*\alpha^2\left(1 + \frac{s^2}{\delta^2}\right)\right] - \frac{r}{r_0}\left(\frac{r}{r_0} - 1\right)\left[A^* + \frac{1}{2}C^{**}\left(\frac{r}{r_0}\right)^2\left(1 + \frac{\phi^2}{\phi_0^2}\right)\right.$$

$$\left.\left.+ D^*\left(\frac{r}{r_0} - 1\right)^2\right]\right\}(\phi_0^2 - \phi^2) \tag{A24}$$

$$F_4(\alpha, r, \phi) = \frac{\beta}{8}\alpha^2\left(\frac{r}{r_0}\right)^2\left[2A^* + C^{**}\left(\frac{r}{r_0}\right)^2\left(1 + \frac{\phi^2}{\phi_0^2}\right)\right.$$

$$\left.+ D^*\alpha^2\left(1 + \frac{s^2}{\delta^2}\right)\right]\left(1 - \frac{s^2}{\delta^2}\right)(\phi_0^2 - \phi^2) \tag{A25}$$

$$\beta = \frac{M_z\alpha^*}{8\phi_0 r_0^3\alpha(1 + \alpha^2 - \alpha^*)} \tag{A26}$$

$$\lambda_{33} = \frac{E_z}{G_z} \tag{A27}$$

With the notation

$$\lambda_{312} = \frac{E_z}{G} \tag{A28}$$

the coefficient γ^* is written as

$$\gamma^* = \frac{-\lambda_{33}S_2 + [(\lambda_{33}S_2)^2 - 16\lambda_{312}\alpha^2\phi_0^2 S_1 S_3/3]^{1/2}}{4\lambda_{312}\alpha^2\phi_0^2 S_1/3} \tag{A29}$$

The stress $\tau_{z\phi}^0$ of the principal stress field given by Eqs. (4) can be represented in a similar manner by

$$\tau_{z\phi}^0 = 2\frac{\beta}{\alpha^*}\left(\frac{r}{r_0} - \frac{\alpha^*}{r/r_0}\right) \tag{A30}$$

Let us note that the material coefficients enter only into the equations representing the quantities E_z^* and γ^*. The quantities A^*, C^{**}, D^*, α^*, and β depend on the single variable α.

A3 THE VISCOELASTIC STRESS FIELD

Inspection of Eq. (A30) shows that the principal stress field $\tau_{z\phi}^0$ does not depend on the elastic constants, and therefore remains the same in the case in which the material of the tube becomes viscoelastic. As far as the auxiliary stress field is concerned, the situation is more complicated: The elastic constants are present in the coefficients λ_{33}, λ_{312}, and γ^*; in the latter they are found in the exponent under the radical sign.

To derive the auxiliary stress system in a viscoelastic body we use the Hilton-Dong elastic-viscoelastic correspondence principle [22], valid for a general anisotropic material. According to this principle, the transforms of the viscoelastic constitutive equations are obtained from the corresponding elastic constitutive equations by replacing the elastic coefficients in the elastic solution with the transformed viscoelastic coefficients.

Assume then that the viscoelastic properties of the body are represented by the standard three-element model defined for uniaxial stress by the differential equation, Eq. (1). We now write this equation in a form more convenient for our purposes,

$$\dot{\sigma}\tau_1 + \sigma h_1 = E_0(\tau_1 \dot{e} + e) \tag{A31}$$

involving explicitly the retardation time $\tau_1 = \eta_1/E_1$, where $h_1 = 1 + E_0/E_1$, E_0 is Young's modulus for the free spring (i.e., for instantaneous response), and E_1 and η_1 are the characteristics of the elements of the Kelvin-Voigt model (i.e., of retarded response). With the Laplace transform denoted by a superposed bar, and in the present three-dimensional case, we get the following correspondence between the elastic and transformed viscoelastic moduli[7]:

$$E_z \rightarrow \bar{E}_{zz} = \frac{1 + s\tau_3}{h_3 + s\tau_3} E_z$$

$$G \rightarrow \bar{E}_{r\phi} = \frac{1 + s\tau_{12}}{h_{12} + s\tau_{12}} G \tag{A32}$$

$$G_z \rightarrow \bar{E}_{rz} = \frac{1 + s\tau_{13}}{h_{13} + s\tau_{13}} G_z$$

where the notation is self-explanatory. As a further specialization, assume that at time $t = 0$ the viscoelastic tube is suddenly subjected to a twisting moment M_z, which remains unchanged with time. The transform of E_z^* in the viscoelastic case now becomes

$$\bar{E_z^*} = \frac{\bar{\lambda}_{33} \sqrt{\gamma^*}}{s} \exp\left(-\sqrt{\gamma^*} \, \frac{z}{r_0}\right) \tag{A33}$$

where

$$\bar{\lambda}_{33} = \frac{\bar{E}_{zz}}{\bar{E}_{rz}}$$

$$\bar{\lambda}_{312} = \frac{\bar{E}_{zz}}{\bar{E}_{r\phi}} \tag{A34}$$

[7] The reader interested in a detailed derivation of this correspondence for a standard three-dimensional model may consult p. 70 of [22] and p. 254 of [23]. The theoretical basis of the correspondence principle (analogy between elastic and viscoelastic problems) is presented in detail in Sec. 8.5 of [11].

$$\bar{\gamma}^* = \frac{-\bar{\lambda}_{33}S_2 + [(\bar{\lambda}_{33}S_2)^2 - 16\bar{\lambda}_{312}\alpha^2\phi_0^2 S_1 S_3/3]^{1/2}}{4\bar{\lambda}_{312}\alpha^2\phi_0^2 S_1/3} \qquad \text{(A34)}$$
$$\text{(Cont.)}$$

The inversion of the transforms obtained above is complicated and requires the evaluation of involved contour integrals. For our purposes it is sufficient to obtain asymptotic solutions for a short time (for which one has to put $s \to \infty$), and a long time (for which one has to put $s \to 0$) using the limit theorems of the Laplace-transform calculus:

$$f(t = 0) = \lim_{s \to \infty} s\bar{f}(s) \qquad f(t = \infty) = \lim_{s \to 0} s\bar{f}(s) \qquad \text{(A35)}$$

With this in mind we first evaluate the λ parameters as follows:

$$\bar{\lambda}_{33}(s = 0) = \frac{h_{13}E_z}{h_3 G_z} \qquad \bar{\lambda}_{33}(s = \infty) = \frac{E_z}{G_z}$$

$$\bar{\lambda}_{312}(s = 0) = \frac{h_{12}E_z}{h_3 G} \qquad \bar{\lambda}_{312}(s = \infty) = \frac{E_z}{G} \qquad \text{(A36)}$$

Clearly, the influence of the auxiliary system reaches its maximum at $z = 0$, which is the location of the discontinuity of the cross sections. It suffices, therefore to invert the transform $\bar{E}_z^*$ assuming $z = 0$.

As already noted, according to the scanty experimental data available, the effect of orientation on the mechanical properties of bone is small in planes perpendicular to the grain. However, in the direction parallel to the grain, Young's modulus E_z was found to be approximately twice the modulus E in directions perpendicular to the grain. We take, therefore,

$$E_z = 2E \qquad \text{(A37)}$$

With regard to the shear modulus, according ot Yamada [24], the ratio of Young's modulus in tension and compression to the shear modulus in torsion is, for wet femur, roughly equal to

$$E_{\text{tens}} : G_{\text{tors}} = 5 \qquad E_{\text{comp}} : G_{\text{tors}} = 3 \qquad \text{(A38)}$$

However, according to Kraus [25], for moderate strain rates there is no perceptible difference between E_{tens} and E_{comp}. For our purposes, which represent in fact rather approximate estimates of plausible situations, we take the average value

$$\lambda_{312} \equiv E_z : G = 4 \qquad \text{(A39)}$$

Actually, in the isotropic case and for $v = 0.26$ (according to experimental findings for the osseous material), this ratio becomes roughly equal to 2.5. In the absence of data, let us now assume for definiteness the following relation among the elastic moduli:

$$E_z : E = G_z : G \qquad \text{(A40)}$$

so that

$$\lambda_{33} \equiv E_z : G_z = 2 \qquad \text{(A41)}$$

With these numbers in mind and using Eqs. (A35) and (A36), we find the inverted moduli of the viscoelastic material from Eq. (A33) as follows:

$$E_z^{*\text{visc}}(t = 0, z = 0) = 2\sqrt{\gamma_0^*} \tag{A42}$$

$$E_z^{*\text{visc}}(t = \infty, z = 0) = 2\,\frac{h_{13}}{h_3}\,\sqrt{\gamma_\infty^*} \tag{A43}$$

where

$$\gamma_0^* = \frac{-S_2 + (S_2^2 - 16\alpha^2\phi_0^2 S_1 S_3/3)^{1/2}}{8\alpha^2\phi_0^2 S_1/3} \tag{A42a}$$

$$\gamma_\infty^* = \frac{-(h_{13}/h_3)S_2 + [(S_2\,h_{13}/h_3)^2 - 16(h_{12}/h_3)\alpha^2\phi_0^2 S_1 S_3/3]^{1/2}}{8(h_{12}/h_3)\alpha^2\phi_0^2 S_1/3} \tag{A43a}$$

We are mostly interested in the stress components $\tau_{zz}^{*\text{visc}}$ and $\tau_{z\phi}^{*\text{visc}}$. Their final representations, based on Eq. (A20) and relations (A42) and (A43), are

$$
\begin{aligned}
\tau_{zz}^{*\text{visc}}\big|_{t=0} &= 2\,\sqrt{\gamma_0^*}\,F_1(\alpha, r, \phi) \\[4pt]
\tau_{zz}^{*\text{visc}}\big|_{t=\infty} &= 2\,\frac{h_{13}}{h_3}\,\sqrt{\gamma_\infty^*}\,F_1(\alpha, r, \phi) \\[4pt]
\tau_{z\phi}^{*\text{visc}}\big|_{t=0} &= \gamma_0^*\,F_3(\alpha, r, \phi) \\[4pt]
\tau_{z\phi}^{*\text{visc}}\big|_{t=\infty} &= \frac{h_{13}}{h_3}\,\gamma_\infty^*\,F_3(\alpha, r, \phi)
\end{aligned}
\tag{A44}
$$

A4 ILLUSTRATIVE EXAMPLE

For a tubular bone with mean radius r_0 equal to unity, and disregarding the layer of spongy bone, we take $a = 0.9$ and $b = 1.1$. Thus, $\delta = 0.1$, $r_0 = 1$, $\alpha = \delta/r_0 = \frac{1}{10}$, and, from Eq. (A18), $\alpha^* \approx 1$. Furthermore, lacking any exact data, we accept the following ratios for the characteristic parameters h_3, h_{12}, and h_{13} appearing in Eqs. (A32): $h_3/h_{13} = E_z/G_z = 2$ and $h_3/h_{12} = E_z/G = 4$ according to Eqs. (A41) and (A39), respectively. Thus, $h_{13}/h_{12} = 2$. We assume for definiteness that the opening in the tube has the form of a longitudinal crack corresponding to $\phi_0 = \pi$. We find from Eqs. (A42a) and (A43a) the parameters

$$\gamma_0^* = 2.141 \qquad \gamma_\infty^* = 4.282 \tag{A45}$$

and from Eqs. (A44), with the notation given by Eqs. (A22) to (A25), the stress components are

$$
\begin{aligned}
\tau_{zz}^{*\text{visc}}\big|_{t=\infty} &= 0.707\,\tau_{zz}^{*\text{visc}}\big|_{t=0} \\[4pt]
\tau_{zz}^{*\text{visc}}\big|_{t=0} &= 2.926 F_1(\alpha, r, \phi) \\[4pt]
\tau_{z\phi}^{*\text{visc}}\big|_{t=\infty} &= \tau_{z\phi}^{*\text{visc}}\big|_{t=0} = 2.141 F_3(\alpha, r, \phi)
\end{aligned}
\tag{A46}
$$

Similarly, we arrive at the following relations, using these same equations:

$$\tau_{zr}^{*\text{visc}}\big|_{t=\infty} = \tau_{zr}^{*\text{visc}}\big|_{t=0} = -2.141 F_2(\alpha, r, \phi) \tag{A47}$$

$$\tau_{r\phi}^{*\text{visc}}\big|_{t=\infty} = 1.414\tau_{r\phi}^{*\text{visc}}\big|_{t=0} \tag{A47}$$
$$\tau_{r\phi}^{*\text{visc}}\big|_{t=0} = 0.783F_4(\alpha, r, \phi) \tag{Cont.}$$

Graphs of the distributions of the stress components $\tau_{z\phi}$, $\tau_{z\phi}^0$ and $\tau_{zz}^{*\text{visc}}$, $\tau_{z\phi}^{*\text{visc}}$ along the outer edge of the cross section ($z = 0$ in terms of the angle ϕ) are displayed in Fig. 10. There, $\tau_{z\phi}$ stands for the shear stress in a complete tube, and $\tau_{z\phi}^0$ for the shear stress in a fractured tube, and $\tau_{zz}^{*\text{visc}}$ and $\tau_{z\phi}^{*\text{visc}}$ are stresses of the auxiliary system.

APPENDIX B: MAJOR CALCULATIONS FOR ANALYSIS IN SEC. 4

B1 NOTATION

a, b	semiaxes of ellipse
a_i, b_i	unknown coefficients in Eqs. (B17)
b	coefficient of permeability
e, ϵ	dilatation of solid and fluid, respectively
e_{ij}	strain components
r, θ	cylindrical coordinates
r_0^2	equal to $K/b\xi$
t	time
x, y	Cartesian coordinates
$\left.\begin{array}{l} z_1 = x_1 + iy_1 = r_1 e^{i\theta} \\ z = x + iy = re^{i\theta} \end{array}\right\}$	complex variable in plane of aperture
A, N, M, Q	material moduli
F	stress function
F_1^*, Σ^*	component stress functions defined by Eqs. (22) to (24)
K	equal to $[(A + 2N)M - Q^2]/[A + M + 2(N + Q)]$
P	external tensile stress
R	parameter [equal to $(a + b)/2$ for ellipse]
R_k	solutions of Eq. (B22)
α	angle between ζ, δ (natural) coordinate lines and r, θ coordinate lines (in actual plane)
$\epsilon = (a - b)/(a + b)$	eccentricity of ellipse
κ	equal to $[(A + 2N)M - Q^2]/2N(Q + M)$
ξ	Laplace parameter
σ_0, q_0	pressures at aperture on solid and fluid, respectively
$\sigma_{rr}, \sigma_{\theta\theta}, \sigma_{zz}, \sigma_{r\theta}, \sigma$	stresses (radial, azimuthal, longitudinal, shear, fluid pressure)

$\sigma_{\rho\rho}, \sigma_{\delta\delta}, \sigma_{\rho\delta}$	stresses in natural coordinates (ρ, δ)
$\zeta = \rho e^{i\delta}$	complex variable in transformed plane (of mapping)
$\phi^*(z), \chi^*(z)$	complex potentials defined by Eq. (B6a)
B, H	subscripts denoting basic stresses (plane with absent hole) and auxiliary stresses (influence of hole)
elast	subscript explained after Eq. (B36)
overbar	denotes complex conjugate
*	denotes Laplace transform
∞	denotes infinite value

B2 GEOMETRY OF THE APERTURE

Consider the $x_1 y_1$ plane as Argand's plane of the complex variable (Fig. 14) in which the opening is located:

$$z_1 = x_1 + iy_1 = r_1 e^{i\theta} \tag{B1}$$

For convenience, nondimensionalize this equation to get

$$z = \frac{z_1}{R} = x + iy = r e^{i\theta} \tag{B2}$$

and

$$r_1 = rR$$

where R characterizes the absolute dimension of the hole, R being real and positive. The mapping function, which we choose in the form

$$z = w(\zeta) = \zeta + \frac{\epsilon}{\zeta} \tag{B3}$$

is, as already noted, the relationship between the exterior of the elliptic hole in the z plane and the exterior of a unit circle in the ζ plane. In the last equation,

$$\zeta = \rho e^{i\delta} \qquad \epsilon = \frac{a-b}{a+b} \tag{B4}$$

with ϵ the eccentricity coefficient, and a and b the major and minor semiaxes of the ellipse.

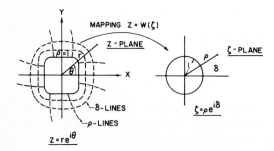

Figure 14 Illustration of conformal mapping.

It is easily found from Eq. (B3) that

$$x = \left(\rho + \frac{\epsilon}{\rho}\right) \cos \delta \qquad y = \left(\rho + \frac{\epsilon}{\rho}\right) \sin \delta \qquad \text{(B5)}$$

Furthermore, as the point ζ moves around the circle with radius $\rho = 1$ in the ζ plane, the point z describes (in the same direction) an ellipse whose semiaxes are now represented by

$$a = R(1 + \epsilon) \qquad b = R(1 + \epsilon) \qquad \text{(B6)}$$

so that the constant parameter $R = (a + b)/2$.

B3 THE STRESS FUNCTION F_1^*

In modeling our reasoning on the approach of Savin [18], it is expedient to split the function F_1^* into two component functions. The first of these F_{1B}^* describes the stress field in an infinite plane with no aperture subjected to the given external load (in the present case, to the tension P). The second component function is the function F_{1H}^* describing the disturbance of the stress distribution produced by the presence of the hole; hence, the subscript H. The first stress field will be called the *basic* field, and the second the *correcting* field.

The biharmonic function F_1^* can be represented in terms of Goursat complex potentials $\phi^*(z)$ and $\chi^*(z)$, analytic[8] in a simply connected domain {see Eq. (31.1) of [26]}

$$F_1^*(r, \theta) = \text{Re} \; [\bar{z}\phi^*(z) + \chi^*(z)] \qquad \text{(B6a)}$$

where an overbar denotes the complex conjugate (here, in particular, $\bar{z} = x - iy$).

In view of the above, the component functions take the form

$$\begin{aligned} F_{1B}^* &= \text{Re} \; [\bar{z}\phi_B^*(z) + \chi_B^*(z)] \\ F_{1H}^* &= \text{Re} \; [\bar{z}\phi_H^*(z) + \chi_H^*(z)] \end{aligned} \qquad \text{(B7)}$$

B3.1 Stresses of the Basic Field

It is easily seen that

$$\phi_B^* = \frac{P}{4\xi} \; z \qquad \chi_B^* = -\frac{P}{4\xi} \; z^2 \qquad \text{(B8)}$$

satisfy the requirements associated with the basic stress field. In fact, using the polar form (B2) of the complex variable z gives

---

[8] A readable and comprehensive presentation of the elements and applications of the theory of complex variables and conformal mapping is given in Muskhelishvili [26]. For a brief account, see Timoshenko and Goodier [19]; see also Fig. 14.

$$F_{1B}^* = \frac{P}{4\xi} \, r^2 \, \mathrm{Re} \, (1 - e^{2i\theta})$$ (B8a)

or
$$F_{1B}^* = \frac{P}{2\xi} \, y^2$$ (B8b)

so that the basic stress field, represented similarly to Eq. (17) but expressed in Cartesian coordinates x, y, becomes

$$\sigma_{xx}^{B*} = \frac{\partial^2 F_{1B}^*}{\partial y^2} = \frac{P}{\xi} \qquad \sigma_{yy}^{B*} = \sigma_{xy}^{B*} = 0$$ (B9)

as desired in the Laplace-transformed space. In "natural" coordinates[9] ρ, δ applied in the ζ plane, on combination of Eqs. (B5) and (B8b), the basic stress function becomes

$$F_{1B}^* = \frac{P}{4\xi} \left(\rho - \frac{\epsilon}{\rho} \right)^2 (1 - \cos 2\delta)$$ (B10)

Clearly, ρ, δ form an orthogonal system because they originate from the polar system r, θ on a conformal mapping that leaves angles unchanged. In the ρ, δ system the stresses of the basic field, according to Sec. 50 of [26], are

$$\sigma_{\rho\rho}^{B*} + \sigma_{\delta\delta}^{B*} = 4 \, \mathrm{Re} \, \frac{\phi_B'^*(\zeta)}{w'(\zeta)}$$

$$\sigma_{\delta\delta}^{B*} - \sigma_{\rho\rho}^{B*} + 2i\sigma_{\rho\delta}^{B*} = \frac{2\zeta^2}{\rho^2 \, \overline{w'(\zeta)}} \left\{ \overline{w(\zeta)} \left[\frac{\phi_B'^*(\zeta)}{w'(\zeta)} \right]' + \psi_B'^*(\zeta) \right\}$$ (B11)

with the notation

$$\psi_B^*(z) = \chi_B'^*(z)$$ (B11a)

The convenience of using stress components in the ρ, δ system consists in the fact that they are normal or parallel to the contour of the actual aperture in the z plane. A longer computation provides the following equations for the basic stress field in the ρ, δ system of coordinates:

$$\sigma_{\rho\rho}^{B*} = \frac{P}{\xi} - \sigma_{\delta\delta}^{B*}$$

$$\sigma_{\delta\delta}^{B*} = \frac{P}{2\xi} \, \frac{(\rho^2 + \epsilon)^2}{\rho^4 - 2\epsilon\rho^2 \, \cos 2\delta + \epsilon^2} \, (1 - \cos 2\delta)$$ (B12)

$$\sigma_{\rho\delta}^{B*} = -\frac{P}{2\xi} \, \frac{\rho^4 - \epsilon^2}{\rho^4 - 2\epsilon\rho^2 \, \cos 2\delta + \epsilon^2} \, \sin 2\delta$$

[9] The polar coordinates ρ, δ in the ζ plane of mappings become natural coordinates in the original z plane in the sense that the δ family envelops the aperture and the ρ family remains orthogonal to the former. For an elliptic aperture this corresponds to the elliptic coordinate system composed of mutually orthogonal ellipses and hyperbolas.

With future procedures in mind, it is convenient to develop these functions into MacLaurin series expressed in terms of the eccentricity parameter ϵ. This leads to the basic stress field in the form

$$\sigma_{\rho\rho}^{B*} = \frac{P}{2\xi}\left(1 + \cos 2\delta - \epsilon\, \frac{1 - \cos 4\delta}{\rho^2} - \epsilon^2\, \frac{\cos 2\delta - \cos 6\delta}{\rho^4} - \cdots\right)$$

$$\sigma_{\delta\delta}^{B*} = \frac{P}{2\xi}\left(1 - \cos 2\delta + \epsilon\, \frac{1 - \cos 4\delta}{\rho^2} + \epsilon^2\, \frac{\cos 2\delta - \cos 6\delta}{\rho^4} + \cdots\right) \quad \text{(B13)}$$

$$\sigma_{\rho\delta}^{B*} = -\frac{P}{2\xi}\left(\sin 2\delta + \epsilon\, \frac{\sin 4\delta}{\rho^2} - \epsilon^2\, \frac{\sin 2\delta - \sin 6\delta}{\rho^4} + \cdots\right)$$

This completes the derivation of the stresses of the basic stress field.

B3.2 The Disturbing Influence of the Aperture

The correcting field describing the disturbing influence of the aperture may be taken, following Savin [18], in the form of the classical correcting field, with the numerical coefficients, however, replaced by unknown coefficients that are determined from additional conditions of the problem under investigation. By the classical correcting field is meant the perturbation field associated with the presence of an elliptic hole in a uniform tension field in which the medium is considered purely elastic. This field is well known, and it is found, following Sec. 32a of [26], by subtracting expressions (B8). In the present case, in the Laplace-transformed space, this leads to the equations

$$\phi_{class}^*(\zeta) = \frac{P}{2\xi}\frac{1 - \epsilon}{\zeta}$$

$$\psi_{class}^*(\zeta) = -\frac{P}{2\xi}\frac{(1 - \epsilon)^2\zeta^2 + \epsilon^2 - 1}{\zeta(\zeta^2 - \epsilon)} \quad \text{(B14)}$$

or, on introduction of the dimensioned variable z_1,

$$\phi_{class}^*(z_1) = \frac{P}{\xi}\frac{1 - \epsilon}{\epsilon(z_1 + \sqrt{z_1^2 - 4\epsilon})}$$

$$\psi_{class}^*(z_1) = -\frac{P}{\xi}\frac{(1 - \epsilon)^2(z_1 + \sqrt{z_1^2 - 4\epsilon})^2 + 4(\epsilon^2 - 1)}{(z_1 + \sqrt{z_1^2 - 4\epsilon})\,[(z_1 + \sqrt{z_1^2 - 4\epsilon})^2 - 4\epsilon]} \quad \text{(B15)}$$

Again the expansion in terms of the parameter ϵ and subsequent integration of the function $\psi_{class}^*(z_1)$ give

$$\phi_{class}^* = \frac{P}{2\xi}\left(\frac{1}{z_1} + \epsilon\,\frac{1 - z_1^2}{z_1^3} + \epsilon^2\,\frac{2 - z_1^2}{z_1^5} + \cdots\right)$$

$$\chi_{class}^* = \frac{P}{2\xi}\left[-\ln z - \frac{1}{2z_1^2} + \epsilon\left(\frac{1}{z_1^4} - \frac{1}{z_1^2}\,2\ln z\right) + \epsilon^2\left(-\ln z - \frac{3}{2z_1^2}\right.\right.$$

$$\left.\left. + \frac{3}{2z_1^4} - \frac{5}{2z_1^6}\right) + \cdots\right] \quad \text{(B16)}$$

As already mentioned, to adapt these classical potentials to the present case, it is necessary to cast them in the following general form involving unknown parameters to be determined later:

$$\phi_{1H}^*(z_1) = \frac{C}{z_1} + \epsilon \left(\frac{b_1}{z_1} + \frac{b_2}{z_1^3} \right) + \epsilon^2 \left(\frac{b_3}{z_1^3} + \frac{b_4}{z_1^5} + \frac{b_5}{z_1} \right) + \cdots$$

$$\chi_{1H}^*(z_1) = A \ln z_1 + \frac{B}{z_1^2} + \epsilon \left(a_1 \ln z_1 + \frac{a_2}{z_1^2} + \frac{a_3}{z_1^4} \right)$$
$$+ \epsilon^2 \left(a_4 \ln z_1 + \frac{a_5}{z_1^2} + \frac{a_6}{z_1^4} + \frac{a_7}{z_1^6} \right) + \cdots$$

$$(B17)$$

Introducing Eqs. (B17) into the second of Eqs. (B7) leads to the final form of the correcting stress function in nondimensional variables:

$$F_{1H}^*(r, \theta; \epsilon) = A \ln rR + \left(\frac{B}{r^2R^2} + C \right) \cos 2\theta + \epsilon \left[a_1 \ln rR \right.$$
$$+ \left(\frac{a_2}{r^2R^2} + b_1 \right) \cos 2\theta + \left(\frac{a_3}{r^4R^4} + \frac{b_2}{r^2R^2} \right) \cos 4\theta \right]$$
$$+ \epsilon^2 \left[a_4 \ln rR + \left(\frac{a_5}{rR^2} + b^5 \right) \cos 2\theta \right.$$
$$+ \left(\frac{a_6}{r^4R^4} + \frac{b_3}{rR^2} \right) \cos 4\theta + \left(\frac{a_7}{r^6R^6} + \frac{b_4}{r^4R^4} \right) \cos 6\theta \right] + \cdots$$

$$(B18)$$

This can be written concisely as

$$F_{1H}^* = \sum_{k=0}^{\infty} \epsilon^k F_{1Hk}^* \qquad (B19)$$

where the meaning of the component functions F_{1Hk}^* is apparent.

This completes the derivation of the function F_1^* as part of the function F^* according to Eqs. (22), both its components now being known: F_{1B}^* from Eq. (B8a) or (B10), and F_{1H}^* from Eq. (B19).

B4 THE STRESS FUNCTION Σ^*

To determine the complete stress function F^* represented by Eqs. (22), we now must find the function Σ^*, which, as mentioned earlier, satisfies the Helmholtz equation (24). As was done before with other functions, it is expanded in terms of ϵ:

$$\Sigma^*(r_1, \theta; \epsilon) = R_0(r_1) + R_1(r_1) \cos 2\theta + \epsilon[R_2(r_1) + R_3(r_1) \cos 2\theta$$
$$+ R_4(r_1) \cos 4\theta] + \epsilon^2 [R_5(r_1) + R_6(r_1) \cos 2\theta$$
$$+ R_7(r_1) \cos 4\theta + R_8(r_1) \cos 6\theta] + \cdots \tag{B20}$$

Substitution of the above equation into Eq. (24) represented in dimensional variables explicitly by

$$\frac{\partial^2 \Sigma^*}{\partial r_1^2} + \frac{1}{r_1} \frac{\partial \Sigma^*}{\partial r_1} + \frac{1}{r_1^2} \frac{\partial^2 \Sigma^*}{\partial \theta^2} - \frac{1}{r_0^2} \Sigma^* = 0 \tag{B21}$$

leads to a set of equations for the functions $R_k(r_1)$ of the form

$$R_k'' + \frac{1}{r_1} R_k' - \left(\frac{1}{r_0^2} + \frac{\nu^2}{r_1^2}\right) R_k = 0 \tag{B22}$$

whose solutions are the modified Bessel functions of the second kind:

$$R_k = K_\nu \left(\frac{r_1}{r_0}\right) \tag{B23}$$

This enables one to transform the function Σ^* into its final form,

$$\Sigma^*(r, \theta; \epsilon) = DK_0 \left(\frac{rR}{r_0}\right) + EK_2 \left(\frac{rR}{r_0}\right) \cos 2\theta + \epsilon \left[c_1 K_0 \left(\frac{rR}{r_0}\right)\right.$$
$$+ c_2 K_2 \left(\frac{rR}{r_0}\right) \cos 2\theta + c_3 K_4 \left(\frac{rR}{r_0}\right) \cos 4\theta \right]$$
$$+ \epsilon^2 \left[c_4 K_0 \left(\frac{rR}{r_0}\right) + c_5 K_2 \left(\frac{rR}{r_0}\right) \cos 2\theta \right.$$
$$\left. + c_6 K_4 \left(\frac{rR}{r_0}\right) \cos 4\theta + c_7 K_6 \left(\frac{rR}{r_0}\right) \cos 6\theta \right] + \cdots \tag{B24}$$

or more concisely into the form

$$\Sigma^*(r, \theta; \epsilon) = \sum_{k=0}^{\infty} \epsilon^K \Sigma_K^* \tag{B25}$$

where the meaning of the component functions Σ_K^* is apparent.

This completes the derivation of the stress function F^* represented by the first of Eqs. (22) as well as the representation of the transformed fluid pressure σ^* by means of the second of Eqs. (22).

B5 STRESSES IN THE VICINITY OF THE APERTURE

To evaluate the stresses in the vicinity of the aperture, which is the location of a maximum stress concentration, it is expedient to write the quantities concerned in terms of the natural coordinates ρ, δ instead of the polar coordinates r, θ (see the z plane in Fig. 14). This enables one to cast the boundary conditions in a form considerably more convenient for effective calculation. This was done with regard to the basic field σ_{ij}^{B*} represented by Eqs. (B13), and it now remains to cast the correcting stress field σ_{ij}^{H*} as well as the fluid pressure σ^* in a similar form.

As follows from Eqs. (22) and (B6), the component F_H^* of the general stress function F^* associated with the correcting system is represented by the equation

$$F_H^* = F_{1H}^* + \frac{r_0^2}{K} \Sigma^* \tag{B26}$$

In this equation, on account of Eqs. (B18) and (B24), the right-hand side depends on the polar coordinates r, θ and, of course, on the Laplace parameter ξ and the eccentricity ϵ of the ellipse.

Following Savin [18], it is first expedient to find the stress field derived from the potential F_H^* in polar coordinates by using the equations

$$\sigma_{rr}^{H*}(r, \theta) = \sum_{k=0}^{\infty} \epsilon^k \left[\frac{1}{R^2} \left(\frac{1}{r} \frac{\partial}{\partial r} + \frac{1}{r^2} \frac{\partial^2}{\partial \theta^2} \right) \left(F_{1HR}^* + \frac{r_0^2}{K} \Sigma_k \right) - \sigma_k^* \right]$$

$$\sigma_{\theta\theta}^{H*}(r, \theta) = \sum_{k=0}^{\infty} \epsilon^k \left[\frac{1}{R^2} \frac{2}{\partial r^2} \left(F_{1Hk}^* + \frac{r_0^2}{K} \Sigma_R^* \right) - \sigma_k^* \right] \tag{B27}$$

$$\sigma_{r\theta}^{H*}(r, \theta) = \sum_{k=0}^{\infty} \epsilon^k \left[\frac{1}{R^2} \left(\frac{1}{r^2} \frac{\partial}{\partial \theta} - \frac{1}{r} \frac{\partial^2}{\partial r \partial \theta} \right) \left(F_{1HR}^* + \frac{r_0^2}{K} \Sigma_k^* \right) \right]$$

These stresses now have to be restructured into functions of the coordinates representing the mapped ζ plane. To this end we use the Taylor expansion whose general form is

$$V(r, \theta) = V(\rho, \delta) + \frac{\partial V}{\partial \rho} (\rho, \delta)(r - \rho) + \frac{\partial V}{\partial \delta} (\rho, \delta)(\theta - \delta)$$

$$+ \frac{\partial^2 V}{\partial \rho \, \partial \delta} (\rho, \delta)(r - \rho)(\theta - \delta) + \frac{1}{2!} \frac{\partial^2 V}{\partial \rho^2} (\rho, \delta)(r - \rho)^2$$

$$+ \frac{1}{2!} \frac{\partial^2 V}{\partial \delta^2} (\rho, \delta)(\theta - \delta)^2 + \cdots \tag{B28}$$

and in which the $r - \rho$ and $\theta - \delta$ terms can be found from the following infinite series (the overbar denoting complex conjugates):

$$r = \rho + \epsilon \left(\frac{\bar{\xi}f + \xi\bar{f}}{2\rho} \right) - \epsilon^2 \left(\frac{\bar{\xi}f - \xi\bar{f}}{8\rho^3} \right)^2 + \cdots \tag{B29}$$

$$\theta = \delta + \epsilon \left(\frac{f - \bar{f}}{2\rho i} \cos \delta - \frac{f + \bar{f}}{2\rho} \sin \delta \right) + \epsilon^2 \left(\frac{f^2 + \bar{f}^2}{4\zeta\bar{\zeta}} \sin 2\delta \right.$$

$$\left. - \frac{f^2 - \bar{f}^2}{4\zeta\bar{\zeta}i} \cos 2\delta \right) + \cdots$$

$$\text{(B29)}$$
$$\text{(Cont.)}$$

In the case of an elliptic hole we have $f = 1/\zeta$ and $\bar{f} = 1/\bar{\zeta}$.

The correcting stresses in the ζ plane, namely the stresses $\sigma_{\rho\rho}^{H*}$, $\sigma_{\delta\delta}^{H*}$, and $\sigma_{\rho\delta}^{H*}$, can be represented by the correcting stresses in the z plane through the well-known transformation formulas

$$\sigma_{\rho\rho}^{H*} = \sigma_{rr}^{H*} \cos^2 \alpha + \sigma_{\theta\theta}^{H*} \sin^2 \alpha + \sigma_{r\theta}^{H*} \sin 2\alpha$$

$$\sigma_{\delta\delta}^{H*} = \sigma_{rr}^{H*} \sin^2 \alpha + \sigma_{\theta\theta}^{H*} \cos^2 \alpha - \sigma_{r\theta}^{H*} \sin 2\alpha \qquad \text{(B30)}$$

$$\sigma_{\rho\delta}^{H*} = \frac{\sigma_{\theta\theta}^{H*} - \sigma_{rr}^{H*}}{2} \sin 2\alpha + \sigma_{r\theta}^{H*} \cos 2\alpha$$

where α is the angle of rotation between the ρ, δ coordinate lines and the r, θ coordinate lines (see Fig. 14).

The trigonometric terms $\cos \alpha$ and $\sin \alpha$ can easily be determined from the real and imaginary parts of the series

$$e^{i\alpha} = 1 + \epsilon \left(\frac{\zeta^2 - \bar{\zeta}^2}{\zeta^2 \bar{\zeta}^2} \right) - \frac{\epsilon^2}{8} \left(\frac{8}{\zeta\bar{\zeta}^2} - \frac{4}{\bar{\zeta}^4} - \frac{4}{\zeta^4} \right) + \cdots \qquad \text{(B31)}$$

With regard to conditions applied at the boundary of the infinite poroelastic plane with an elliptic hole,[10] it is assumed for definiteness that at time $t = +0$ the elliptic contour is subjected to a normal pressure q_0 acting on the solid elastic skeleton of the material. The surface of the hole is unsealed, and the fluid is subjected to a pressure σ_0. Far from the hole the pressure of the liquid σ is assumed to vanish, while the skeleton remains under uniform tensile tractions such that at large values of the radius r,

$$\sigma_{xx} = P \qquad \sigma_{yy} = \sigma_{xy} = 0 \qquad \text{(B32)}$$

The boundary conditions imposed on the elliptic contour as well as those far from it have to be transformed by means of Laplace transformation and mapped into the complex ζ plane. After these two operations, the boundary conditions at the infinitely large distance ρ become

$$\sigma^*(\infty, \delta; \xi) = 0$$

$$\sigma_{\rho\rho}^*(\infty, \delta; \xi) = \frac{P}{2\xi} (1 + \cos 2\delta) \qquad \text{(B33)}$$

[10] The boundary conditions adopted here are similar to those applied in the case of a circular hole in [27].

$$\sigma_{\delta\delta}^*(\infty, \delta; \xi) = \frac{P}{2\xi}(1 - \cos 2\delta)$$

$$\sigma_{\rho\delta}^*(\infty, \delta; \xi) = -\frac{P}{2\xi}\sin 2\delta$$

(B33)
(Cont.)

Similarly, at the contour of the aperture where $\rho = 1$, we get

$$\sigma_{\rho\rho}^*(1, \delta; \xi) = -\frac{q_0}{\xi}$$

$$\sigma_{\rho\delta}^*(1, \delta; \xi) = 0$$

$$\sigma^*(1, \delta; \xi) = \frac{\sigma_0}{\xi}$$

(B34)

The two sets of equations (B33) and (B34) can also be imagined as expanded in powers of the parameter ϵ with only the zeroth-order[11] terms remaining.

We now use Eqs. (B33) and (B34) in conjunction with the complete stress expressions to generate a system of algebraic equations required to evaluate the unknown constants appearing in the correcting stresses. Let us repeat that the complete stresses are represented as the sums of the basic stresses, Eqs. (B13), and the correcting stresses, Eqs. (B30). The resulting equations are unwieldy, and to save space we refrain from giving them explicitly. Instead, we turn to the procedure of retransformation from the Laplace space to the physical space in which the problem is set. The inverse Laplace transforms are found using two limit theorems of the operational calculus:

$$f(t = +0) = \lim_{\xi \to \infty} \xi f(\rho, \delta; \xi)$$

(B35)

$$f(t = \infty) = \lim_{\xi \to 0} \xi f(\rho, \delta; \xi)$$

(B36)

The first of these equations serves to supply the stresses and the fluid pressure at the moment of application of the load, i.e., at time $t = +0$; the second supplies the values of the functions after a long (theoretically infinite) period of time. After multiplication of both sides of the corresponding equations (not written here) by the parameter ξ, some terms become independent of this parameter; this implies their independence of time, and they are referred to as $\sigma_{ij\text{elast}}$, because their values may be reproduced from known elastic solutions. Symbolically, in this notation the stresses are expressed as follows:

$$\sigma_{\rho\rho}(\rho, \delta; t = 0) = \sigma_{\rho\rho\,\text{elast}}^0 + \frac{\sigma_0}{\rho^2} + \epsilon\left[\sigma_{\rho\rho\,\text{elast}}^1 + 4\cos(2\delta)\,\sigma_0\left(\frac{1}{\rho^4} - \frac{1}{\rho^2}\right)\right] + \cdots$$

(B37)

[11] The zeroth-order terms are those terms associated with the zeroth power of the eccentricity parameter.

$$\sigma_{\rho\rho}(\rho, \delta; t = \infty) = \sigma_{\rho\rho\,\text{elast}}^0 + \sigma_0 \left(\frac{1}{\rho^2} - 1 \right) + \epsilon \left\{ \sigma_{\rho\rho\,\text{elast}}^1 \right. \tag{B37}$$
$$\text{(Cont.)}$$

$$\left. + \cos(2\delta) \left[\frac{3\sigma_0}{\kappa} \left(\frac{1}{\rho^2} - \frac{1}{\rho^4} \right) + 4\sigma_0 \left(\frac{1}{\rho^4} - \frac{1}{\rho^2} \right) \right] \right\} + \cdots$$

$$\sigma_{\delta\delta}(\rho, \delta; t = 0) = \sigma_{\delta\delta\,\text{elast}}^0 + \frac{\sigma_0}{\rho^2} + \epsilon \left[\sigma_{\delta\delta\,\text{elast}}^1 - 4 \cos(2\delta) \frac{\sigma_0}{\rho^4} \right] + \cdots \tag{B38}$$

$$\sigma_{\delta\delta}(\rho, \delta; t = \infty) = \sigma_{\delta\delta\,\text{elast}}^0 + \frac{\sigma_0}{\rho^2} + \sigma_0 \left(\frac{1 - \kappa}{\kappa} \right) + \epsilon \left\{ \sigma_{\delta\delta\,\text{elast}}^1 \right.$$

$$\left. + \cos(2\delta) \left[-\frac{4\sigma_0}{\rho^4} + \frac{\sigma_0}{\kappa} \left(\frac{3}{\rho^4} - \frac{1}{\rho^2} \right) \right] \right\} + \cdots$$

$$\sigma_{\rho\delta}(\rho, \delta; t = 0) = \sigma_{\rho\delta\,\text{elast}}^0 + \epsilon \left[\sigma_{\rho\delta\,\text{elast}}^1 + 2 \sin(2\delta) \sigma_0 \left(\frac{1}{\rho^4} - \frac{1}{\rho^2} \right) \right] + \cdots \tag{B39}$$

$$\sigma_{\rho\delta}(\rho, \delta; t = \infty) = \sigma_{\rho\delta\,\text{elast}}^0 + \epsilon \left[\sigma_{\rho\delta\,\text{elast}}^1 + \sin(2\delta) \sigma_0 \left(\frac{3 - 2\kappa}{\kappa} \right) \left(\frac{1}{\rho^2} - \frac{1}{\rho^4} \right) \right] + \cdots$$

REFERENCES

1. J. E. Koch, The Laws of Bone Architecture, *Am. J. Anat.,* vol. 21, pp. 177–298, 1917.
1a. J. H. McElhaney, Dynamic Response of Bone and Muscle Tissue, *J. Appl. Physiol.,* vol. 21, pp. 1231–1236, 1966.
2. V. H. Frankel and A. H. Burstein, "Orthopaedic Biomechanics," Lea & Febiger, Philadelphia, 1970.
3. R. F. S. Hearmon, "An Introduction to Applied Anisotropic Elasticity," Oxford University Press, London, 1961.
4. S. W. Laird and H. B. Kingsbury, Complex Viscoelastic Moduli of Bovine Bones, *J. Biomed.,* vol. 6, pp. 59–67, 1973.
5. E. D. Sedlin, A Rheological Model for Cortical Bone, *Acta Orthop. Scand. Suppl.,* vol. 83, pp. 3–77, 1965.
6. J. M. Zarek and J. Edwards, Dynamic Considerations of the Human Skeleton System, in R. Kenedi (ed.), "Biomechanics and Related Bioengineering Topics," pp. 187–203, Pergamon, New York, 1965.
7. Y. N. Rabotnov, "Creep Problems in Structure Members," North-Holland, Amsterdam, 1969.
8. N. A. Biot, General Solutions of the Equations of Elasticity and Consolidation for a Porous Material, *J. Appl. Mech.,* vol. 23, pp. 91–96, 1956.
9. G. Heinrich and K. Desoyer, Theory of Three-Dimensional Consolidation Phenomena in Clay Layers, *Ing. Arch.,* vol. 30, pp. 225–253, 1961 (in German).
9a. A. Lubinski, The Theory of Elasticity for Porous Bodies Displaying a Strong Pore Structure, *Proc. 2d U.S. Nat. Congr. Appl. Mech.,* pp. 247–256, 1954.
10. G. Paria, Flow of Fluids through Porous Deformable Solids, in H. N. Abramson, H. Liebowitz, J. M. Crowley, S. Juhash (eds.), "Applied Mechanics Surveys," pp. 901–907, Spartan Books, Washington, D.C., 1966.
11. W. Flugge, "Viscoelasticity," Blaisdell, Waltham, Mass., 1967.

12. J. Prescott, "Applied Elasticity," p. 172, Dover, New York, 1961.

13. M. T. Huber, "Theory of Elasticity," vol. 1, p. 322, P.W.N., Warsaw, 1954 (in Polish).

14. J. L. Nowinski, Torsion of a Bar of Rectangular Cross-Section Whose One Cross-Section Remains Plane, *Arch. Mech. Stosow.,* vol. 1, pp. 47–66, 1953 (in Polish).

15. J. L. Nowinski, Bielayev's Point in Poroelastic Bodies in Contact, *Int. J. Mech. Sci.,* vol. 15, pp. 145–155, 1973.

15a. A. A. Griffith, The Phenomena of Rupture and Flow in Solids, *Phil. Trans. Roy. Soc. London,* A221, p. 163, 1920.

16. T. V. Baughn and J. L. Nowinski, Stress Fields Around Cylindrical Holes of Arbitrary Form in Poroelastic Media Simulating the Osseous Tissue, *Dept. Mechanical and Aerospace Engineering Tech. Rept.* 165, University of Delaware, Newark, Dela., 1973.

17. G. N. Savin, "Concentration of Stress around Holes," Gosudavstviennoye Izdatelstvo Tekhniko-Teoreticheskoy Literatury (State Publication of Technical Theoretical Literature), Moscow, 1951 (in Russian).

18. G. N. Savin, "Distribution of Stress around Holes," Naukova Dumka, Kiev, 1968 (in Russian).

19. S. Timoshenko and J. N. Goodier, "Theory of Elasticity," McGraw-Hill, New York, 1951.

20. A. I. Lurie, "Statics of Thin Elastic Shells," Gostekhizdat, Moscow, 1948 (in Russian).

21. O. M. Guz, Torsion of Cylindrical Shells Weakened by Equilateral Triangular Holes with Rounded Corners, Dokl. Akad. Nauk URSR, vol. 1, 1965 (in Ukranian).

22. H. H. Hilton and S. B. Dong, An Analogy for Anisotropic, Nonhomogeneous, Linear Viscoelasticity Including Thermal Stresses, in vol. 2, "Developments in Mechanics," Proc. 8th Midwest Mech. Conf., pp. 58–73, Pergamon, 1963.

23. M. Bieniek, W. R. Spillers, and A. M. Freudenthal, Nonhomogeneous Thick-walled Cylinder under Internal Pressure, *ARS J.,* pp. 1249–1255, 1962.

24. H. Yamada, pp. 20–29 in F. G. Evans (ed)., "Strength of Biological Materials," Williams and Wilkins, Baltimore, 1970.

25. H. Kraus, On the Mechanical Properties and Behavior of Human Compact Bone, *Adv. Biomed. Eng. Med. Phys.,* vol. 2, pp. 169–204, 1968.

26. N. I. Muskhelishvili, "Some Basic Problems of the Mathematical Theory of Elasticity," trans. by J. R. M. Radok, Noordhoff, Groningen, 1963.

27. J. L. Nowinski, Stress Concentration around Holes in a Class of Rheological Materials Displaying a Poroelastic Structure, in "Developments in Mechanics," Proc. *12th Midwestern Mechanics Conf.,* vol. 6, pp. 445–458, 1972.

THREE

ON THE MECHANISM OF LUBRICATION
OF HUMAN ARTICULAR JOINTS

R. Collins
H. B. Kingsbury

Extremely low coefficients of friction in weight-bearing human joints are explained by a combined fluid film-boundary lubrication theory. Simplified analyses are formulated for pressure and synovial fluid flow fields in cartilage and the joint space. Results of preliminary tests of human joints using an articulation machine constructed for this purpose tend to justify the lubrication model proposed and unify interpretations of previous researchers' results. Further work should suggest improvements in the therapeutic treatment of arthritis and prosthesis design.

1 INTRODUCTION

Articulation of the weight-bearing human joints, such as the hip, knee, and ankle, leads to coefficients of friction of about 0.01, significantly lower than the majority of engineering bearings [1 to 3]. The present investigation is directed toward a quantitative understanding of the mechanisms by which such low friction is achieved, with a view to both improved treatment of arthritis and the design of prostheses.

The configuration of the hip and knee joints is shown in Fig. 1. The joint consists of a pair of convex and concave articular surfaces coated with cartilage, and the whole is immersed in synovial fluid encapsulated by a synovial membrane, as

The authors acknowledge the contribution of Harry McKellop whose M.S. thesis, "Lubrication Mechanisms in Human Joints," formed the basis of the experimental study described in Secs. 4 and 5.

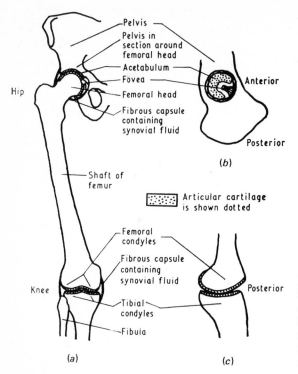

Figure 1 Schematic diagrams of the hip and knee joints. (*a*) Front view of the hip and knee joints; (*b*) view looking into the acetabulum showing the horseshoe-shaped bearing area; (*c*) side view of the knee. *(From Dowson et al. [3a].)*

illustrated in Fig. 2. The anatomy of the principal joints differs somewhat in the geometry of the articular surfaces. The knee (Fig. 3) consists of a two-ridged cylinder that moves upon a nearly flat socket, whereas the hip corresponds to a closely conforming ball and socket, while the ankle possesses the simplest geometry of a cylinder articulating upon a cylindrical socket of slightly larger radius of curvature.

1.1 The Articular Cartilage

The articular surfaces are coated with a layer of cartilage of thickness of about 1 to 2 mm, with surface irregularities of order 2 to 3 μm as measured by Talysurf traces (Fig. 4). Transmission electron microscope studies by Davies et al. [4] indicated smooth surfaces with asperities less than 0.2 μm in height. Walker et al. [5] measured acrylic castings of cartilage and reported asperities on the order of 40 μm. Clarke [6], using a scanning electron microscope, found 2- to 10-μm-deep depressions in the surface. The Young's modulus of the porous cartilage has been estimated by McCutchen [2] to lie in the range 10^6 to 10^8 dyn/cm^2, a value that is observed to decrease with continued application of a load.

Permeability experiments by McCutchen have led to estimates of the pore size of the cartilaginous matrix of about 60 Å (see also [7]). The cartilage has been estimated by Edwards [8] to contain 70 to 80 percent liquid when fully saturated, with two-thirds contained within the matrix. McCutchen [9] has shown that cartilage specimens, when placed between two porous glass plates and compressed, lose about 40 percent of their volume in expressed water. The porosity has been measured by Linn; in youth, the dry weight of cartilage represents 18 percent of its wet weight, rising to 22 percent after 25 to 30 yr of age, and remaining constant thereafter. Measurements of the permeability of cartilage with depth, as well as its variation with age, have been made by Maroudas [10], the results of which are shown in Figs. 5 and 6. It is clear that the permeability decreases in an almost linear fashion with depth. Cartilage permeability has been measured by McCutchen [2, 11], Edwards [8] and Maroudas [12, 13]. It is nearly the same in all directions

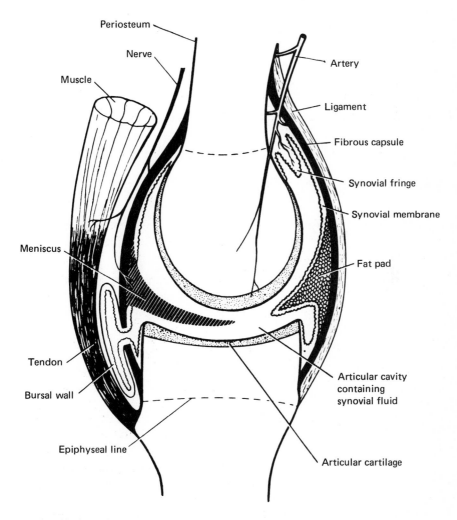

Figure 2 Schematic representation of a synovial joint. *(From Barnett et al. [13a]. Courtesy of Charles C Thomas, Springfield, Ill.).*

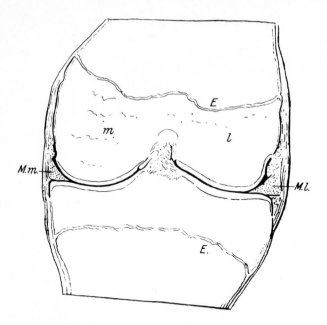

Figure 3 Anatomy of knee joint. *(From Strasser [44].)*

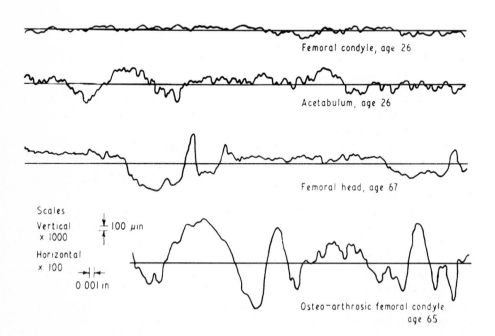

Figure 4 Typical Talysurf traces from acrylic castings of cartilage. *(From Dowson et al. [3a].)*

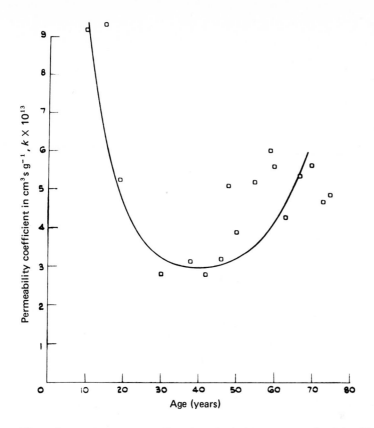

Figure 5 Variation of permeability of cartilage with age. Depth $d = 0.15$. *(From Maroudas [10].)*

at a given depth. The decrease in permeability in the region extending from just below the surface to the deep regions of the cartilage was shown to vary inversely with the fixed charge density of the cartilage matrix.

Since the pressure applied *in vivo* is substantially greater than pressure used in these *in vitro* permeability tests, and since cartilage is a relatively soft material, Mansour and Mow [14] carried out experiments to determine the effect of compressive strain and pressure on cartilage permeability. They found that permeability decreases with increasing compressive strain for all pressure gradients.

Cartilage consists of a matrix of collagen fibers in a hydrated-gel ground substance. Cells called chondrocytes are distributed throughout the cartilage to within 1 μm of the surface. The size and orientation of fibers varies with depth in the cartilage. The surface zone is composed of densely packed sheets on bundles of fibrils oriented predominantly parallel to the surface. In the middle zone the fibrils become more randomly oriented. In the deeper zone the fibrils are generally larger, less dense, and anchored radially into the subchondral bone [15].

The surface layer of the cartilage has been examined separately by Maroudas [12] and has been found to exhibit an anomalous behavior because of the closer

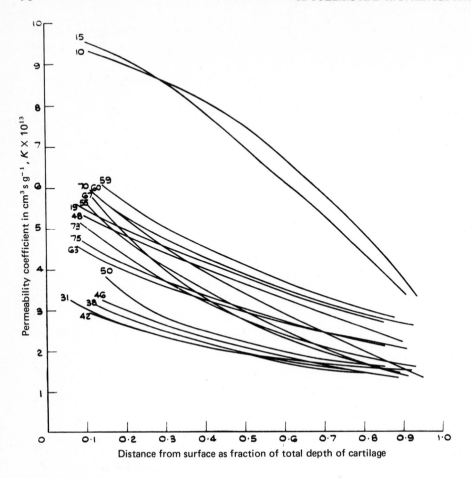

Figure 6 Permeability of human cartilage from the femoral condyle. The numbers refer to age in years. *(From Maroudas [10].)*

weave of collagen fibers near the surface which inhibits the outflow of mucopoly-saccharides and inflow of hyaluronic acid; both substances are important con-stituents of the synovial fluid that bathes the articular surfaces. According to Mow, Lai, and Redler [16, 15], the superficial tangential zone is composed of layers of sheets of tightly woven fibers parallel to the articular surface. There is an abrupt transition to the middle and deep zones in which the collagen fibers are randomly oriented. The variation in permeability of articular cartilage with depth from the surface as first mentioned by McCutchen [17] and confirmed by Maroudas and Bullough [12] seems to support these findings. From this ultrastructural informa-tion, the superficial tangential zone may be assumed to be transversely isotropic, while the middle and deep zones may be considered to be isotropic as proposed by Mow et al. [16].

As reported by Hayes and Mockros [18] and others, typical response of articular cartilage to a suddenly applied load is an instantaneous elastic response followed by a long-term viscoelastic response.

The short-time "elastic" response of cartilage to load by means of indenter tests analyzed by using solutions to various contact problems of elasticity has been reported by several investigators.

Hirsch [19] was one of the first to appeal to the Hertz solution for contact between two elastic spheres to model the contact between a rigid spherical indenter and the curved articular surface. Zarek and Edwards [20] used as their model the Hertz solution generalized for the case of contact between a rigid sphere and the flat surface of an elastic half-space. The solution for the indentation of an elastic half-space by a plane cylindrical indenter was used by Sokoloff [21]. In each of these cases the layered geometry of the articular joint, an important consideraton, was neglected.

In order to account for the layered geometry of the articular joint, Kempson et al. [22] employed as a model the results of indentation tests on thin rubber sheets lying on a rigid surface. Simon [23] reported, however, that he was unable to obtain consistent results with the theoretical models of either Kempson et al. [22] or Sokoloff [21].

Hayes et al. [24] presented a solution for the contact problem of the indentation by either a spherical or a cylindrical punch pressed normally into an elastic layer bonded to a rigid half-space. Their solution, based on classical theory of elasticity, assumed material isotropy and homogeneity. Using the values for the elastic material properties of mildly osteoarthritic cartilage previously published [18], these authors were able to obtain a correspondence between indentations as predicted by their model and the results of Hirsch [19].

Recently Hori and Mockros [25] determined the short-time shear and bulk moduli of articular cartilage using torsional shear and uniaxial confined compression tests. Their results are compared to the values of shear moduli predicted by using data from independent indenter tests. They conclude the predicted and measured values correlate but with considerable dispersion. The short-time shear modulus of articular cartilage, including both healthy and diseased samples, was found to vary over the range 4-35×10^5 N/m^2 and the short-time bulk modulus over the range 9-170×10^6 N/m^2. The method of tissue storage was found to have a major effect on the measured mechanical properties.

The indentation characteristics of cartilage subjected to enzymatic attack have been studied by Harris et al. [26].

Tests to determine elastic properties of articular cartilage in tension were carried out by Woo et al. [27]. Using specimens from each of the surface, middle, and deep zones, stress-strain curves were obtained and fitted to nonlinear constitutive equations of the form $\sigma = A(e^{B\epsilon} - 1)$.

The viscoelastic nature of the articular cartilage has been discussed by Mow [20] who proposed a Voigt-linear spring model for the cartilage and a constitutive equation expressible in the form

$$\tau_{ij} + \lambda_1 \frac{\partial \tau_{ij}}{\partial t} = 2\eta_0 \left(e_{ij} + \lambda_2 \frac{\partial e_{ij}}{\partial t} \right)$$

where $\eta_0, \lambda_1, \lambda_2$ are constants.

Experiments performed by Linn and Sokoloff [29] and Edwards [30] on the rate of expression and resorption of fluid from cartilage have shown that the quantity of expressible fluid for any given loading tends towards an asymptotic value. The expressed fluid has been shown to be essentially extracellular by Linn and Sokoloff [29]. Linn [31] devised an experiment enabling the variation of normal deformation of articular cartilage to be determined as a function of time, which suggests a strong relation between the exudation of interstitial fluid and the apparent viscoelasticity of the material. Hayes and Mockros [18] conducted a series of experiments to determine the viscoelastic material properties of human articular cartilage, specifically the shear and bulk creep compliances. Their investigation also suggests that flow processes are not important in the initial stage of deformation of normal tissue.

Parsons and Black [32] applied a theoretical solution for the indentation of a layered medium to the indentation of the articular surface of the distal femur of the rabbit. Experimental results yield shear moduli and retardation spectra which are invariant with respect to cartilage thickness and applied stress within the stress range used. Values for these mechanical properties are presented in this paper.

1.2 The Synovial Fluid

The synovial fluid is a clear or yellowish viscous fluid similar in appearance to egg white or saliva, present only in minute quantities. The human knee contains 0.2 to 0.3 ml of free fluid [33], whereas the ox ankle contains about 25 ml. The concentration of the long-chain polymer mucopolysaccharide (hyaluronic acid) is of the order of 3.5 mg/g, providing a molecular weight of about 10^6, the linear length of the long chain molecules being approximately 10^4 Å[34]. It is the hyaluronic acid that accounts for the slipperiness and stringy quality of synovial fluid. This constitutent was first isolated by Meyer et al. [35] in 1939. It is found also in the vitreous humor of the eye and in the umbilical cord. Passage of synovial fluid through a 0.22-μm filter removes the hyaluronate, leaving a watery filtrate [36]. In solution, hyaluronic acid molecules combine with protein in a weak bond. The complex possesses a high negative charge. According to Maroudas [13, 37], ion transport in the cartilage is important in governing flow properties and the nutrition of the cartilage. Synovial fluid exhibits a non-Newtonian character as a result of its hyaluronic acid content. The variation of relative viscosity with shear rate is indicated in Fig. 7. Figure 8 indicates shifts in the viscosity curves for synovial fluid in rheumatoid arthritis cases. However, most data have been obtained for shear rates below 100 s^{-1}, whereas Tanner [38] estimates that in normal walking at 4 mi/h, articular surfaces are subjected to shear rates of the order of 2500 s^{-1}.

Hyaluronic acid is degraded (depolymerized) by the enzyme hyaluronidase, whereupon synovial fluid becomes Newtonian (as in arthritic patients). Burch et al.

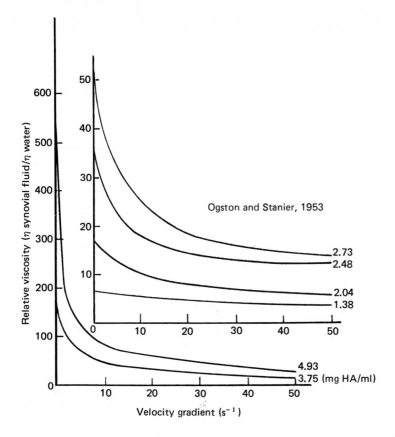

Figure 7 Dependence of viscosity of synovial fluid on velocity gradient. *(From Mow [52].)*

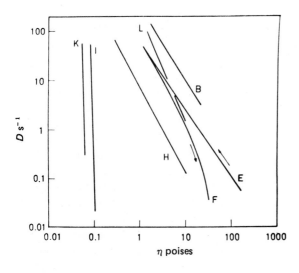

Figure 8 Dependence of viscosity of synovial fluid on shear rate *D*. *K* and *I* represent synovial fluid from rheumatoid arthritis cases; *B*, *E*, and *F* from traumatic arthritis cases. Note that the viscosity of the fluid depends on the rheological history, as illustrated by curves *E* and *F*, determined consecutively and in the opposing direction of rates of shear. Curve *H* is after Ogston and Stanier and represents ox synovial fluid. Curve *L* is after Sundblad and represents a 0.24 percent solution of hyaluronic acid. *(From Dintenfass [57].)*

[39] point out that this may well be due to a reduction in the concentration of hyaluronic acid in the synovial fluid of such patients.

Swann [40] has discussed the roles of the various constitutents of synovial fluid relating to joint function. He points out that the two primary functions of synovial fluid are joint lubrication and nutrition of the joint tissues.

Two different constituents of synovial fluid, both synthesized by the synovial lining cells, are responsible for two different lubricating functions. The hyaluronic acid constituent is the lubricant for the soft tissue of the synovial membrane [41], while boundary lubrication of the cartilage is provided by a specific lubricating glycoprotein, LGP-1.

Rheological models for synovial fluid that describe various aspects of its non-Newtonian viscoelastic behavior have been proposed by Mow [28] and Kuei and Mow [42] and have been recently reviewed by Lai et al. [43].

1.3 The Motion and Loading of Articular Joints

The motions of articulation of human joints have been investigated most thoroughly in a monograph by Strasser [44], in which the locus of instantaneous centers of rotation has been determined for the knee joint as an example (Fig. 9). Shinno [45] and Morrison [46] provide further details. Figure 10 depicts the initial rolling and subsequent sliding motions occurring during normal joint articulation, the motions consisting of three degrees of freedom: rotation about an axis normal to the mating surfaces, rolling, and sliding. These may be isolated in various regimes of the loading cycle (Fig. 11) in such a manner that each degree of freedom may be analyzed separately.

The articular surfaces may be subjected to local loads varying between 0 and 150 kg/cm, with maximum pressures of 570 lb/in^2 [47] for a 175-lb human. Standing load corresponds to approximately twice body weight [47]. Dynamic loads transmitted by joints may be as high as five times body weight [48], with corresponding pressures on the articular surfaces reaching several hundred pounds per square inch. For example, Greenwald and O'Connor [49] estimate that, during walking, the peak pressure in the human hip is over 300 lb/in^2. This is an average value, calculated by dividing the load by the contact area. The local pressures may be even greater. The contact area between the articular surfaces is generally horseshoe shaped (Fig. 12), measuring 0.75 to 1 in^2 for the knee. At a normal walking speed of 4 mi/h, with a ratio of radius of curvature of femur surface to length of leg of 1:30, a motion pivoted about the center of the ball of the femur produces a linear surface velocity at the articular cartilage of 2.5 in/s, whereas a velocity of the order of 25 in/s may occur in the shoulder of a baseball pitcher throwing a ball at 100 mi/h. It is important, therefore, to recognize that a variety of load-speed combinations occurs: high load at low speed (standing, jumping), high load at high speed (contact phase of running), and low load at high speed (swing phase of running).

Defining an effective radius of curvature $\bar{R}$ as

$$\bar{R} = \frac{R_1 R_2}{R_1 \pm R_2} \tag{1}$$

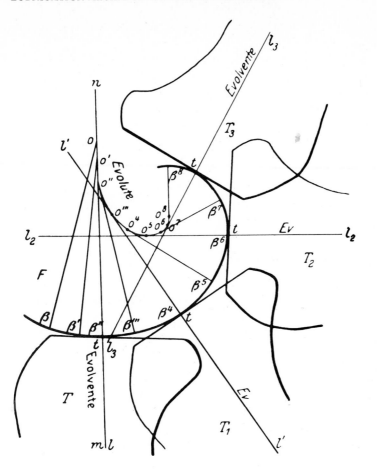

Figure 9 Articulation of knee joint. *(From Strasser [44].)*

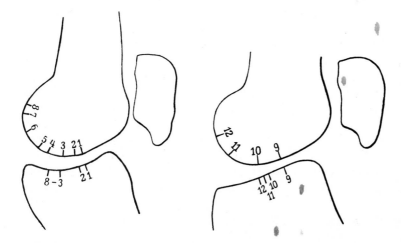

Figure 10 Sliding and rolling motions of knee joint. *(From Strasser [44].)*

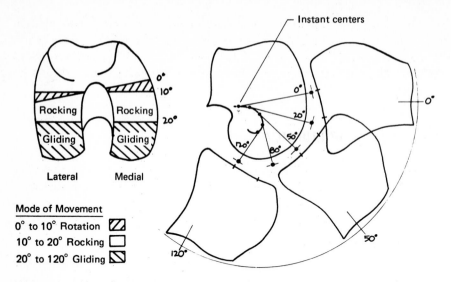

Figure 11 Normal knee movement. *(From F. H. Gunston, Polycentric Knee Arthroplasty, J. Bone J. Surg., vol. 53-B, 1971.)*

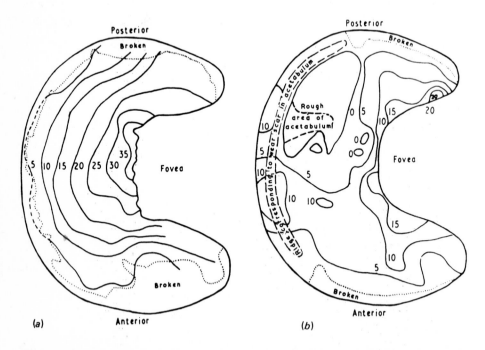

Figure 12 Contour maps of hip-joint surfaces. (*a*) 26-yr-old healthy hip; (*b*) osteoarthrosic hip. *(From D. Dowson, M. D. Longfield, P. S. Walker, and V. Wright, An Investigation of the Friction and Lubrication in Human Joints, Proc. Inst. Mech. Eng., vol. 182, pt. 3N, 1967-1968.)*

where the minus sign obtains if the centers of curvature of the two articular surfaces lie on the same side of the contact interface, Dowson [50] quotes Tanner [51], who estimates $\bar{R}$ for the knee as 2 to 10 cm, and for the hip and ankle as 10 to 100 cm. These estimates have apparently been misquoted by Mow [52] in his review article.

2 MECHANISMS OF LUBRICATION

A number of mechanisms have been suggested in the literature to explain the low friction observed in healthy joints (Figs. 13 and 14). Each will now be described briefly.

2.1 Hydrodynamic Lubrication

Studies of lubrication span the last 98 yr, beginning with the first recorded study by Petroff [53], who proved that a journal must ride eccentrically in its bearing, followed by the friction experiment of Tower [54], and the first formulation by Reynolds [55] based upon these experiments. MacConaill [56] suggested adaptation of Reynolds' theory of hydrodynamic lubrication to joints, where the menisci were thought to provide the convergent channels into which the fluid is dragged by the friction between the fluid and the moving channel wall. The pressure then would

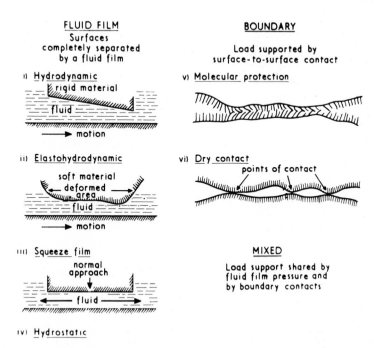

Figure 13 Lubrication modes proposed for synovial joints. *(From Walker et al. [5].)*

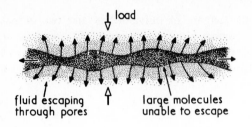

fluid escaping
through pores   large molecules
                 unable to escape

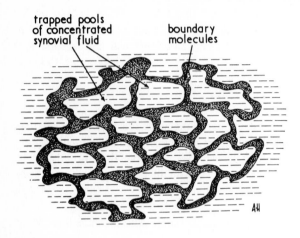

Figure 14 Schematic of trapped pool lubrication of cartilage with synovial fluid. *(From Walker et al. [5].)*

rise in such a channel, furnishing the force necessary to separate the opposing surfaces.

The motion is similar to that between two parallel plates, except that, as a result of the slight inclination of the two opposing surfaces, the convective term $u\, \partial u/\partial x \neq 0$. However, the Reynolds number $(Ul/v)(h/l)^2 \ll 1$ if the gap $h \ll l$, the length of the plates. Here U is the relative velocity, and v the kinematic viscosity. In this case (as for biological joints), the convective term may be neglected in spite of the divergence of the articular surfaces, so that one obtains the problem for Couette flow:

$$p' \equiv \frac{\partial p}{\partial x} = \mu\, \frac{\partial^2 u}{\partial y^2}$$

with

$$u = \begin{cases} U & \text{at } y = 0 \\ 0 & \quad\ y = h \end{cases}$$

$$p = p_0 \quad \text{at } \begin{cases} x = 0 \\ x = l \end{cases} \tag{2}$$

The solution in terms of the velocity distribution is

$$u = U\left(1 - \frac{y}{h}\right) - \frac{h^2}{2}\, \frac{p'}{\mu}\, \frac{y}{h}\left(1 - \frac{y}{h}\right) \tag{3}$$

The ratio of gap width h_0 to radius of curvature $\bar{R}$, defined above, for two surfaces moving with relative velocity U_R under a normal load P is then given by

$$\frac{h_0}{\bar{R}} = 4.9 \frac{\mu U_R}{P} \tag{4}$$

where μ is the viscosity of the fluid. For the knee, with $\bar{R} = 5$ cm, $\mu = 0.01$ p, $U_R = 2.5$ cm/s, and $P = 50$ kg/cm, the gap width h_0 is calculated to be 0.0125×10^{-6} cm, much less than the characteristic surface roughness depicted in Fig. 4. Under these conditions it is doubtful that hydrodynamic lubrication would succeed in producing a stable film that would not be pierced by surface irregularities. It appears that the relative surface velocities of the articular cartilage are not high enough to drag in sufficient fluid to produce the desired film. Furthermore, it is noted from the above that the corresponding frictional force will depend upon the fluid viscosity and the relative speed of the surfaces.

With a view to remedying this difficulty, it was subsequently suggested by Dintenfass [57] and others that greater film thicknesses would be achieved if one were to take into account the deformability of the cartilage, leading to a theory of elastohydrodynamic lubrication. Taking a mean elastic modulus E' of 10^7 dyn/cm^2, and neglecting the effect of pressure on fluid viscosity, one obtains a gap-width ratio of

$$\frac{h_m}{\bar{R}} \approx 1.35 \left(\frac{2\mu U_R}{E'\bar{R}}\right)^{1/2} \tag{5a}$$

For the knee, $h_m \approx 2 \times 10^{-4}$ cm, which is of the order of the surface roughness. Elastohydrodynamic lubrication is therefore still considered by a number of researchers today to be a plausible mechanism for joint lubrication. Again we note the dependence of friction upon fluid viscosity and relative speed. Further refinements of this theory include consideration of the non-Newtonian character of the fluid under the name elastorheodynamics.

Fein [58] has considered the role of deformation of the cartilage in enhancing the formation of squeeze films in joints. The problem of the deformation and pressure exerted between two spherical and deformable bodies in contact was solved by Hertz [59] and its adaptation to cartilage-coated articular surfaces yields an estimate of the "squeeze film" thickness h_s corresponding to an applied load P,

$$h_s = 2.86 \frac{\mu^{1/2} P^{1/6}}{t^{1/2}} \left(\frac{\bar{R}}{E}\right)^{2/3} \tag{5b}$$

as a function of the time t after application of the load. For example, with $\bar{R} = 1$ cm, $\mu = 0.1$ p, and $P = 30$ kg, one obtains $h_s = 3.5$ μm at $t = 1$ s and 0.058 μm after 1 h, indicating the relatively slow rate of expulsion of the film. The above result agrees well with film measurements of oil between a convex glass lens and a deformable methacrylate plate. Fein proposes the possibility that joints at rest under load are lubricated by this principle.

2.2 Boundary Lubrication

Repeated failures of artificial hip joints in England led Charnley [1] to propose the mechanism of boundary lubrication. (An excellent review of this subject may be found in a chapter by Rowe [60].) One considers the sliding of one surface over another, both possessing microscopic surface roughness. It is then postulated that

$$F = A_c \bar{s} \qquad W = A_c \bar{p} \tag{6}$$

where F = frictional (tangential) force
$\quad W$ = normal load
$\quad A_c$ = contact area
$\quad \bar{s}$ = mean shear strength
$\quad \bar{p}$ = mean yield stress of all contact points
Then the coefficient of friction η is given by

$$\eta = \frac{F}{W} = \frac{\bar{s}}{\bar{p}} \tag{7}$$

Work done in compressing the material will modify the above estimate of the frictional force. For metals, $\bar{s}$ is determined by measuring F and A_c. It is found that the mean shear strength at an interface where sliding occurs over surface asperities is of the same order of magnitude as in bulk materials, lending support to the existence of a "cold-welding" process for surface asperities.

The frictional force $F = A_c \bar{s}$ may be reduced by reducing both the contact area A_c and the shear strength $\bar{s}$ at the interface. Copper has a relatively lower value of $\bar{s}$, but owing to its ductility, the contact area A_c under load is high. For steel, the opposite is true: $\bar{s}$ is high and A_c low, in such a manner that the frictional force of copper sliding past copper is of the same order of magnitude as for steel sliding upon steel. However, interposing a monomolecular layer of copper between two steel surfaces leads to markedly reduced values of friction, since, for the combination, A_c corresponds to that of the steel substrate, while the shear strength $\bar{s}$ is that of the weaker component, copper. The same reduction in coefficient of friction may be demonstrated dramatically with soap films. For thick soap films, $\mu = 0.2$ to 0.3, whereas thin soap films on a metal substrate exhibit a coefficient of 0.05! However, reductions in friction are mitigated by the tendency of $\bar{s}$ to increase with pressure. A refinement of the above theory to take this into account has been described by McFarlane and Tabor [61]. A brief summary of the important ideas is given next.

Combined stress theory If $\bar{p}$ and $\bar{s}$ may be considered uniform across a junction, a shear-strain energy criterion gives

$$p^2 + \alpha \bar{s}^2 = \text{constant} = \bar{p}_0^2 = \alpha \bar{s}_m^2 \tag{8}$$

where $\bar{s}_m$ = shear strength of metal
$\quad \bar{p}_0$ = plastic deformation strength
The exact value of α varies from metal to metal, having little effect on the

coefficient of friction η. The interfacial shear stress is $\bar{s}_i = \beta \bar{s}_m$, where $0 < \beta < 1$. Then

$$\bar{p}^2 + \alpha \bar{s}_i^2 = \frac{\alpha \bar{s}_i^2}{\beta^2} \tag{9}$$

and

$$\eta = \frac{F}{W} = \frac{A^* \bar{s}_i}{A^* \bar{p}} = \left[\alpha \left(\frac{1}{\beta^2} - 1 \right) \right]^{-1/2} \tag{10}$$

where A^* is the deformed area of contact under load. When one exceeds the limiting shear strength that the interface can transmit from one surface to the other, the film fails and microscopic sliding occurs. For physiological joints, $\beta < 0.2$ and the above expression for the coefficient of friction simplifies to

$$\eta \approx \beta [\alpha(1 - \beta^2)]^{-1/2} \approx \frac{\beta}{\alpha} = \frac{\bar{s}_i}{\bar{p}_0} = \frac{\text{Critical shear stress of film}}{\text{Plastic yield stress of substrate}} \tag{11}$$

The more general theory accounts for changes in A_c with the load W. It is the intended role of the lubricant to restrict the contact area A_c. A noteworthy feature of boundary lubrication is total independence of the coefficient of friction on viscosity or relative speed. It is currently conjectured that boundary lubrication may be important in the functioning of biological joints, the interfacial film being established by the long-chain mucopolysaccharide molecules "washed" out to the superficial layers of the cartilage where they bond to the surfaces.

Maroudas [10] has suggested that a gel of concentrated synovial fluid forms under pressure on the surface of the cartilage. The experiments of Walker et al. [5] provide data to substantiate this possibility, which is further confirmed by electron microscope studies of the cartilage surface. Anchoring of long-chain molecules into the cartilaginous surfaces ("lubricating factor") decreases the coefficient of friction η because expulsion of the mucopolysaccharide film is inhibited when sliding occurs. Such bonding is established for inorganic materials by chemical reaction of the film with its substrate. Cameron [62] has calculated the force required to break the bonds between hydrocarbon chains of the lubricant. The result implies a coefficient of friction η of the correct order of magnitude. For example, in engineering bearings functioning on this principle, the addition of oleic acid to the boundary lubricant calcium stearate assures the desired chemical reaction, which has been observed to result in a significant reduction in the coefficient of friction [60]. On the other hand, silicones, which are inert and exclude water vapor and hence oxidation, constitute very poor boundary lubricants, even leading sometimes to increased coefficients of friction. Synovial fluid is highly corrosive to metals and may also react with the cartilaginous surfaces. It has been suggested by Wilkins [63] that protein components of synovial mucin anchor the mucin to the surface, a feature essential to boundary lubrication.

Experiments by Linn [3, 64] using mechanically articulated dogs' ankles (Fig. 15) indicate that apparent severalfold changes in the controlled viscosity of the bathing fluid resulted in only small changes in the coefficient of friction, of the same order as accompanying alterations in the molecular weight. The measured friction was not sensitive to relative speed of the joint surfaces. These features alone

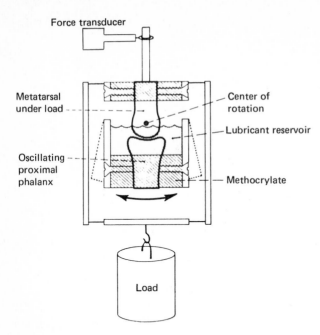

Figure 15 Schematic diagram of arthrotripsometer. Friction measuring device based on Linn's arthrotripsometer. The bottom half of the joint is oscillated by a motor. The top half, although loaded, is free to move. If the joint's center of rotation is properly aligned with respect to the center of the drive shaft of the motor, the frictional force at the joint interface can be obtained by subtracting the tare values of the machine from the "drag" on the top half of the joint, measured by a transducer and corrected for the geometry of the joint and the machine. *(From Radin et al. [122].)*

would normally be sufficient to rule out dominant influences of hydrodynamic or elastohydrodynamic lubrication in the functioning of biological joints.

An osmotic pressure gradient develops as the mucopolysaccharides, which exist in higher concentrations near the outer layer of the cartilage, tend to migrate inward toward more dilute levels. Tension may develop in the long chains. This aspect has been discussed by McCutchen [65].

As pointed out by Swann [40], boundary lubrication of cartilage appears to be caused by the action of specific lubricating glycoproteins LPG-1. It had earlier been suggested by Roberts [66] that electrical repulsive forces may be of significance in the boundary lubrication of surfaces by synovial fluid. In effect, the main molecules bear a slight negative change, and seem to occupy the largest possible volume.

Davis et al. [67] have recently presented a general model for boundary lubrication of joint cartilage by synovial fluid as the basis of friction tests employing both cartilage and several artificial surfaces. It postulates that one portion of the synovial lubricating glycoprotein (LGP) is adsorbed to the surface. Reduction in surface shear is accomplished by formation of hydration shells about the polar portions of the adsorbed LGP creating a thin layer of viscous structured water at the surface. Mutual electrostatic repulsion between charged polysaccharide moieties aids in separation of the adsorbed surface layers. The hydration shell also serves as a check valve to control the movement of water out of and into the cartilage matrix during motion.

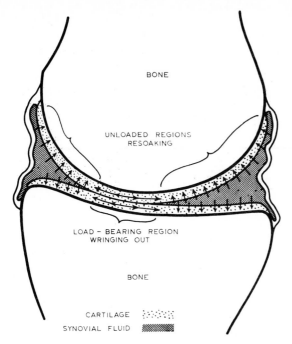

BONE

UNLOADED REGIONS
RESOAKING

LOAD - BEARING REGION
WRINGING OUT

BONE

CARTILAGE
SYNOVIAL FLUID

Figure 16 Fluid flow in articular cartilage. *(From McCutchen [9].)*

2.3 Weeping Lubrication

It was shown in Sec. 2.1 that the relative velocities of the articular surfaces are not high enough to draw in sufficient fluid to separate the surfaces. However, McCutchen [68] demonstrated experimentally that lubrication may be achieved in a hydrostatic bearing by "pumping" in fluid between the two joint surfaces. In this case, the pump is introduced through the mechanism of *weeping* (Fig. 16).

Consider two cartilaginous sponges pushed together. The fluid contained in the pores may be considered incompressible. When these are in contact, no room exists for the displacement of fluid. Hence, the cartilage cannot deform initially, and therefore can bear no load. That is, in the initial stages of contact before a significant amount of fluid has time to leak out of the cartilage, all the load is borne by fluid, the cartilaginous matrix being relatively weak in compression. The frictional force between the lightly rubbing matrices is low during this stage, and the joint operates as a "self-pressuring bearing," called a weeping bearing.

Owing to subsequent tangential leaking of fluid, the bearing will not maintain its low friction indefinitely under continous load. The cartilage wrings out, deforms, and supports an increasing fraction of the load. Then, as the load is released, the cartilaginous matrix swells, drawing in new fluid.

To illustrate the weeping mechanism, McCutchen [9] performed a simple experiment in which cartilage was rubbed against a glass plate. The measured friction increased with time, as the fluid was expressed from the cartilage (Fig. 17). Brief periods of resoaking (1 to 10 s) lowered the friction only momentarily, as a

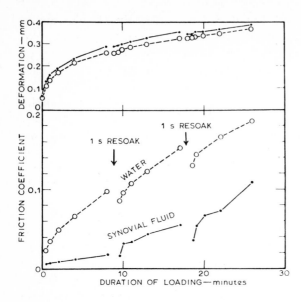

Figure 17 Friction and deformation of excised cartilage on glass versus duration of loading. *(From McCutchen [9].)*

new surface film was temporarily reestablished. Upon subsequent rubbing, the coefficient of friction rapidly assumed the value it had prior to resoaking, indicating that the surface lubricant had been worn off without the interior fluid content having been altered significantly. Had the cartilage been resoaked for 30 min (the time for almost complete resaturation), the friction would have dropped to its original value at time zero, and the whole history would have repeated itself. The weeping process may therefore be interpreted in this experiment as a means of supplying long-chain molecules to the outer surface of the cartilage by "weeping" from the interior. In the normally functioning joint, the rate of supply of fluid to the articular surfaces should not be less than its rate of wear if an equilibrium state is to be realized.

The time required for complete wring-out of cartilage has been estimated, on the basis of a simple squeeze-film analysis, to be of the order of 24 h. Figure 16 indicates that fluid is imbibed across a relatively short, broad path normal to the cartilage when load is released, whereas leaking must occur over a longer tangential path, a feature that may explain the ability of a joint to retain its fluid for such long periods.

The importance of "boosted lubrication" has been put forth by Walker et al. [5, 69–71]. It is suggested that as the joint is loaded and unloaded, synovial fluid escapes through the matrix pores, with pools of fluid collecting in superficial pockets on the surfaces of the cartilage (Fig. 14). The watery components are squeezed out, but the hyaluronic acid molecules remain in the collagenous fibrils to form a "gel" that provides subsequent lubrication.

2.4 Earlier Experiments

Jones [72] employed a pendulum apparatus in an attempt to determine whether joints are lubricated by fluid film or boundary mechanisms. His experiment was based on the principle that the coefficient of friction in a fluid film-lubricated bearing varies with the relative sliding speed of the bearing surfaces; whereas, in a boundary-lubricated bearing the coefficient of friction is independent of the sliding speed.

Excised human finger joints were mounted in a pendulum apparatus, so that the joint formed the fulcrum of the pendulum. It was reasoned that frictional losses at the fulcrum determine the rate of decay of the amplitude of the swinging pendulum. If the finger joint was lubricated by a fluid film mechanism, the decay rate should be proportional to the swing velocity. If, however, the joint was boundary lubricated, the decay rate should be independent of swing velocity. This principle was first elaborated by Stanton [73]. Jones' results indicated a nonlinear rate of decay, corresponding to fluid film lubrication, with some boundary lubrication at very low speeds.

Further evidence of fluid film lubrication in joints was provided by Barnett [47], who reported that rabbit ankles that had been injected with hyaluronidase and articulated under a spring-applied load produced more cartilage wear than ankles that had not been injected. Hyaluronidase reduces the viscosity of synovial fluid by breaking up the long-chain hyaluronic acid molecules [34, 74]. Barnett attributed the accelerated wear to a breakdown in hydrodynamic lubrication due to the reduced viscosity of the synovial fluid.

Charnley [1] suggested that physiological articulation speeds were too low for hydrodynamic action to produce a significant fluid film in joints, and attributed the speed-dependent friction effects observed by Jones [72] to the presence of connective tissues on the specimens and the shifting center of rotation in finger joints. Charnley performed pendulum experiments with human ankles devoid of any such connective tissues and found that the friction was indeed independent of speed, indicating boundary lubrication.

Barnett and Cobbold [75] tested dogs' ankle joints in a pendulum device and also found that the friction was not speed dependent. However, further experiments with pressurized hydrostatic mechanical bearings in the pendulum apparatus demonstrated that these bearings also exhibited an apparent speed-independent friction. It was concluded, therefore, that speed-independent friction was *not* proof of a boundary lubricating mechanism.

Faber et al. [76] suggested that the freely swinging pendulum devices failed to produce evidence of speed-dependent friction in joints because they operated in a lower than physiological speed range. Faber used a spring-driven pendulum device to measure the friction in rabbit knees, producing cartilage surface sliding speeds greater than 6 cm/s, which should exceed the maximum speed for a running rabbit. The experimental results indicated that, at these higher velocities, at least 80 percent of the total frictional stress was due to velocity-dependent fluid film friction.

The results of the various pendulum experiments are compared in Table 1.

3 FLOW IN POROUS MEDIA

Treating the articular cartilage as a fluid-filled porous medium, one can use the well-known consolidation theory to calculate in full detail the history of matrix

Table 1 Summary of pendulum experiments

Study	Joint tested	Device	Load (lb)	Maximum amplitude (degrees)	Oscillation frequency	Coefficient of friction reported (with synovial fluid)	Conclusions regarding nature of lubrication mechanism
Jones [47]	Human finger	Free-swinging pendulum	13	±2	–	0.022–0.114	Primarily fluid film with some boundary
Charnley [1]	Human ankle	Free-swinging pendulum	30	–	–	0.01–0.02	Boundary only
Barnett and Cobbold [50]	Human finger	Free-swinging pendulum	–	±15	32	0.0075–0.0180	Primarily fluid film; boundary may occur
Faber et al. [51]	Rabbit knee *in vivo*	Spring-driven pendulum	0–55	±10	240–600	–	80% of friction due to fluid shearing; 20% due to solid contact

deformations and fluid flow in time. In general, the calculation is extremely complex [77] and must be resolved numerically. The philosophy adopted in this chapter is to use a number of greatly simplified formulations leading to closed-form approximate expressions for physical quantities such as pressure and flow velocity distributions in the cartilage under load. These preliminary solutions will serve to point out the dependence on and sensitivity to physical parameters such as fluid viscosity and matrix porosity and permeability and to establish a framework for the design of simple controlled experiments in the laboratory. When the physical model has been justified, one may then proceed with refined calculations, which may include more complex geometries and material constitutive relations. On this basis, a simplified analysis is now given for wring-out and uptake of fluid in a porous medium under load, based upon the work of McCutchen [11], in which it is assumed according to Fig. 16 that wring-out takes place tangentially, and liquid uptake normally, to the articular surfaces.

3.1 Wring-out of Cartilage: One-Dimensional Analysis

Consider only radial outflow through a stationary elemental porous cylindrical volume (Fig. 18) whose height h is decreasing under load at velocity $\dot{h}$. The law of Darcy [78] for flow in a porous medium relates the fluid velocity linearly to the pressure gradient,

$$v = -K \frac{\partial p}{\partial r} \tag{12}$$

with a proportionality factor [79]

$$K = \frac{\text{permeability of matrix}}{\text{fluid viscosity}}$$

The decrease in volume per unit time is

$$\Delta V = -\pi r^2 \dot{h} \tag{13}$$

causing fluid to flow radially outward through an area $2\pi r h$ at radius r, so that the outflow velocity is

$$v = -\frac{r}{2} \frac{\dot{h}}{h} \tag{14}$$

The law of Darcy then gives the radial pressure gradient as

$$\frac{dP_r}{dr} = \frac{r}{2K} \frac{\dot{h}}{h} \tag{15}$$

where $P_r(r = R) = 0$ is the reference state, and

$$P_r = \frac{-1}{4K} \frac{\dot{h}}{h} (R^2 - r^2) \qquad \dot{h} < 0 \tag{16}$$

if the permeability K can be considered constant during the deformation. The total

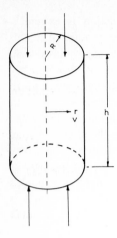

Figure 18 Flow lines in loaded cylindrical cartilage element. *(From Zarek and Edwards [87].)*

force on a disk perpendicular to the loading direction due to this pressure distribution is then

$$F_p = \int_{r=0}^{R} 2\pi r P_r \, dr = -\frac{\pi}{8K} \frac{\dot h}{h} R^4 \tag{17}$$

The elastic force on a cross-sectional area A due to a compression ϵ of the matrix is

$$F_e = E\epsilon A = E\pi R^2 \frac{h_0 - h}{h_0} \tag{18}$$

For small deformations,

$$\frac{\dot h}{h} \approx \frac{\dot h}{h_0} \tag{19}$$

The total imposed load W, being $F_p + F_e$, gives us

$$W = F_p + F_e = \pi R^2 \left[-\frac{\dot h}{h_0} \frac{R^2}{8K} + \left(1 - \frac{h}{h_0} \right) E \right] \tag{20}$$

or

$$a\dot H + bH + c = 0 \tag{21}$$

where

$$H = \frac{h}{h_0} \qquad a = -\frac{\pi R^4}{8K} \qquad b = -\pi R^2 E \qquad c = E\pi R^2 - W \tag{22}$$

The above equation has a particular integral

$$H = -\frac{c}{b} \tag{23}$$

and hence a general solution

$$H = -\frac{c}{b} + A' e^{\alpha t} \tag{24}$$

where α is determined from the corresponding homogeneous equation as

$$\alpha = -\frac{8EK}{R^2} \tag{25}$$

There remains the constant A', which is determined by the initial condition $h(t = 0) = h_0$. Hence,

$$\frac{h}{h_0} = \frac{W}{\pi R^2 E} \, (e^{-8EKt/R^2} - 1) + 1 \tag{26}$$

The net radial outflow of fluid per unit time under a constant compressive load W is then

$$\Delta V = -\pi r^2 \dot{h} = \frac{8h_0 WK}{\pi R^4} \, e^{-8EKt/R^2} \tag{27}$$

It is clear that this relation could provide estimates of the average permeability K of cartilage under load, from measurements of the radial fluid outflow with time.

3.2 Liquid Uptake: One-Dimensional Analysis

Reabsorption of liquid is considered to occur primarily in the direction normal to the articular surfaces when the load is released (Fig. 16).

For a cylindrical element of volume, u denotes displacement in the direction of the axis of symmetry z (Fig. 19). If the swelling time of the matrix is large compared with the time of application of the load, then

$$\frac{\partial u}{\partial z} \ll 1$$

The fluid velocity (in the z direction) relative to the moving matrix is given by Darcy's law:

$$v = -K \frac{\partial P}{\partial z} \tag{28}$$

where P is the liquid pore pressure. Swelling of the matrix in the positive z direction causes displacement of absorbed liquid in the negative z direction. If a

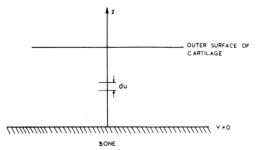

Figure 19 Swelling of a layer of cartilage.

fraction f of the matrix is occupied by solid, and if no voids form during swelling, then the velocity of the fluid relative to the moving cartilage is

$$v = -(1 + f)\dot{u} \tag{29}$$

and the corresponding pressure gradient developed as a result of fluid motion is given by Darcy's law as

$$\frac{dP}{dz} = \frac{1 + f}{K} \dot{u} \tag{30}$$

If there is no significant acceleration of the matrix during swelling, this force is just balanced by the elastic forces developed in the matrix due to its displacements u at each point z:

$$F_e = E \frac{\partial u}{\partial z} \tag{31}$$

The net force across an infinitesimal thickness dz of the cartilage is

$$\Delta F_e = E \frac{\partial^2 u}{\partial z^2} dz = -\frac{\partial P}{\partial z} dz \tag{32}$$

so that, for equilibrium,

$$E \frac{\partial^2 u}{\partial z^2} = -\frac{1 + f}{K} \dot{u} \tag{33}$$

Equation (33) shows that the rate of swelling of the cartilage as it imbibes fluid is governed by a diffusion-type equation, similar to the diffusion of temperature into a semi-infinite slab whose surface is heated. The solution of Eq. (33) is well known in terms of the error function, and for this case indicates that after 1 s, synovial fluid would be absorbed into the cartilage to a depth of 10^{-2} mm, while complete resoaking would take 40 min (based on the above simplified theory). These ideas are in qualitative agreement with McCutchen's experiments (Fig. 17).

The above simple one-dimensional models of cartilage deformation under load serve to develop the physical concepts that are utilized in the more general two-dimensional unsteady flow analysis that follows.

3.3 Fluid Motion in Cartilage under Compressive Load: Two-Dimensional Unsteady Analysis

It has been estimated by Linn [64] and McCutchen [2, 11] that nearly all the load imposed on the joint is borne by the interstitial fluid contained in the cartilage, and not by the matrix itself. However, as the cartilage is progressively compressed, matrix resistance becomes increasingly important, and classical consolidation theory as usually applied to soil mechanics may come into play (Fig. 20). In this section, an exact analytic solution is obtained for the time-dependent distribution of pressure and fluid velocity in an infinitely long layer of cartilage of finite thickness subjected to a nonstationary load whose area of application also varies in time.

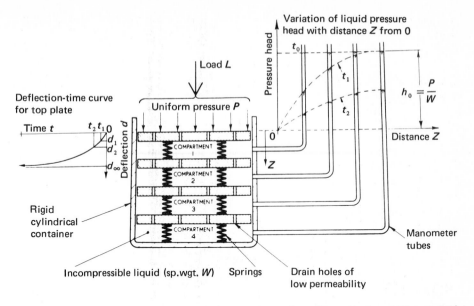

Figure 20 Simple analogy for consolidation of articular cartilage. *(From Zarek and Edwards [98].)*

Consider a layer of cartilage of thickness h, loaded as in Fig. 21. The bone is assumed impermeable to fluid, and Darcy's law then indicates that the normal derivative of pressure must vanish at the subchondral surface (cartilage-bone interface). For an incompressible fluid,

$$\text{div } v = 0 \tag{34}$$

which, when combined with Darcy's law for flow in a porous medium, leads to the Laplace equation for the fluid pore pressure:

$$\frac{\partial^2 p}{\partial x^2} + \frac{\partial^2 p}{\partial y^2} = 0 \tag{35}$$

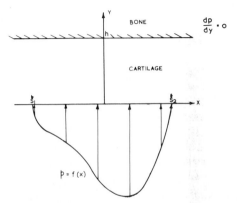

Figure 21 Boundary-value problem for a loaded cartilage layer.

with
$$p = f(x) \qquad \text{at } y = 0$$

$$\frac{\partial p}{\partial y} = 0 \qquad \text{at } y = h \tag{36}$$

The problem may be solved in a straightforward manner by taking the Fourier transform with respect to x:

$$\tilde{p}(\omega, y) = \frac{1}{(2\pi)^{1/2}} \int_{-\infty}^{\infty} e^{-i\omega x} \, p(x, y) \, dy \tag{37}$$

so that
$$\frac{d^2\tilde{p}}{dy^2} - \omega^2\tilde{p} = 0 \tag{38}$$

with
$$\tilde{p}(0) = \tilde{f} \qquad \frac{d\tilde{p}}{dy}(h) = 0 \tag{39}$$

The solution in the transformed place is simply

$$\tilde{p} = \tilde{f}(\omega) \frac{\operatorname{ch}(h - y)\omega}{\operatorname{ch} h\omega} \tag{40}$$

Inverting to return to the physical xy plane gives

$$p(x, y) = \frac{1}{\sqrt{2\pi}} \int_{-\infty}^{\infty} e^{i\omega x} \frac{\operatorname{ch}(h - y)\omega}{\operatorname{ch} h\omega} \, \tilde{f}(\omega) \, d\omega$$

$$= \frac{1}{\sqrt{2\pi}} \int_{-\infty}^{\infty} f(\xi) \, d\xi \int_{-\infty}^{\infty} e^{i\omega(x-\xi)} \frac{\operatorname{ch} \omega(h - y)}{\operatorname{ch} h\omega} \, d\omega \tag{41}$$

A table of Fourier transforms [80] gives

$$\frac{2 \cos(a/2) \operatorname{ch}(\bar{y}/2)}{\cos a + \operatorname{ch} \bar{y}} = \int_{-\infty}^{\infty} e^{ixy} \frac{\operatorname{ch} ax}{\operatorname{ch} \pi x} \, dx \tag{42}$$

from which one obtains the pressure distribution

$$p(x, y) = \frac{1}{h} \sin \frac{\pi y}{2h} \int_{-\infty}^{\infty} f(\xi) \frac{\operatorname{ch}(\pi/2h)(x - \xi)}{\operatorname{ch}(\pi/h)(x - \xi) - \cos(\pi y/h)} \, d\xi \tag{43}$$

If the load $f(\xi) = A(t)$ for $\xi_1(t) < x < \xi_2(t)$ and equals zero otherwise, then

$$p(x, y; t) = \frac{A}{h} \sin \frac{\pi y}{2h} \int_{\xi_1}^{\xi_2} \frac{\operatorname{ch}(\pi/2h)(x - \xi)}{\operatorname{ch}[(\pi/h)(x - \xi)] - \cos(\pi y/h)} \, d\xi \tag{44}$$

Make the substitutions

$$\frac{\pi}{2h}(x - \xi) = u \qquad \cos \frac{\pi y}{h} = b$$

to obtain

$$p(x, y; t) = -\frac{2A}{\pi} \sin \frac{\pi y}{2h} \int_{u_1}^{u_2} \frac{\text{ch } u}{\text{ch } 2u - b} \, du \qquad (45)$$

and the substitutions

$$\text{ch } 2u = 2 \text{ ch}^2 u - 1 \qquad \frac{1 + b}{2} = \tau$$

to get

$$p(x, y; t) = -\frac{A}{\pi} \sin \frac{\pi y}{2h} \int_{\text{sh}u_1}^{\text{sh}u_2} \frac{dw}{w^2 + 1 - \tau} \qquad (46)$$

where

$$1 - \tau \geqslant 0 \qquad 0 \leqslant y \leqslant h$$

whence $p(x, y; t) = \dfrac{A}{\pi} \left[\arctan \dfrac{\text{sh } (\pi/2h)(x - \xi_1)}{\sin (\pi y/2h)} - \arctan \dfrac{\text{sh } (\pi/2h)(x - \xi_2)}{\sin (\pi y/2h)} \right]$ (47)

If u and v denote the fluid velocity components in the x and y directions, respectively, then Darcy's law leads (Fig. 23) to

$$u = -\frac{KA}{2h} \sin^2 \frac{\pi y}{2h} \left[\frac{\text{ch } (\pi/2h)(x - \xi_1)}{\sin^2 (\pi y/2h) + \text{sh}^2 (\pi/2h)(x - \xi_1)} \right.$$

$$\left. - \frac{\text{ch } (\pi/2h)(x - \xi_2)}{\sin^2 (\pi y/2h) + \text{sh}^2 [\pi(x - \xi_2)/2h]} \right] \qquad (48)$$

$$v = -\frac{KA}{2h} \cos \frac{\pi y}{2h} \left[\frac{\text{sh } (\pi/2h)(x - \xi_2)}{\sin^2 (\pi y/2h) + \text{sh}^2 (\pi/2h)(x - \xi_2)} \right.$$

$$\left. - \frac{\text{sh } (\pi/2h)(x - \xi_1)}{\sin^2 (\pi y/2h) + \text{sh}^2 (\pi/2h)(x - \xi_1)} \right] \qquad (49)$$

As $y \to 0$, $u \to 0$ and

$$v = v_n \to -\frac{KA}{2h} \left[\frac{1}{\text{sh } (\pi/2h)(x - \xi_2)} - \frac{1}{\text{sh } (\pi/2h)(x - \xi_1)} \right] \qquad (50)$$

Mathematical singularities exist at the edges $x = \xi_1, \xi_2$ of the loading zone.

The analysis may be extended to slightly curved surfaces for which the layer thickness $h \ll R$, the radius of curvature. The results of Linn [3] as reproduced by Mow [52] (see Fig. 22) indicate that the normal deflection of the cartilage is almost constant under an oscillatory load, and hence one is justified in assuming $h = $ constant in the above analysis, corresponding to the deformed thickness.

3.4 Synovial Fluid Concentration in the Joint Space

The results of the previous section for the fluid flow field in the cartilage [Eqs. (47 to 50)] may be applied directly to an analysis of the distribution of synovial fluid in the joint space, as a means of estimating the concentration of long-chain molecules available for lubrication of the apposing articular surfaces. The synovial fluid circulating in the joint spaces contains hyaluronic acid dissolved in an aqueous solution, whereas the cartilage pores are filled with chondroitin sulphate and keratan sulphate. In the preliminary analysis below, the joint space is idealized as a thin

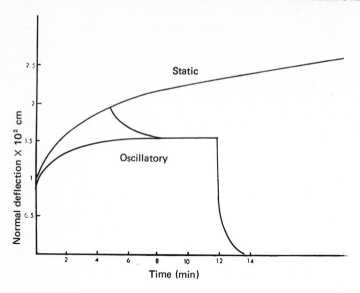

Figure 22 Time-dependent deformation of loaded cartilage for a load of 40 lb. *(From Mow [52].)*

uniform channel of height h, and no distinction is made between the identities of the synovial fluid components, other than to separate them into solute and solvent parts. By denoting the average value of the axial fluid velocity component in the channel as $u(x)$, where x is the distance along the channel measured from the momentary point of nearest contact of the apposing joint surfaces, and as $v_n(x)$ the inflow velocity component normal to the cartilaginous free surface (as in Fig. 23), the time rate of change of long-chain molecules (solute) in the joint gap h may be expressed as

$$2N(x)\,\Delta x + D\,\frac{d^2c}{dx^2}\,\Delta x\,h - h\,\Delta x\,\frac{d}{dx}\,[u(x)C(x)] = 0 \tag{51}$$

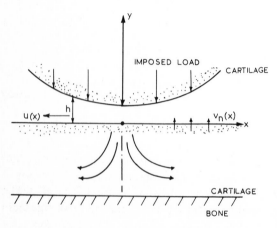

Figure 23 Fluid balance in joint space during loading.

in the steady state, where $N(x)$ is the distribution of solute deposited into the channel, D the diffusion coefficient of long-chain molecules in synovial fluid, and C the osmolarity. Ionic transport in the cartilage was not considered in the preliminary analysis. The three terms in the above balance represent, respectively, the active transport of solute across the channel walls and transport along the length of the channel due to diffusion and convection.

Aqueous solution will enter the joint space by osmosis across the channel walls at a rate given by

$$Q_{osm}(x) = 2 \, \Delta x \, P \, [C(x) - C_0] \tag{52}$$

where P is a factor of proportionality. This flow rate Q_{osm} combines with the inflow Q_n of aqueous solution given by pressure loading of the cartilage from the previous section,

$$Q_n(x) = 2v_n \, \Delta x \tag{53}$$

where v_n is the normal velocity component at the cartilage free surface, given by Eq. (50).

The total inflow rate of aqueous solution must equal the axial flow rate in the channel, if no fluid is to be accumulated. Hence the total rate of flow of aqueous solution into the channel per elemental length Δx is

$$Q(x) = h \, \Delta x \, \frac{du}{dx} = Q_{osm}(x) + Q_n(x) = 2 \, \Delta x \, P[C(x) - C_0] + 2v_n \, \Delta x \tag{54}$$

One may eliminate C between Eqs. (51) and (54) to obtain a single third-order nonlinear differential equation for the channel flow $u(x)$

$$2N(x) + \frac{Dh^2}{2P} \frac{d^3u}{dx^3} - \frac{h^2u}{2P} \frac{d^2u}{dx^2} + \left(\frac{hv_n}{P} - hC_0 \right) \frac{du}{dx}$$
$$- \frac{h^2}{2P} \left(\frac{du}{dx} \right)^2 - \left(\frac{Dh}{P} \frac{d^2v_n}{dx^2} - \frac{hu}{P} \frac{dv_n}{dx} \right) = 0 \tag{55}$$

with the following boundary conditions at $x = 0$, the nearest point of approach of the articular surfaces, and at $x = L$, sufficiently removed from $x = 0$ to achieve an undisturbed state:

At $x = 0$:

$$\frac{dC}{dx} = 0 = \frac{d^2u}{dx^2} \qquad u = 0 \tag{56a}$$

At $x = L$:

$$C(x) = C_0 \Rightarrow \frac{du}{dx} = 0 \tag{56b}$$

The solute distribution $N(x)$ in the channel must be estimated (cf [81]), whereupon Eq. (55) may be integrated numerically, in a marching procedure from

$x = 0$, with boundary conditions (56a) and a guess for $(du/dx)_{x=0}$, toward $x = L$, where condition (56b) must be satisfied approximately. An overshoot or undershoot at $x = L$ allows one to correct the initial estimate for $(du/dx)_{x=0}$, and the procedure is repeated to convergence. The concentration $C(x)$ is subsequently determined from Eq. (54). This trial-and-error method is necessitated by the nature of the "split" boundary conditions (56).

The solution may, however, also be achieved by converting Eqs. (55) and (56) to a system of first-order differential equations

$$\frac{du}{dx} = \frac{2}{h}\left[P(C - C_0) + v_n(x)\right] \qquad\qquad u(0) = 0$$

$$\frac{dC}{dx} = B \qquad\qquad\qquad\qquad\qquad C(L) = C_0 \qquad (57)$$

$$\frac{dB}{dx} = \left[uB + C\frac{du}{dx} - \frac{2N(x)}{h}\right]\frac{1}{D} \qquad B(0) = 0$$

and the numerical integration in the interval $0 \leqslant x \leqslant L$ again proceeds by successive guesses of $C(0)$.

Although the time dependence of v_n can be carried rigorously throughout, the convective changes in solute concentration have been assumed to dominate over time rates of change in Eq. (51). The foregoing analysis is therefore quasi-stationary.

The results of this section establish a relatively simple framework that may serve to guide the planning of careful experiments aimed at evaluating the parametric influence of cartilage permeability, synovial fluid properties, etc., on the buildup of lubricating gel on the articular joint surfaces. Nonetheless, as will be clear in the following section, experimental measurements in the intact joint are not simple, and one must limit oneself to much less information from experimental measurements than would be adequate for full verification of the theoretical analysis.

3.5 Other Analytical Studies of Synovial Joint Lubrication and Cartilage Deformation Response

In addition to the preceding analysis, a number of analytical models of joint lubrication and fluid flow in cartilage have been formulated in order to examine the various theories of joint lubrication or to explain the observed time-dependent response of joint cartilage to load.

Dinnar [82] has presented an analysis of the load-carrying capacity of the joint for sliding motion based on hydrodynamic lubrication theory. Flow in the fluid layer between joint surfaces is governed by the Reynolds equation for hydrodynamic bearings and that within the cartilage by Darcy's law and continuity. The cartilage is rigid and consists of two layers of different permeability. Using this model, he concludes the load-carrying capacity of the joint depends on fluid film viscosity, geometry, and thickness, and on cartilage thickness and permeability.

This model incorporates end effects due to finite length and considers the interaction between flow in the cartilage and flow in the joint space. However, since it neglects cartilage deformation and, as pointed out by Radin and Paul [83] and McCutchen [84], assumes a mode of lubrication that is probably seldom operative, its usefulness is somewhat limited.

Dowson et al. [85] investigated the effectiveness of boosted lubrication by carrying out an analysis of squeeze film lubrication for normal approach of various models of joint geometry. The "boosting" action in their model is obtained by requiring the fluid film viscosity to increase as opposing surfaces approach one another, rather than by allowing flow into the cartilage; the latter is considered impermeable.

Although the analysis predicts lengthening of squeeze film times under these conditions (because of increased viscosity), it does not really address the problem of imbibation of fluid by cartilage which is a required mechanism of boosted lubrication.

Another analysis of hydrodynamic squeeze film lubrication of articular surfaces has recently been carried out by Rybicki et al. [86] in which the joint is represented as a squeeze film bearing having low modulus linear elastic compliant surfaces separated by a Newtonian viscous fluid. The fluid pressure in the squeeze film is governed by Reynold's equation and the cartilage and underlying bone by a finite element mesh.

The compliant surface bearing is found to maintain a fluid film longer than does a rigid one, although the results are highly sensitive to synovial fluid viscosity.

In 1964 Zarek and Edwards [87] employed concepts based on the principles of soil consolidation to investigate energy dissipation in synovial joints. Using qualitative but elegant arguments and a parallel spring-dashpot model of the joint, they conclude that in the early stages of loading, the load is to a large extent supported by the excess fluid pressure rather than the solid matrix; that fluid is forced to the surface of the cartilage (weeping lubrication); and that energy is efficiently dissipated by flow of the liquid through the cartilage.

The one-dimensional theory of consolidation formulated in soil mechanics to study the settling of water-soaked soils under load was the basis of a more general theory of fluid-filled porous elastic, or poroelastic, solids formulated in a series of papers by Biot [88, 89, 90, 91, 92, 93]. Since the mechanisms governing friction, lubrication, load distribution and energy dissipation in synovial joints involve interactions among the synovial fluid, the articular cartilage, and the underlying bone, the theory of poroelastic media would appear to be well suited for use in the study of these phenomena.

Mow [94] and Mow and Ling [95] have modeled a bone articulation as a poroelastic layer (cartilage) on a semi-infinite elastic foundation (bone) subject to a moving load. Quasistationary solutions were obtained for displacements and stresses with shear-free surface and perfect interface continuity conditions. Upon examining the variation of these quantities with porosity of the layer and velocity of the moving load, he concluded that the major portion of friction loss must be either adhesive or viscous losses as opposed to deformation loss; that fluid flow within the cartilage is along the layer and away from the loading; and that the effect of load velocity on deformation is small.

To model the inhomogeneous and large deformation characteristics of joint cartilage, Ling [96] introduced a three-element model of the fluid-filled cartilage. This nonlinear model consists of a rigid substrate (bone); a porous pseudomatric layer that is fluid-filled and offers resistance to flow in its plane and mechanical resistance to the swelling of the layer but whose matrix material has no stiffness in compression and no resistance to reduction of thickness; and a porous pseudoskin with permeability distinct from that of the layer. This model was used to predict response of the cartilage surface to a rigid indenter and also to determine flow patterns when a fluid layer is compressed between two cartilaginous layers under squeeze film lubrication. Predicted displacement response to indenter loading showed good agreement with results of an experiment presented by McCutchen [97, 17]. The second analysis indicated that both boosted and weeping lubrication modes are operative during the initial phase of loading, with the fluid being circulated within the contact zone from the gap to the cartilage and then returning to the gap. After a certain period, however, the weeping lubrication mechanism appeared to dominate.

Higginson and Norman [98] present an analysis of squeeze film lubrication of a joint during normal approach of joint surfaces. This model employs a porous elastic layer on one joint surface whose resistance to compressive deformation depends solely on local fluid pressure. Anisotropic permeability and its dependence on matrix deformation is accounted for in the formulation of Darcy's law for flow through the cartilage. The interaction between the fluid lubricant film and the deformed articular surfaces is also considered.

Calculations are carried out for the case of zero layer permeability parallel to the cartilage surface; and the resulting predictions for film thickness and fluid pressure are compared with corresponding measured values obtained from a simple experimental model.

Although these calculations indicate a weeping lubrication mechanism may be present, the authors conclude that cartilage layer permeability has only a marginal effect on lubrication performance.

In an investigation of synovial joint lubrication by Wijesinghe and Kingsbury [99] joint cartilage in the underlying bone was modeled as a poroelastic layer supported on a poroelastic half-plane and subjected to a fluid pressure distribution at its surface. The response both to a spatially fixed but harmonically time-dependent surface pressure distribution and to a distribution moving uniformly along the surface but otherwise independent of time, is presented. A time-dependent dynamic solution was obtained for the former case, while a quasistatic solution was obtained for the latter.

In the case of a harmonically varying pressure distribution the interstitial fluid was shown to cause viscous damping caused by the phase difference between surface displacement and surface load. The cartilage layer was found to imbibe fluid at times of low surface pressure and to exude fluid at high surface pressure selectively over its surface in a manner dependent on frequency. Thus if it is assumed that lubrication of the surface is necessary at times of high surface pressure, then the flow across the surface was consistent with boosted lubrication at one frequency and with weeping lubrication at another. In the case of the moving pressure distribution the effect of the velocity of the load on the displacements, pore pressure, and total stress is small. The flow was directed into the cartilage in a central region under the load, which is consistent with boosted lubrication, but beyond the central region the flow was out of the layer. Thus, expression and resorption of fluid at the surface of the layer was found to be consistent in different regions under the loading zone with both weeping and boosted lubrication.

The system of equations governing the interaction of fluid flow and deformation of porous solid phase has been rederived by Torzilli and Mow [100] based on thermodynamic mixture theory. The equations of motion for each phase and for the total mixture were derived from the extended Hamilton's principle. The general equations yield for special cases Biot's consolidation equations and Darcy's law for flow through a permeable rigid solid. These equations are employed in a second paper [101] to study the flow of synovial fluid in cartilage subject to a spatially fixed but harmonically time-varying surface traction. This solution, like that of Wijesinghe and Kingsbury, showed the fluid transport mechanism to be strongly dependent upon frequency through a parameter representing the ratio of force required to deform the tissue as a whole to the frictional resistance due to the rate of fluid flow relative to the solid matrix. Upon using values of cartilage stiffness and porosity corresponding to levels measured for normal and pathological cartilage, investigators found consolidation effects dominate the system response for normal cartilage, whereas for more porous degenerative cartilage, direct pressure effects governed by Darcy's law of filtering become relatively more important.

Arthrosis of the articular joints may ensue following important modifications of the mechanical and biochemical properties of the cartilage and synovial fluid. It is now clear that the dynamic interaction between these two components is responsible for the momentary formation of a protective gel of mucin of molecular dimensions on the cartilaginous surfaces within the zone of current contact [102, 103]. This tenuous layer of reversible gel is formed by a net exclusion of the aqueous component of synovial fluid and a concomitant concentration of mucopolysaccharides within by "trapping" as the intraarticular channel height decreases during loading, to dimensions comparable to those of the long-chain solute molecules of synovial fluid. Preliminary analysis by Collins [104, 105] of the evolution of the channel concentration of mucin indicates a critical dependence on the permeability and elasticity of the cartilaginous matrix, modeled as a porous deformable medium, and the diffusion coefficient for mucin in synovial fluid. A pathological perturbation of this delicate state of equilibrium may indeed inhibit the spontaneous formation of gel. Under such conditions, the collagen fibers will rupture as the outer layers of the articular surfaces are subjected to excessively high shear stresses. This state, known as *fibrillation*, is often considered the first indication of the onset of *arthrosis*. As additional collagen fibers break, water-containing proteoglycans escape progressively from the cartilage matrix. Articular loads are then brought to bear directly on the deforming matrix tissue more deeply within the cartilage. An inevitable aggravation of this state of affairs may lead to a new initiation of fibrillation at the junction with the subchondral bone. Under attack from both sides, the cartilage matrix can do little to resist the accelerating cycle of deterioration. In time the subchondral bone itself will be damaged as progressive *osteoarthrosis* sets in.

It is for this reason that physiological conditions conducive to the maintenance of a reversible mucin gel must be preserved. These have been analyzed by Collins [106] by means of a fluid mechanical model to determine the buildup of mucin molecules in the intraarticular gap as a result of three physical processes: convection, diffusion, and ultrafiltration. The latter is found to play an important role in returning the local mucin concentrations to their ambient level toward the extremities of the loading zone. As the zone of contact translates along the articular surfaces during body motion, the local gel layer is rapidly reabsorbed into the dilute synovial bath to which it is suddenly exposed, while a new gel is laid down in the subsequent contact region.

The moving load problem was examined by Mansour and Mow [107] using Biot's poroelasticity equations for a three-layer model of articular cartilage and its underlying subchondral bone. The calculated flow field shows that for normal cartilage properties a naturally lubricated surface is created. The movement of the interstitial fluid at the surface is circulatory: it is exuded in front and near the leading half of the moving surface load and is imbibed behind and near the trailing half of the moving load. Flow fields for pathological tissue are found to be incapable of sustaining a fluid film at the articular surface.

Mow and Mansour [108] employ the two-phase mixture theory derived by Torzilli and Mow [100, 101] to study the creep response of a cartilage layer to a suddenly applied spatially uniform normal surface traction. In this one-dimensional model of the indenter response problem, the permeability is assumed to depend on the matrix dilatation [14]. Time dependent response of the fluid-matrix system is determined both by viscous flow through the matrix and by viscoelastic matrix deformation.

The model is found to display classical creep response with short-time surface displacement depending substantially on the (unknown) matrix viscoelastic parameter; whereas the long-time equilibrium configuration depends only on the elastic properties of the matrix. The nonlinear, dilatation-dependent aspect of matrix permeability is found to exert a relatively small effect on creep response.

Measurements carried out to verify the analytical model have been described by Kuei et al. [109].

Mow and Mansour [108] used their model to study cartilage stress relaxation. Further, Mow et al. [110] show that the relaxation time is independent of the rate of compression, and that the rate of relaxation depends only on the magnitude of compressive strain.

Prompted perhaps by comments by McCutchen [111] concerning the results obtained by Torzilli and Mow [100, 101], Kuei [112] again formulated constitutive equations for fluid-filled cartilage using the mixture theory of Bowen [113]. This derivation of a biphasic rheological model of articular cartilage is summarized in a recent review article by Mow and Lai [114].

Kuei's equations have been used in a specialized form considering the matrix elastic and the fluid incompressible (Kuei et al. [115]) to study the effect of fluid motion on cartilage creep response. The authors conclude that fluid exudation and fluid redistribution inside the cartilage tissue is the main mechanism contributing to the apparent viscoelastic behavior of articular cartilage.

The same mathematical model is used by Lai and Mow [116] to study sliding articulation. The results of this investigation are qualitatively similar to those of Mansour and Mow [107] in that fluid exudation occurs in advance of the load traveling over the surface while fluid is imbibed by the cartilage after the passage of the load. Some experimental confirmation of these results has been obtained by Mow and Lai [117] using sliding indenter apparatus.

It has now become apparent that mechanical behavior of cartilage such as swelling and creep response is affected by ionic concentration. This effect is described by Lipshitz et al. [118], Maroudas [119] and is further studied and explained by Parsons and Black [120].

Swenson et al. [12] have recently discussed a new mechanical-electrochemical model in which fluid-filled articular cartilage is considered to be a multiphasic mixture of an ion-exchangeable matrix with diffusing interstitial fluids consisting of water and cations and anions of an electrolyte. This model, which is based on the mixture theory of Bowen [113], recognizes cartilage as an ion exchange material in which solute and fluid transport depend on the concentration and distribution of glycosaminoglycans' (GAG) fixed charge density.

Results are presented for the case of a spatially fixed, harmonically varying surface pressure applied to a cartilage layer. The model is shown to predict the effects of time-dependent cartilage swelling on surface displacement and water pressure within the cartilage.

In summary, it may be concluded that analytical models for the fluid-filled cartilage have been quite successful in illuminating the mechanisms of time-dependent, or "viscoelastic," response of cartilage under indenter load. The path of these investigations indeed proceeds almost directly from the early conceptual model proposed by Zarek and Edwards [87] to recent studies by Kuei et al. [109, 115].

It appears that by means of porous, deformable material models of cartilage, the debate over whether the interstitial fluid is forced into or forced out of the cartilage is well on its way to being resolved. These models also seem capable of being used to distinguish the differences in joint lubrication mechanisms between normal and pathological cartilage and synovial fluid. Still to be answered however, is the question of how these mechanisms are related to the apparently dominant boundary lubrication mode and under what conditions of loading and motion the other lubrication modes become operative.

4 LABORATORY EXPERIMENTS

Articulation experiments have been performed by Linn [64], Radin et al. [122], and others as described above. Similar experiments have been carried out by the present authors, R. Collins and H. B. Kingsbury, using a specially constructed

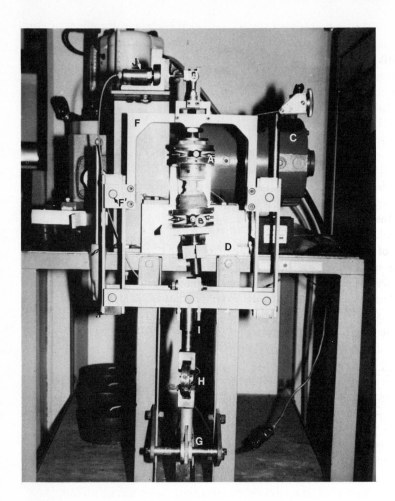

Figure 24 Articulation machine with dog ankle mounted for test.

machine (Fig. 24) of the general configuration employed initially by Linn [3].
Friction was measured under conditions of pure sliding without rotation of the joint
surfaces in an intact joint under a range of levels of physiological loading. Such
measurements have not been made previously and could form the basis of further
studies. For pure controlled sliding motions under a compressive load, the surface film
will be worn without the possibility of a simultaneous formation process. For pure
oscillatory motions normal to the articular surfaces, the surface film will grow without
the possibility of a simultaneous wearing process. The coefficient of friction was
monitored by a force transducer during the loading cycle. The use of an intact joint is
essential in ensuring that the chemical environment, upon which depends the process
of bonding of the mucopolysaccharides to the articular surfaces and hence the value of
the coefficient of friction, is not altered.

Using the known loading cycles, one may determine from the analysis of the previous section the complete pressure and fluid velocity distributions [Eqs. (47) to (49)] in the cartilage. From the latter may be calculated the volume flow rate [Eq. (50)] of fluid across the outer surface of the cartilage. This volume flow rate of synovial fluid, a mixture of mucopolysaccharides in a watery solution, should then be proportional to the flow rate of long-chain molecules normal to the surface [Eq. (53)], and hence to the rate of formation of surface gel. The rate of accumulation of this hyaluronic acid component of synovial fluid on the articular surfaces depends parametrically upon the cartilage porosity and fluid viscosity, as indicated by Eqs. (5a), (50), and (55).

In a normally functioning joint, the rates of wear and formation of surface gel must be of comparable magnitude in order to maintain a lubricant layer. If the porosity of the cartilage were to decrease or the fluid viscosity to increase, the rate of supply of mucopolysaccharides to the articular surfaces would diminish below the rate of wear. On the other hand, abnormal surface irregularities may increase the rate of wear above that of an otherwise normal rate of formation of boundary lubricant. The sensitivity of these rates to change in the parameters characterizing the cartilage and synovial fluid may be assessed from the analysis of the previous section by solving the system (55), (56), or (57) for sets of specified values of C_0, K, μ, D, $N(x)$.

4.1 Experimental Apparatus

The friction-measuring device constructed for these tests was of the arthro-tripsometer type [3]. The design permits complete freedom of control of such variables as load, speed, and angle of articulation, while providing a continuous record of the frictional force.

The experiments reported here involve the measurement of joint friction as a function of axial load and oscillation frequency in Ringer's solution and synovial fluid. These parameters have been investigated previously [64, 122]. Since large differences in measured values of the coefficient of friction have been reported in the literature, the previous tests were repeated to establish the base values for the coefficient of friction for this machine and to allow comparisons with earlier published results.

The joint articulation machine is illustrated in Figs. 24 to 27. The tibia is held in the upper universal mount A, the talus in the lower universal mount B. The motor and gear reductor C drive an off-center crank mechanism (Fig. 27) connected to the lower mount through the bearing support block D. The motor provides continuously variable oscillation speeds up to 300/min. The crank mechanism allows oscillation amplitudes to $100°$ (i.e., $±50°$) centered over any portion of the surface of the talus. A transducer (E in Fig 27), connected to the support shaft by a cable, records the instantaneous angular velocity and displacement. The loading frame F, containing five knife-edge bearings F', is attached to the upper mount. Load is applied to the frame by weights hung on the lever arm G attached to the loading frame through the load-ring transducer H and a thrust bearing I. The axial load is

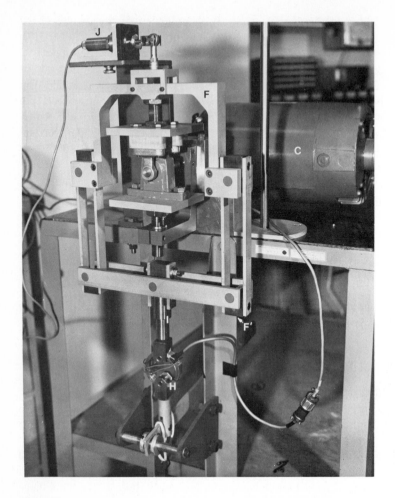

Figure 25 Articulation machine with journal bearing mounted for test.

monitored with strain gauges attached to the load ring. The thrust bearing I allows the entire load frame to rotate about the vertical axis in response to the spinning component of ankle joint motion. The friction transducer J records the force generated on the tibia assembly by the friction at the cartilage interface. The load, friction, speed, and displacement signals are recorded simultaneously on a multichannel oscillograph (Fig. 26). During operation, the joint is enclosed by a flexible rubber bag. The rubber bag is supported by a copper ring through which hot water from a water heater is circulated. This allows the lubricant bath temperature to be controlled without circulating the lubricant.

When the talus is oscillated about its center by the crank mechanism, frictional stress at the interface tends to rotate the tibia. The alignment of the loading frame must ensure that the only resistance applied to the tibia comes from the friction transducer itself (cf. Sec. 4.2). Thus, the force generated at the friction transducer is proportional to the coefficient of friction of the joint.[1]

4.2 Procedure

Preparation of joints The joints and fluids tested are listed in Table 2. Unless used immediately, the joint was stored frozen and intact. Prior to experimentation, the joint was thawed and completely dissected so that no membrane or connective tissue remained (Fig. 28). The talus and calcaneus were rigidly connected by

---

[1] The relationship between this force and the coefficient of friction is discussed in App. A. Calibration of the transducers is described in App. B.

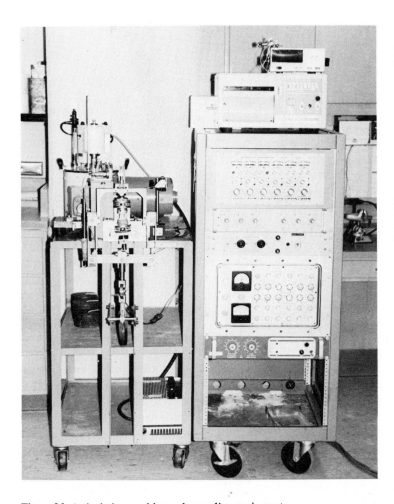

Figure 26 Articulation machine and recording equipment.

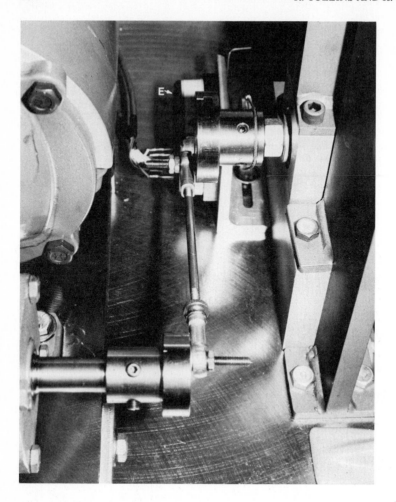

Figure 27 Off-center crank mechanism.

insertion of a screw through the subtalar joint (Fig. 29). To minimize dehydration during the preparation process, the exposed cartilage was covered with gauze soaked in Ringer's solution.

The axis of rotation of the joint was located by means of a metal collar attached to the shaft of the tibia (Fig. 30). Two metal wires extending from this collar were bent so that their ends almost touched the medial and lateral faces of the talus. When the tibia was articulated, the tips of these wires described small arcs on the faces of the talus. The center of each arc was marked, providing two points on the axis of rotation. A clamp with two pointed metal rods was attached to the talus with the points on the marked centers. This positioned the rods along the axis of rotation of the joint (Fig. 31). The centered rods provided a visual reference for prealigning the talus in the mold, ensuring that the initial misalignment did not

Table 2 Specimens

Specimen	Description
	Joints
D-1	Dog ankle joint, stored frozen for 1 mo prior to use
D-2	Dog ankle joint, stored frozen for 1.5 mo prior to use
D-3	Dog ankle joint, stored frozen for 2 weeks prior to use
D-4	Dog ankle joint, stored frozen for 5 weeks prior to use
	Fluids
S-1	Human synovial fluid (rheumatoid arthritic), stored frozen for 4 mo prior to use
S-2	Human synovial fluid (traumatic effusions), fresh
S-3	Human synovial fluid (traumatic effusions), fresh
S-4	Bovine synovial fluid (normal), pooled from several joints, fresh
S-5	Bovine synovial fluid (normal), pooled from several joints, fresh

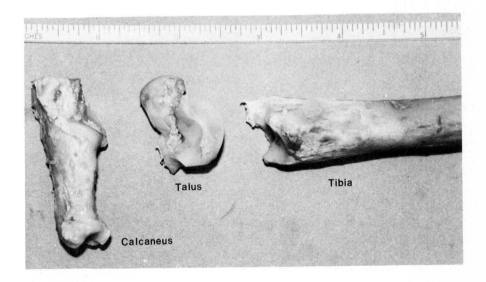

Figure 28 Dissected joint.

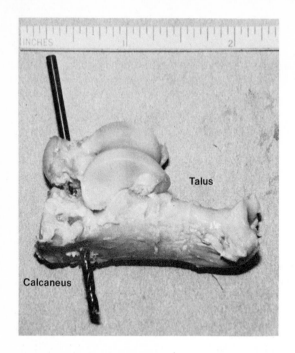

Figure 29   Drill indicating hole through subtalar joint.

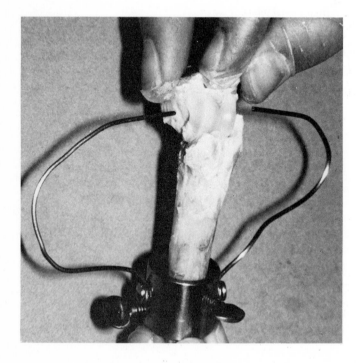

Figure 30 Collar with wires to locate joint axis.

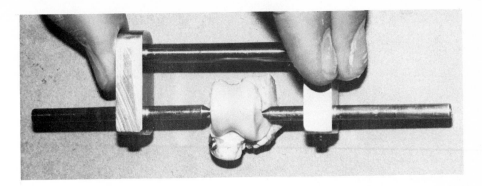

Figure 31 Talus centering rod.

exceed the range of adjustment on the universal mounts (Fig. 32). The excess shaft of the tibia was then cut off, and the two halves of the joint were cast in a magnesium silicate-based polyester resin.[2] This compound cured at temperatures less than 40°C, causing minimal degradation of the tissues. After being removed from the rubber molds (Fig. 33), the potted joints were inserted into the universal mounts of the machine and locked in place with setscrews. Between experiments the joints could be removed from the machine and stored in a refrigerator without necessitating realignment.

Alignment of the machine and joint axis The degree of misalignment of the joint axis could be determined by monitoring the resulting motion of the loading frame

[2] Woodhill Chemical Sales Corp., Cleveland, Ohio.

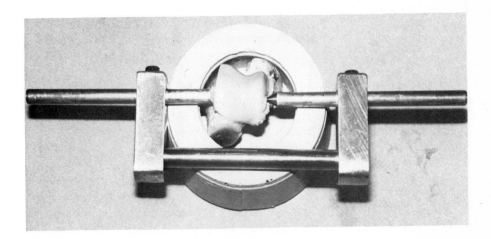

Figure 32 Talus in mold with centering rod attached.

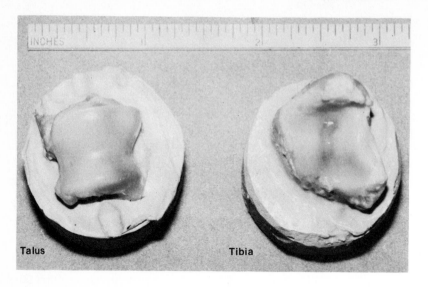

Figure 33 Joint potted in resin.

when the joint was oscillated, and adjusting the lower mount accordingly. When the joint axis and the machine axis coincided, the loading frame remained stationary during articulation. Relative to the coordinates of Fig. 34, the alignment was accomplished according to the following scheme:

Motion of loading frame during joint articulation	Required adjustment on lower mount
Rise and fall along y axis	Move in $\pm x$ direction
Horizontal translation	Move in $\pm y$ direction
Rocking about x axis	Rotate in $\pm\psi$ direction
Rotation about y axis	Rotate in $\pm\phi$ direction

Neither the alignment errors nor the resultant motions were totally independent of each other. However, consecutive adjustments soon minimized the error. The final adjustment was accomplished using a dial indicator to detect the motion of the loading frame (Fig. 24). When the alignment was complete, the loading frame moved less than 0.001 in in any direction.

Two degrees of adjustment were necessary to align the loading frame. The frame was adjusted in the x and y directions such that a line through the center of the upper knife-edge bearings passed through the axis of the joint and was bisected by it (Fig. 35). This adjustment was necessary to ensure that the line of action of the axial load remained stationary when the loading frame rotated; (a slight rotation was necessary to activate the friction transducer). Fine adjustment of the loading frame was accomplished by connecting the friction transducer, applying a high axial

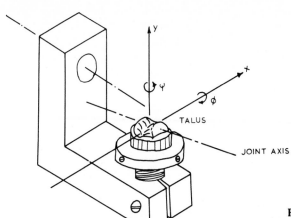

MACHINE AXIS

TALUS

JOINT AXIS

Figure 34 Alignment of axes of articulation machine and joint.

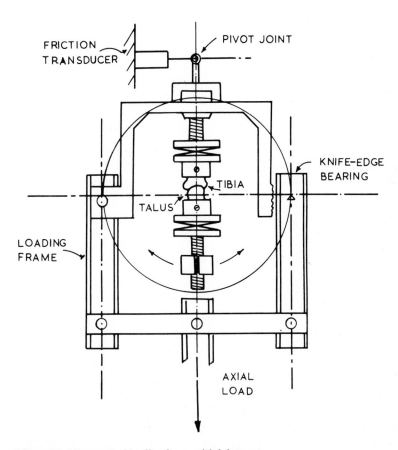

FRICTION
TRANSDUCER

PIVOT JOINT

KNIFE-EDGE
BEARING

TIBIA

TALUS

LOADING
FRAME

AXIAL
LOAD

Figure 35 Alignment of loading frame with joint center.

load, and moving the loading frame in the $\pm x$ direction until no deflection was indicated by the friction-force recorder. This completed the alignment procedure.

5 RESULTS AND DISCUSSION

The magnitude and variation of the measured coefficients of friction are shown in Figs. 36 to 39, and a comparison with results obtained by other researchers in Table 3. The designation of joint and fluid specimens follows the description in Table 2.

Synovial fluid lubricated better than Ringer's solution throughout the load range tested (13 to 60 lb); however, this advantage diminished after synovial fluid was stored for a few days (Figs. 36 and 37) and later tests exhibited increased levels of friction. A sample of specimen S-1 (see Table 2), examined under a microscope after a week of testing, showed evidence of extensive bacteriological activity, accounting for the deterioration of the lubricating properties of the synovial fluid-cartilage interface.

When synovial fluid was substituted for Ringer's solution in the lubricant bath, the coefficient of friction dropped gradually over a period of 2 to 3 min. This effect was reversible; after the articular surfaces were wiped several times with gauze soaked in Ringer's solution, the previous higher coefficient of friction was regained.

The coefficient of friction ($0.005 > \eta < 0.019$) decreased with increasing load, both for Ringer's solution and synovial fluid (Figs. 36 and 37). When the load on the joint was suddenly applied (or increased), the coefficient of friction rose slowly over 2 min (Fig. 38) from 0.009 to 0.013. For this reason, the joint was oscillated for 3 min at each load before the friction was recorded.

The frictional force (and, therefore, the coefficient of friction) was found to decrease to $\eta = 0.007$ with increasing oscillation frequency up to 132 cycles/min (Fig. 39). Unfortunately, resonant vibrations in the experimental apparatus

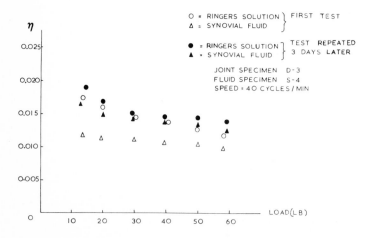

Figure 36 Coefficient of friction versus load (constant speed).

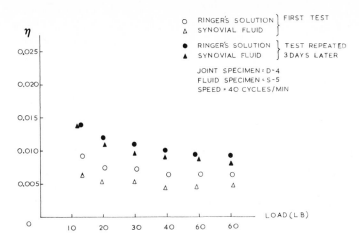

Figure 37 Coefficient of friction versus load (constant speed).

prevented testing above this level. The variation of the coefficient of friction suggests that it might begin to increase at higher frequencies. Improvements in the design of the articulation machine will allow future tests to include this higher range of frequencies.

5.1 Magnitude of the Coefficient of Friction

The coefficients of friction measured in these tests tended to be somewhat higher than the values reported by previous experimenters using arthrotripsometer devices [64, 122]. Table 3 gives a comparison of the coefficients of friction reported here

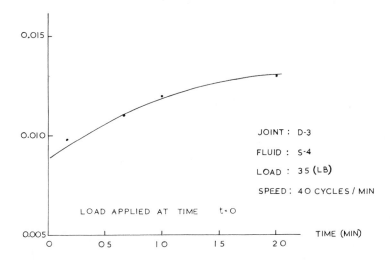

Figure 38 Coefficient of friction versus time (constant speed and load).

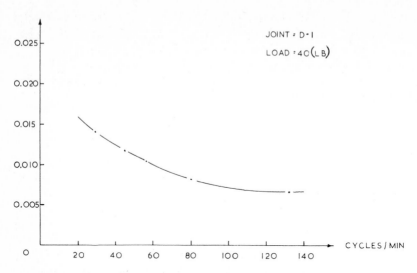

Figure 39 Coefficient of friction versus speed (constant load).

with those of other investigations. The coefficient of friction has been generally found to lie within the range 0.001 to 0.020, indicating that the joints are lubricated by a combination of mechanisms. The following sample calculations illustrate this.

Dowson [50] has shown that elastohydrodynamic theory predicts a fluid film thickness of over 2 μm. However, if a film of this thickness were produced between the cartilage surfaces, and if no solid friction occurred, the resultant coefficient of friction would be well below the observed range. For example, the expression for the shear stress τ transmitted by a fluid film of thickness h and viscosity μ is

$$\tau = \mu \frac{U}{h} \tag{58}$$

where U is the relative velocity of the two opposing surfaces. The total transmitted friction force F is then

$$F = \tau A = A\mu \frac{U}{h} \tag{59}$$

where A is the contact area. In the current experiment using dogs' ankles, with a relative velocity of approximately 10 cm/s, a contact area of about 1 cm^2, and a fluid viscosity of $\mu = 0.01$ p, Dowson's estimate of the film thickness $h = 2$ μm ($= 2 \times 10^{-4}$ cm) leads to a frictional force $F = 500$ dyn $= 1.1 \times 10^{-3}$ lb. For an axial load L of 40 lb, the coefficient of friction η is given by

$$\eta = \frac{F}{L} \tag{60}$$

or
$$\eta = \frac{1.1 \times 10^{-3} \text{ lb}}{40 \text{ lb}} = 0.000028$$

Thus, a dog's ankle lubricated by a 2-μm film would have a coefficient of friction less than one-hundredth of the observed value. A higher coefficient of friction would result if the fluid film were much thinner, or if some solid friction occurred. It is suggested here that both cases apply.

Let us critically examine Dowson's estimate of the film thickness. Recalling the equation for the elastohydrodynamic film thickness [Eq. (5a)],

$$h_m = 1.35 \left(\frac{2\mu}{E} U_R \bar{R} \right)^{1/2} \tag{61}$$

we see that the film thickness varies inversely as the square root of the elastic modulus of the bearing liner. Dowson based his calculation on the elastic modulus of the cartilage matrix as measured by McCutchen [2], that is, $E = 1 \times 10^7$ dyn/cm^2. Elastohydrodynamic theory predicts that the fluid film thickness is enhanced as a result of the deformation of the bearing material, which in turn results from the fluid hydrostatic pressure. However, the saturated cartilage layers are not likely to deform significantly under fluid pressure, as the hydrostatic pressure will be transmitted through the cartilage and applied directly to the substrate of impermeable bone. It is rather this subcondral bone that will deform and whose elastic modulus should be used in calculating the augmented film thickness, and not the modulus of the cartilage. Radin et al. [122] report the modulus for subchondral bone to be about 10^{10} dyn/cm^2, or about 100 times that of cartilage. From Eq. (61) it is seen that increasing E by a factor of 100 reduces the film thickness h_m by a factor of 10, giving $h_m = 0.2$ μm. In Sec. 1.1 it is noted that this modified estimate of the film thickness corresponds to the smallest reported height for the cartilage surface asperities [4]. From this comparison, significant solid contact is predicted. That is, elastohydrodynamic theory predicts a substantial fluid film, but not enough to eliminate cartilage-cartilage contact, a situation that would produce a coefficient of friction in the observed range.

Linn [64] found that synovial fluid that had been mildly digested in hyaluronidase lubricated dogs' ankles as well as did normal synovial fluid. Since the digested synovial fluid had a much lower viscosity, and the elastohydrodynamic film thickness depends on the fluid viscosity [Eq. (61)], Linn concluded that elasto-hydrodynamic action was not essential to joint lubrication. However, Ogston and Stanier [123] have shown that synovial fluid is thixotropic (i.e., shear thinning)

Table 3 Measured values of the coefficient of friction η

Study	Experimental system	Value of η reported
Jones [47]	Horse knee in articulation device	0.02
Charnley [1]	Human ankle in pendulum	0.01–0.02
Linn [64]	Dog ankle in arthrotripsometer	0.004–0.010
Barnett [75]	Human finger in pendulum (in vivo)	0.0057–0.0106
Radin et al. [90]	Bovine metatarsal phalangeal joint in arthrotripsometer	0.0014–0.0039
Present	Dog ankle in arthrotripsometer	0.005–0.020

such that, at physiological shear rates, it is only slightly more viscous than water (Figs. 7 and 8). Thus, one would not expect prethinning of the fluid by hyaluronidase digestion to necessarily affect the film thickness at the high shear rates. In view of this, Linn's conclusion does not appear to be justified.

But the magnitude of the coefficient of friction indicates that the load is not supported entirely by the boundary lubricated solid contacts, as was suggested by Charnley [1] and others. McCutchen [68] and Walker et al. [5] demonstrated that cartilage specimens pressed against a glass plate for a long period of time exhibited high coefficients of friction in the range 0.1 to 0.4. Since this corresponds to the range generally measured for engineering bearings lubricated solely by boundary mechanisms, it was concluded by those authors that the cartilage specimens were operating in a pure boundary lubrication mode, the fluid film mechanism having been defeated by side leakage (Fig. 16) during the long loading period. The coefficients measured here are much less than those for the glass plate experiments, indicating that fluid film lubrication was also present here.

5.2 Variation of the Coefficient of Friction with Speed at Constant Load

If the mixed lubrication model (boundary and fluid lubrication) is an accurate representation of the cartilage lubrication process, then the variation of the net coefficient of friction should depend on the speed range tested due to the fluid film contribution. At low speeds the friction arises primarily from the boundary-lubricated asperities that come into contact and is not strongly dependent on the cartilage sliding speed. As the speed increases, the thickness of the elastohydro-dynamic fluid film increases, progressively unloading the asperities and decreasing the coefficient of friction. At the highest speeds it is possible that most of the friction arises from fluid shearing. At this point the coefficient of friction would eventually increase with further increases in velocity.

As illustrated by Fig. 39, the coefficient of friction was observed to decrease with increasing speed. This same effect was reported by Linn [64]. However, most experimenters using pendulum-type devices reported no variation in the coefficient of friction with speed. The apparent contradiction in the results may result from overlapping of the friction mechanisms as described above. Faber et al. [76] pointed out that the free-swinging pendulum devices, driven only by gravitational forces, produced cartilage sliding speeds in the very low end of the physiological range, from zero to less than 1 in/s. In this range, boundary lubrication, whose frictional coefficient is speed independent, should predominate. In contrast to this, in the tests reported here, the sliding speeds ranged from 0.5 in/s to nearly 2.5 in/s. This is roughly the same range tested by Linn, who also reported a decrease in the coefficient of friction with increasing speed. Faber employed a spring-driven pendulum device to produce cartilage sliding speeds up to 2.5 in/s in rabbit knees. He reported that at the highest speeds tested over 80 percent of the total frictional force arose from fluid shearing, and this proportion increased with increasing speed. Thus, when considered on the basis of the speed range tested, the various experimental results all follow the pattern predicted by the mixed lubrication model.

There is a further complication to the interpretation of the dependence of friction on sliding speed. As Linn [64] pointed out, the arthrotripsometer measures the total resistance to joint articulation, including a resistance due to the process Linn called cartilage "plowing." When a loaded joint is articulated, mechanical work must be done to compress the cartilage as the load moves across the surface (rolling friction). At the same time the previously loaded cartilage expands and must be recompressed when the joint motion reverses direction. It is not obvious whether this plowing component of joint friction decreases or increases with speed. Linn maintained that the plowing effect diminishes at higher oscillation frequencies because the cartilage has less time to expand as the unloaded phase becomes progressively shorter. However, McCutchen [9] and others have shown that, because of its high water content, cartilage is much stiffer at high compression rates. Thus the resistance of the joint cartilage to recompression will increase with oscillation frequency. In view of these effects, a more quantitative evaluation of the variation of the coefficient of friction with speed will depend on a determination of the precise relationship between such factors as the expected film thickness, the height of cartilage surface asperities, and the compression and expansion rates of the cartilage.

5.3 Variation of the Coefficient of Friction with Load at Constant Speed

The friction force was observed to increase with increasing load, but not in direct proportion to the load, so that the coefficient of friction exhibited a net decrease (Figs. 36 and 37). A similar effect was observed by McCutchen [68] and Linn [64]. Radin et al. [122] reported that the coefficient of friction decreased with increasing load in joints lubricated with saline solution, but *increased* in joints lubricated with synovial fluid.

From Eq. (7) for the coefficient of friction in boundary lubrication,

$$\eta = \frac{\bar{s}}{\bar{p}}$$

it is seen that the coefficient of friction depends on the mean shear strength of the lubricant layer and the mean yield strength of the contacting asperities (substrate), and therefore is not a direct function of the load. With elastohydrodynamic lubrication, the frictional *force* (rather than the coefficient of friction) is nearly constant. From the expression for the frictional stress transmitted by a fluid film [Eq. (59)],

$$F = A\mu \frac{U}{h}$$

it is seen that the frictional force does not depend directly on the load. As was shown in Sec. 5.1, the film thickness h in an elastohydrodynamic bearing is nearly independent of the load. Although the contact area A and viscosity μ can increase slightly with load, these effects are generally assumed to be negligible [50]. Thus in a pure elastohydrodynamic bearing the friction is nearly constant, so the coefficient of friction varies inversely with the load. The predicted variations in the coefficient of friction for boundary and fluid film mechanisms are illustrated in Fig. 40, along with the experimentally observed variation. It is seen that the observed variation lies between the two extremes, a behavior that again suggests a combination of the two fundamental mechanisms.

McCutchen [2] suggests that the decrease in the coefficient of friction is due to the weeping process. He claims that when the load is increased, fluid flows out of the cartilage matrix and into the gap between the surfaces. This forces contacting asperities apart and reduces the friction. In contrast, Walker et al. [5] maintain that the opposite process occurs. That is, with increased load the watery portion of the synovial fluid is forced *into* the porous cartilage. The concentration of the synovial mucin is increased in the fluid remaining in the gap, forming a viscous gel between the cartilaginous surfaces, which "boosts" the lubrication process and reduces the friction. The two processes are illustrated schematically in Fig. 41. Neither of these theories seems adequate to explain the observed behavior of the coefficient of friction. The weeping hypothesis requires that the fluid flow into the highly loaded regions. However, the pressure gradient would surely induce flow in the opposite direction. The boosted lubrication theory requires the presence of synovial mucin. But it fails to explain why the coefficient of friction also decreases when no mucin is present, as occurred in the tests with Ringer's solution (Figs. 36 and 37). The slow increase in friction following a sudden increase in load (Fig. 38) at constant speed suggests that the increased load shifts the equilibrium in the direction of the squeeze film process, causing a gradual decrease in the film thickness accompanied by an increase in friction from the contacting asperities.

For mixed lubrication, it is proposed that maintenance of the fluid film depends on an interplay between the elastohydrodynamic and squeeze film processes. That is, the fluid film is replenished by elastohydrodynamic action when the joint is in motion, while it leaks away through squeeze film action when the joint is at rest. It is the squeeze film process that maintains the film during the zero velocity points of each cycle (i.e., when the motion reverses direction).

5.4 Lubricating Advantage of Synovial Fluid

As is shown by Figs. 36 and 37, synovial fluid lubricates better than Ringer's solution. The percentage reduction in the coefficient of friction when synovial fluid

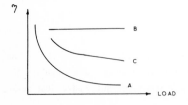

Figure 40 Variation of coefficient of friction with load. A, Variation of η in a pure elastohydrodynamic bearing; η varies inversely with load. B, Variation of η in a pure boundary lubricated bearing; η constant. C, Observed variation of η for dog ankle.

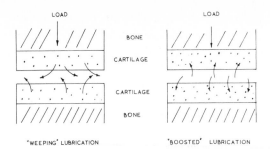

Figure 41 Comparison of weeping and boosted lubrication theories.

is used instead of Ringer's solution is commonly referred to as synovial fluid's lubricating advantage. McCutchen [11], Linn [64], Radin et al. [124], and others have reported a lubricating advantage of 50 percent. The largest lubricating advantage measured in the present experiment was about 30 percent (Fig. 37). This test was performed with the ankle joint D-4 and fluid specimen S-5 (see Table 2), which had been stored for the shortest time. Radin et al. [124] have shown that the magnitude of the lubricating advantage depends strongly on the condition of the protein component of the synovial mucin. It is suspected that the reduced lubricating advantage measured in these tests resulted from the degradation of the protein component by bacteriological activity. To obtain more reliable results in future tests, it will be necessary to use fresh specimens in an environment that is as sterile as possible.

McCutchen [2] and others have suggested that the lubricating advantage of synovial fluid results from a boundary lubricating component of the synovial mucin. This idea seems to explain best the observed phenomenon, and it provides a strong argument for the mixed lubrication theory. If joint lubrication resulted totally from the boundary lubricating mechanism, the low coefficient of friction in Ringer's solution would then be unexplained. On the other hand, if joints are lubricated completely by a fluid film mechanism, then the lubricating advantage of synovial fluid is unexplained.

However, the effect is reconcilable on the basis of the mixed lubrication model. Since the load is principally supported by the fluid film hydrostatic pressure, the friction is low even when the joint is lubricated with Ringer's solution. The addition of the boundary lubricating factor serves to reduce the total friction further by lubricating those asperities that do come into direct contact. This accounts for the lubricating advantage of synovial fluid. The observations of Radin et al. [124] suggest that it is a protein component of synovial mucin that acts as the boundary lubricating factor.

6 GENERAL REMARKS AND CONCLUSIONS

The joint articulation machine provides a useful method for studying joint lubrication phenomena at loads and speeds representative of physiological conditions. The rapid increase in the coefficient of friction over successive test days, which was probably a result of bacteriological degradation of the specimens, illustrates the need to design laboratory procedures with a view to testing fresh specimens under more sterile conditions.

The magnitude of the coefficient of friction for fresh joints was found to lie in the range 0.005 to 0.020. The magnitude decreased with increasing load and speed. The measured coefficients of friction were 10 to 30 percent higher when the joints were lubricated with Ringer's solution instead of synovial fluid, the differences becoming smaller on successive test days owing to bacterial degradation of the protein component of the stored synovial fluid. The coefficient of friction increased slowly with time to a level of 0.013 during application of a constant load.

A mixed lubrication model combining fluid-film and boundary lubrication best resolves the apparently conflicting interpretations of earlier experiments and provides consistent agreement with the present results. Elastohydrodynamic lubrication alone gives a coefficient of friction of 0.000025, which is only 1 percent of the measured values, indicating that solid-contact boundary lubrication must also be present. The calculated film thickness of 0.2 μm (based on Dowson's elasto-hydrodynamic model with Radin's estimate of the modulus of elasticity of the subchondral bone of 10^{10}) corresponds to the order of magnitude of the surface asperities, also confirming the probability of solid contacts during articulation. But the loaded joint is not supported only by boundary-lubricated solid contacts as in McCutchen's experiments with cartilage between glass plates which yielded co-efficients of friction between 0.1 and 0.4, far above the range of 0.005 to 0.020 measured here. Hence the physiological mechanism of lubrication lies between that for pure elastohydrodynamic and pure boundary lubrication, and instead combines the two. This conclusion is further corroborated by the test results reported here.

It has been shown, on the one hand, that the coefficient of friction decreases with increasing speed of articulation. The higher friction at low speeds obtains from solid contact of the asperities, which are boundary lubricated; the lower coefficient of friction at higher speeds reflects the establishment of an elastohydrodynamic fluid film that takes up part of the load from the asperities. The additional effect of rolling friction and its dependence upon speed have not been studied here.

On the other hand, the present experiments show that the coefficient of friction decreases with increasing load. But for boundary lubrication the coefficient of friction is theoretically independent of load, whereas for elastohydrodynamic lubrication the coefficient of friction varies inversely with load. The present results are shown to lie between these two extremes of variation.

The weeping lubrication mechanism has been demonstrated to yield fluid flow *into* the contact zone of the joint space, violating basic physical principles of flow from high to low pressure. The boosted lubrication model implies trapping of mucin on the cartilaginous surface during flow *into* the cartilage, which would not in itself explain the observed decrease in coefficient of friction with increasing load, even with Ringer's solution replacing synovial fluid. One must therefore discard these two models in favor of a mixed lubrication model combining elastohydrodynamic replenishment of the lubricating fluid film at higher velocities of articulation with boundary lubrication of solid-solid asperities at the lower velocities, while hydrostatic pressure is maintained at zero velocity by a squeeze film that leaks very slowly as fluid escapes tangentially past the contact zone.

A simplified analysis has been presented for the pressure and flow fields in the cartilage and joint space and the resulting distribution of macromolecular concentration in the channel separating the two opposing articular surfaces. It is hypothesized that in the zone of impending contact, the aqueous solvent is expulsed tangentially, leaving a relatively higher solute concentration of mucopolysaccharide molecules, which then adhere to the adjacent cartilage as a gel. The osmotic pressure of the gel gradually increases until it becomes equal to the applied pressure, at which point all flow of water from the gel ceases, and the film remains stable. As the zone of contact passes by, the molecular lubricating gel layer deposited upon the cartilage (estimated to be 0.02 to 0.03 μm thick [125]) is redissolved into the now lower concentration synovial fluid that bathes it; whereas ahead of the advancing contact region the same process is repeated. Hence the everdisplacing contact region deposits and then reabsorbs its lubricating surface as it travels by. The corroboration of this hypothesis requires much additional carefully controlled experimentation of the type performed by Maroudas [81], in which the rates of deposition of gel at various filtration pressures were measured.

Load bearing under prolonged loads depends on the rate at which fluid escapes from cartilage, which is affected by the permeability of the cartilage matrix, the applied pressure distribution in the cartilage, and the internal pressure field; the pressure field in turn is influenced by osmosis, matrix elasticity, and ionic transport. These parameters are very difficult to measure. The permeability and elasticity of cartilage do not have the same values in the horizontal and vertical directions because the material is structurally anisotropic. Osmosis, ionic transport, and other factors are influenced by a very complex range of biochemical phenomena.

The main components of connective tissue, the polysaccharides or glycosaminoglycans, possess unusual physiochemical properties that must not be altered during experimentation. Hence the joint tested must remain intact to preserve this biochemical environment, upon which boundary lubrication also critically depends.

However, the measurements of frictional force in an intact joint will necessarily include contributions from stretching of soft tissue around the joints (ligaments, tendons, muscles, subcutaneous tissues) and from the frictional resistance of the parts of the joint that slide across one another (cartilage, synovium, ligaments, tendons). The energy expended to overcome stretching is almost 100 times greater than that required to overcome frictional resistance of the cartilage [126]. These forces must be isolated in obtaining net values of the cartilage friction. Clinical joint stiffness in fact may be primarily a result of soft-tissue resistance!

In addition, pathological and biochemical changes complicate our understanding of joint lubrication because they control the concentration of chondroitin sulphate and thereby the elasticity of the cartilage, for example. Progression of this process could lead to the sequence of pathological changes seen in osteoarthritis, with fraying and softening of cartilage, necrosis of exposed cells, thinning, and finally total erosion of the cartilage and secondary changes in underlying bone. Also, aging and genetic factors influence cartilage polysaccharide metabolism and hence the possible degeneration of cartilage, during which stress distributions are markedly altered, leading to uneven wearing. The synovial fluid may be depolymerized, its long chains shortened in a way similar to treatment by hyaluronidase, and its ability to anchor into the cartilaginous surfaces thus greatly impaired. Excellent reviews of this subject have been given by Bollet [127, 128] and Hamerman et al. [129].

Mechanical factors may also be responsible for osteoarthritis. It recently has been suggested by Radin et al. [130] that repetitive impulsive loading, rather than rubbing, can lead to joint degeneration by the successive steps of trabecular microfracture of the subchondral bone and subsequent increased stiffness of the healed bone, resulting in increased stresses in the articular cartilage which eventually breaks down. Although such mechanical factors could be studied in the articulation machine described here, the biochemical and pathological changes must be monitored by extremely delicate measurements. The results might then be introduced into the preliminary analysis of Sec. 3, the latter being refined to account for better-known variations of material properties of the fluid and matrix components.

Such research may lead to improved therapeutic measures to combat arthritis and to new possibilities in the design of joint prostheses. In fact, synthetic cartilage has been prepared from composite hydrophilic materials by substituting freshly precipitated cellulose fibers in place of collagen and carboxymethyl cellulose in place of protein polysaccharide. Gellike materials have been prepared by a different approach, which diffuses polyvalent cations into solutions of linear polyanions that may be somewhat cross linked [129]. Studies with a view to developing an artificial lubricant have been reported by Seller et al. [131].

A comprehensive understanding of the basic mechanisms of joint lubrication is of direct value in the interpretation of clinical examinations of pathological joints and may lead to a clarification of current explanations for elevated coefficients of friction in arthritis. Furthermore, it may be found possible and advantageous to pattern the design of joint prostheses upon the natural mechanisms of lubrication revealed in the course of the present investigation.

GLOSSARY *(From Radin and Paul [83])*

Boosted lubrication: According to this model for joint lubrication, the effectiveness of the lubricant separating two cartilage surfaces is boosted by pools of concentrated hyaluronate that are filtered out of the synovial fluid as it is forced through the pores of the cartilage under conditions of high loading. The effectiveness of the fluid film is also potentiated by the natural undulations of the cartilage surface and elastic deformation of cartilage, which tend to trap the film in the area of impending contact. During normal loading without sliding, the trapped puddles act as a squeeze film; when sliding is added a combination of boundary and elastohydrodynamic lubrication can occur at the edges of the trapped puddles.

Boundary lubrication occurs when each bearing surface is coated or impregnated with a thin layer of molecules that keep the surfaces apart and slide on the opposing surface much more readily than they are sheared off the underlying one, as is the case with a polytetrafluoroethylene (Teflon) coating on a frying pan.

Coefficient of friction is the shear force needed to make one surface slide on another divided by the normal force pressing them together. If it takes a 15-kg force to slide a 45-kg box across the floor, the coefficient of friction is 0.3. A low coefficient of friction implies low resistance to sliding.

Elastic lubrication mechanisms lower the coefficient of friction in joints because of the elasticity of articular cartilage. These mechanisms include elastohydrodynamic effects and potentiation of squeeze films. The effect on the squeeze film occurs because one cartilage surface tends to penetrate the other, so that at the margins of the zone of impending contact the peripheral gap through which trapped fluid can flow out is narrowed.

Elastohydrodynamic lubrication is a form of fluid lubrication that occurs when bearing surfaces are elastic enough for the lubricant pressure generated by motion under a given load to depress the surfaces a distance greater than the height of their asperities, thereby facilitating the maintenance of a fluid film.

Fluid lubrication is a class of mechanisms of lubrication having in common a film of fluid that completely separates the opposing bearing surfaces.

Hyaluronate, or hyaluronic acid, is a straight-chain polymer of N-acetyl glucosamine and glucuronic acid with a molecular weight of about 1,000,000 and a length of about 10^4 Å. Hyaluronate macromolecules give synovial fluid its viscosity.

Hydrodynamic lubrication is a form of fluid lubrication in which relative motion of two bearing surfaces forces lubricant in the form of a wedge between the surfaces, keeping them apart. This mechanism, which requires uninterrupted motion in the same direction to maintain the integrity of the wedge, is especially effective in high-speed journal bearings.

Hydrostatic lubrication is a form of fluid lubrication in which the bearing surfaces are held apart by a film of lubricant that is maintained under pressure, usually supplied by an external pump. This mechanism is especially suited to oscillating bearings and heavily loaded bearings in low-speed applications.

Lubricating glycoprotein fraction is the fraction of synovial fluid that gives it its advantage over buffer and other solutions in lubricating the cartilage-on-cartilage system. This substance is not hyaluronate, and its effectiveness is not dependent on hyaluronate.

Squeeze-film lubrication is a form of fluid lubrication in which the approaching surfaces generate pressure in the lubricant as they squeeze it out of the area of impending contact between them; the resulting pressure keeps the surfaces apart. In the cartilage-on-cartilage system the film that forms in the transient area of impending contact may be referred to as the squeeze film.

Thixotropy is the property of fluids that causes their viscosity, or resistance to shear, to diminish as their flow rate, or shear rate, increases. Fluids containing large molecules exhibit thixotropy; ketchup and synovial fluid are thixotropic. The viscosity and hence the thixotropy of synovial fluid are related to the concentration and molecular weight of the hyaluronic acid present.

Weeping lubrication is a form of hydrostatic lubrication in which interstitial fluid of hydrated articular cartilage flows out onto its surface when a load is applied to it. The cartilage acts as a self-pressurizing sponge; when the pressure is released, the fluid flows back into the cartilage.

APPENDIX A: RELATION OF TORQUE ON TIBIA TO COEFFICIENT OF FRICTION

Consider the ankle joint illustrated schematically in Fig. 42. The joint surfaces are pressed together by the axial load L, giving rise to the pressure distribution $P(\theta)$ acting across the cartilage interface over the range of contact θ_1 to θ_2. The talus articulates about a center O with radius R. The normal force dF_n across an element of surface $R\, d\theta$ is given by

$$dF_n = P(\theta)R\, d\theta \tag{A1}$$

and the vertical component dF_y of this force is given by

$$dF_y = dF_n \cos\theta = P(\theta) \cos\theta\, R\, d\theta \tag{A2}$$

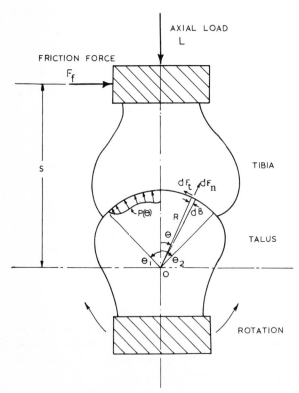

Figure 42 Forces acting on the joint.

The total vertical force is equal to the applied load, or

$$L = \int_{\theta_1}^{\theta_2} dF_y = \int_{\theta_1}^{\theta_2} P(\theta) \cos \theta \, R \, d\theta \qquad \text{(A3)}$$

When the talus is rotated about the center, friction forces act tangentially at the cartilage interface. We assume that the frictional force dF_t generated over the surface of the element is related to the normal force by the local coefficient of friction η_l, such that

$$dF_t = \eta_l \, dF_n = \eta_l P(\theta) R \, d\theta \qquad \text{(A4)}$$

Summing the torque about the point O gives

$$F_f S = \int_{\theta_1}^{\theta_2} R \, dF_t = \int_{\theta_1}^{\theta_2} R \eta_l P(\theta) R \, d\theta \qquad \text{(A5)}$$

where F_f is the force applied at the friction transducer, and S is the vertical distance of this force above the joint center O. If R and η_l do not vary with θ, Eq. (A4) gives

$$L = R \int_{\theta_1}^{\theta_2} P(\theta) \cos \theta \, d\theta \qquad \text{(A6)}$$

and Eq. (A5) gives

$$F_f S = R^2 \eta_l \int_{\theta_1}^{\theta_2} P(\theta) \, d\theta \qquad \text{(A7)}$$

Combining and solving for η_l result in

$$\eta_l = \frac{F_f}{L} \frac{S}{R} \frac{\int_{\theta_1}^{\theta_2} P(\theta) \cos \theta \, d\theta}{\int_{\theta_1}^{\theta_2} P(\theta) \, d\theta} \qquad \text{(A8)}$$

In calculating the coefficient of friction from the experimental data, the ratio of the two integrals was taken to be unity; i.e.,

$$\eta = \frac{F_f}{L} \frac{S}{R} \qquad \text{(A9)}$$

The error in this approximation depends on the relative magnitudes of the two integrals. If the pressure is concentrated near the center of the contact area, i.e., near $\theta = 0$, then the two integrals will be about equal and Eq. (A9) will hold. However, if the pressure is more evenly distributed, significant error is introduced. For example, taking $\theta_1 = \theta_2 = \pi/4$ and $P(\theta) = \text{constant} = P$ gives

$$\eta_l = \frac{F_f}{L} \frac{S}{R} \frac{\int_{-\pi/2}^{\pi/2} P \cos\theta \ d\theta}{\int_{-\pi/2}^{\pi/2} P \ d\theta} \approx 0.9\eta \tag{A10}$$

That is, for an even pressure distribution over a 90° contact area, the coefficient of friction as measured by the machine is about 10 percent greater than the local coefficient of friction. It is especially important to consider this effect in attempting to determine the coefficient of friction as a function of load because the pressure distribution is likely to change with the magnitude of the load.

APPENDIX B: CALIBRATION OF INSTRUMENTS

B1 ANGULAR–POSITION TRANSDUCER

The angular-position transducer[3] was calibrated by attaching a graduated spirit level to the lower mount and rotating through 5° increments. The displacement amplifier on the recorder was then adjusted to give 1 cm of displacement for each 25° of rotation. The error in the readout was estimated to be ±3°, resulting primarily from noise in the recorder trace.

B2 ANGULAR–VELOCITY TRANSDUCER

The angular-velocity transducer[3] was calibrated by operating the machine at a known input frequency and adjusting the displacement of the recorder tracing, at the point corresponding to maximum angular velocity, such that 1 cm of displacement corresponded to 0.7 rad/s.

The instantaneous angular velocity could also be determined by drawing a tangent to the angular-displacement curve. This was employed as a method of checking the accuracy of the velocity transducer. The values for angular velocity as determined by the two methods agreed to within 5 percent.

B3 FRICTION

The friction-force transducer[4] was calibrated, both in tension and compression, using 10-g chemical balance weights accurate to ±0.001 g. The resultant calibration

---

[3] Permalink Corp., King of Prussia, Pennsylvania, model FA 1.10.
[4] Stathan Instruments Inc., Los Angeles, California, model UC-3 transducer with model UL-4-10 load cell accessory.

curve was linear to within 3 percent. However the friction signal was very sensitive to the vibration of the drive motor. As a result the friction trace could only be read to ±0.5 g. At axial loads smaller than 15 lb, this represented an error of 25 to 50 percent. The variation of the coefficient therefore was only determined for loads above this range. It is hoped that this problem can be eliminated in future tests by removing the drive motor from the machine frame and by using a friction transducer with a lower spring constant.

B4 AXIAL LOAD

The axial-load transducer consisted of a brass ring 0.5 cm thick, 1.3 cm wide, and 4.5 cm inside diameter. Four semiconductor strain gauges[5] were attached to the ring, forming a Wheatstone bridge sensitive only to axial loads. In addition, the ring mounts were constructed such that they transmitted only axial loads to the ring. The ring was calibrated directly using a set of weights in the range 5 to 50 lb. The calibration weights were accurate to ±0.005 lb. The resultant force-deflection curve was plotted and a linear approximation was determined using the method of least squares. The final calibration was given by

$$\text{Load} = 5.3 \text{ lb/cm} \times \text{deflection (cm)} - 0.9 \text{ lb}$$

with a standard error of 0.5 lb.

REFERENCES

1. J. Charnley, The Lubrication of Animal Joints, *Proc. Inst. Mech. Eng.*, vol. 181, pt. 3J, pp. 12–22, 1959.
2. C. W. McCutchen, Animal Joints and Weeping Lubrication, *New Sci.*, vol. 301, pp. 412–415, 1962.
3. F. C. Linn, Lubrication of Animal Joints: 1, The Arthrotripsometer, *J. Bone J. Surg.*, vol. 49A, no. 6, pp. 1079–1098, 1967.
3a. D. Dowson, M. D. Longfield, P. S. Walker, and V. Wright, An Investigation of the Friction and Lubrication in Human Joints, *Proc. Inst. Mech. Eng.*, vol. 182, pt. 3N, 1967–1968.
4. D. V. Davies, C. H. Barnett, W. Cochrane, and A. V. Palfrey, Electron Microscopy of Articular Cartilage in the Young Adult Rabbit, *Ann. Rheum. Dis.*, vol. 21, pp. 11–22, 1962.
5. P. S. Walker, D. Dowson, M. D. Longfield, and V. Wright, Boosted Lubrication in Synovial Joints by Fluid Entrapment and Enrichment, *Ann. Rheum. Dis.*, vol. 27, pp. 512–518, 1968.
6. I. C. Clarke, Quantitative Measurement of Human Articular Surface Topography in Vitro by Profile Recorder and Stereomicroscope Techniques, *J. Microsc.*, vol. 97, pt. 3, 1973.
7. P. R. Lewis and C. W. McCutchen, Experimental Evidence for Weeping Lubrication in Mammalian Joints, *Nature*, vol. 184, no. 4695, p. 1285, 1959.
8. J. Edwards, Physical Characteristics of Articular Cartilage, *Proc. Inst. Mech. Eng.*, vol. 181, pt. 3J, pp. 16–24, 1967.

[5] Kulite Semi-conductor Products, Inc., Ridgefield, New Jersey, type DEP-350-500.

9. C. W. McCutchen, Physiological Lubrication, *Proc. Inst. Mech. Eng.,* vol. 181, pt. 3J, pp. 55–62, 1967.

10. A. Maroudas, Hyaluronic Acid Films, *Proc. Inst. Mech. Eng.,* vol. 181, pt. 3J, pp. 122–124, 1967.

11. C. W. McCutchen, The Frictional Properties of Animal Joints, *Wear,* vol. 5, pp. 1–17, 1962.

12. A. Maroudas and P. Bullough, Permeability of Articular Cartilage, *Nature,* vol. 219, no. 5160, pp. 1260–1261, 1968.

13. A. Maroudas, Physicochemical Properties of Cartilage in the Light of Ion Exchange Theory, *Biophys. J.,* vol. 8, pp. 575–595, 1968.

13*a.* C. H. Barnett, D. V. Davies, and M. A. MacConaill, "Synovial Joints: Their Structure and Mechanics," Longmans, Green, and Co., London, 1961.

14. J. M. Mansour and V. C. Mow, The Permeability of Articular Cartilage Under Compressive Strain at High Pressures, *J. Bone J. Surg.,* vol. 58A, pp. 509–516, 1976.

15. V. C. Mow, W. M. Lai, and L. Redler, Some Surface Characteristics of Articular Cartilage I. A Scanning Electron Microscope Study and a Theoretical Model for the Dynamic Interaction of Synovial Fluid and Articular Cartilage, *J. Biomech.,* vol. 7, pp. 449–456, 1974.

16. V. C. Mow, W. M. Lai, and L. Redler, A Scanning Electron Microscope Study of the Articular Surface and a Theoretical Model of Articular Cartilage–Synovial Fluid Interaction: Part I., *J. Biomech.* vol. 7, pp. 449–456, 1973.

17. C. W. McCutchen, The Frictional Properties of Animal Joints, *Wear,* vol. 5, pp. 1–17, 1962.

18. W. C. Hayes and L. F. Mockros, Viscoelastic Properties of Human Articular Cartilage, *J. Appl. Physiol.,* vol. 31, pp. 562–568, 1971.

19. C. Hirsch, The Pathogenesis of Chondromalacia of the Patella, *Acta Chir. Scand.,* vol. 90, Suppl. 83, pp. 1–106, 1944.

20. J. M. Zarek and J. Edwards, The Stress-Structure Relationship in Articular Cartilage, *Med., Electron. Biol. Eng.,* vol. 1, pp. 497–507, 1963.

21. L. Sokoloff, Elasticity of Aging Cartilage, *Fed. Proc.,* vol. 25(3), pp. 1089–1095, 1966.

22. G. E. Kempson, M. A. R. Freeman, and S. A. V. Swanson, The Determination of a Creep Modulus for Articular Cartilage from Indentation Tests as the Human Femoral Head, *J. Biomech.,* vol. 4, pp. 239–250, 1971.

23. W. H. Simon, Scale Effects in Animal Joints II, Thickness and Elasticity in the Deformability of Articular Cartilage, *Arthritis Rheum.,* vol. 14, pp. 493–502, 1971.

24. W. C. Hayes, L. M. Kerr, G. Herrmann, and L. F. Mockros, A Mathematical Analysis for Indentation Tests of Articular Cartilage, *J. Biomech.,* vol. 5, pp. 541–551, 1972.

25. R. Y. Hori and C. F. Mockros, Indentation Tests of Human Articular Cartilage, *J. Biomech.,* vol. 9, pp. 259–269, 1976.

26. E. D. Harris, H. G. Parker, E. L. Radin, and S. M. Kane, Effects of Proteolytic Enzymes in Structural and Mechanical Properties of Cartilage, *Arthritis Rheum.,* vol. 15, pp. 497–503, 1972.

27. S. L-Y. Woo, W. H. Akeson, and G. F. Jemmott, Measurement of Nonhomogeneous Directional Mechanical Properties of Articular Cartilage in Tension, *J. Biomech.,* vol. 9, pp. 785–791, 1976.

28. V. C. Mow, The Role of Lubrication in Biomechanical Joints, *J. Lubr. Technol., Trans. ASME,* vol. 91-F, no. 2, pp. 320–328, 1969.

29. F. C. Linn and L. Sokoloff, Movement and Composition of Interstitial Fluid of Cartilage, *Arthritis Rheum.,* vol. 8, p. 4, 1965.

30. J. Edwards, Physical Characteristics of Articular Cartilage, *Proc. Inst. Mech. Eng.,* vol. 181, pp. 16–24, 1967.

31. F. C. Linn, Lubrication of Animal Joints, *J. of Lubr. Technol., Trans. ASME,* vol. 91-F, no. 2, pp. 329–341, 1969.

32. J. R. Parsons and J. Black, The Viscoelastic Shear Behavior of Normal Rabbit Articular Cartilage, *J. Biomech.*, vol. 10, pp. 21–29, 1977.

33. W. S. C. Copeman, "Textbook of the Rheumatic Diseases," 3d ed., pp. 60–70, Livingston, Edinburgh, 1964.

34. A. G. Ogston and J. E. Stanier, The Dimensions of the Particle of the Hyaluronic Acid Complex in Synovial Fluid, *Biochem. J.*, vol. 49, pp. 585–590, 1951.

35. K. Meyer, E. M. Smyth, and M. H. Dawson, The Isolation of a Mucopolysaccharide from Synovial Fluid, *J. Biol. Chem.*, vol. 128, pp. 319–327, 1939.

36. F. C. Linn and E. L. Radin, Lubrication of Animal Joints: III, The Effect of Certain Chemical Alterations of the Cartilage and Lubricant, *Arthritis Rheum.*, vol. 11, no. 5, pp. 674–682, 1968.

37. A. Maroudas, Distribution and Diffusion of Solutes in Articular Cartilage, *Biophys. J.*, vol. 10, pp. 365–379, 1970.

38. R. I. Tanner, Calculation of the Shear Rate in the Hip Joint Lubricant, *Proc. Symp. Biomech.*, p. 21 (Appendix IV to paper by J. Charnley, 1959).

39. G. E. Burch, W. D. Love, and W. R. Jeffrey, The Waning Joint, *Prog. Med. Sci.*, 1960.

40. D. A. Swann, Macromolecules of Synovial Fluid, in "The Joints and Synovial Fluid," M. Sokoloff (ed.), vol. 1, pp. 407–435, Academic Press, N.Y., 1978.

41. D. A. Swann, E. L. Radin, M. Nazimiec, P. A. Weisser, N. Curran, and G. Lewinnek. Role of Hyaluronic Acid on Joint Lubrication, *Ann. Rheum. Dis.*, vol. 33, pp. 318–326, 1974.

42. S. C. Kuei and V. C. Mow, The Rheological Model for Synovial Fluid, *Orthop. Res. Soc. Trans. 23*, vol. 2, p. 136, 1977.

43. W. M. Lai, S. C. Kuei, and V. C. Mow, Rheological Equations for Synovial Fluids, *J. of Biomech. Eng., Trans. ASME*, vol. 100, pp. 169–186, 1978.

44. H. Strasser, "Lehrbuch der Muskel und Gelenkmechanik," vol. III, pp. 34–52, 335–359, Springer-Verlag, Berlin, 1917.

45. N. Shinno, Statico-Dynamic Analysis of Movement of the Knee: I, Modes of Movement of Knee, *Tokushima J. Exp. Med.*, vol. 8, pp. 101–110, 1961.

46. J. B. Morrison, The Mechanics of the Knee Joint in Relation to Normal Walking, *J. Biomech.*, vol. 3, no. 1, pp. 51–61, 1970.

47. C. H. Barnett, Wear and Tear in Joints, *J. Bone J. Surg.*, vol. 38B, no. 2, pp. 567, 1956.

48. J. P. Paul, Forces Transmitted by Joints in the Human Body, *Proc. Inst. Mech. Eng.*, vol. 181, pt. 3J, 1966.

49. A. S. Greenwald and J. J. O'Connor, The Transmission of Load through the Human Hip Joint, *Univ. of Oxford, Dept. of Eng. Sci. Lab. Rept.* 1002/71, 1971.

50. D. Dowson, Modes of Lubrication in Human Joints, in "Lubrication and Wear in Living and Artificial Joints: A Symposium," *Inst. Mech. Eng. Proc.*, vol. 181, pt. 3J, pp. 45–54, 1967.

51. R. I. Tanner, An Alternative Mechanism for the Lubrication of Synovial Joints, *Phys. Med. Biol.*, vol. 11, no. 1, p. 119, 1966.

52. V. C. Mow, The Role of Lubrication in Biomechanical Joints, *J. Lubr. Technol.*, vol. 2, pp. 320–329, 1969.

53. N. Petroff, Friction in Machines and the Effect of the Lubricant, *Eng. J.*, 1883.

54. B. Tower, Second Report on Friction Experiment, *Proc. Inst. Mech. Eng.*, p. 58, 1885.

55. O. Reynolds, On the Theory of Lubrication and Its Application to Mr. Beauchamp Tower's Experiments, *Philos. Trans. R. Soc. London*, vol. 177, pt. 1, p. 157, 1886.

56. M. A. MacConail, The Function of Intra-Articular Fibro-Cartilages, *J. Anat.*, vol. 66, p. 210, 1932.

57. L. Dintenfass, Rheology of Synovial Fluid and Its Role in Joint Lubrication, *Symp. Biorheology*, Copley, 1963.

58. R. S. Fein, Are Synovial Joints Squeeze-film Lubricated?, *Proc. Inst. Mech. Eng.*, vol. 181, pt. 3J, pp. 125–128, 1967.

59. H. Hertz, "Gesammelte Werke von Heinrich Hertz," vol. 1, p. 155, Leipzig (1895), also H. Hertz (1881) On the Contacts of Elastic Solids. *J. reine angew. Math.*, vol. 92, p. 56.

60. G. W. Rowe, Boundary Lubrication, in A. Cameron (ed.), "Principles of Lubrication," chap. 20, pp. 450–467, Wiley, New York, 1966.

61. J. S. McFarlane and D. Tabor, Relation between Friction and Adhesion, *Proc. R. Soc.,* vol. 202A, pp. 244–253, London, 1956.

62. A. Cameron, A Theory of Boundary Lubrication, *ASLE Trans.,* vol. 2, no. 2, pp. 195–198, 1959.

63. J. F. Wilkins, Proteolytic Destruction of Synovial Boundary Lubrication, *Nature,* vol. 219, no. 5158, pp. 1050–1051, 1968.

64. F. C. Linn, Lubrication of Animal Joints: II, The Mechanism, *J. Biomech.,* vol. 1, pp. 193–205, 1968.

65. C. W. McCutchen, Why Did Nature Make Synovial Fluid Slimy?, *Clin. Orthop.,* vol. 64, pp. 18–20, 1969.

66. A.D. Roberts, The Role of Electrical Repulsive Forces in Synovial Fluid, *Nature,* vol. 231, pp. 434–436, 1971.

67. W. H. Davis Jr., S. L. Lee, and L. Sokoloff, A Proposed Model of Boundary Lubrication by Synovial Fluid: Structuring of Boundary Water, *J. Biomech. Eng., Trans. ASME,* vol. 101, pp. 185–192, 1979.

68. C. W. McCutchen, Mechanism of Animal Joints, *Nature,* vol. 184, no. 4695, pp. 1284–1285, 1959.

69. P. S. Walker, J. Sikorski, D. Dowson, M. D. Longfield, V. Wright, and T. Buckley, Behaviour of Synovial Fluid on Surfaces of Articular Cartilage: A Scanning Electron Microscope Study, *Ann. Rheum. Dis.,* vol. 28, no. 1, pp. 1–14, 1969.

70. P. S. Walker, A. Unsworth, D. Dowson, J. Sikorski, and V. Wright, Mode of Aggregation of Hyaluronic Acid Protein Complex on the Surface of Articular Cartilage, *Ann. Rheum. Dis.,* vol. 29, pp. 591–602, 1970.

71. P. S. Walker, J. Sikorski, D. Dowson, M. D. Longfield, and V. Wright, Features of the Synovial Fluid Film in Human Joint Lubrication, *Nature,* vol. 225, no. 5236, pp. 956–957, 1970.

72. E. S. Jones, Joint Lubrication, *Lancet,* vol. 1, pp. 1043–1044, 1936.

73. T. E. Stanton, Boundary Lubrication in Engineering Practice, *Engineer,* vol. 135, pp. 678–680, 1923.

74. A. G. Ogston and J. E. Stanier, On the State of Hyaluronic Acid in Synovial Fluid, *J. Biochem.,* vol. 46, p. 364, 1950.

75. C. H. Barnett and A. F. Cobbold, Lubrication with Living Joints, *J. Bone Jt. Surg.,* vol. 44B, no. 3, pp. 662–674, 1962.

76. J. J. Faber, G. Williamson, and N. Feldman, Lubrication of Joints, *J. Appl. Physiol.,* vol. 22, pp. 793–799, 1967.

77. J. L. Nowinski, Bone Articulations as Systems of Poroelastic Bodies in Contact, *AIAA J.,* vol. 9, no. 1, pp. 62–67, 1971.

78. H. P. G. Darcy, "Les fontaines publiques de la ville de Dijon," Dalmont, Paris, 1856.

79. R. B. Bird, W. E. Stewart, and E. N. Lightfoot, "Transport Phenomena," p. 150, Wiley, New York, 1966.

80. W. Magnus, F. Oberhettinger, and R. P. Soni, "Formulas and Theorems for the Special Functions of Mathematical Physics," 3d ed., Springer-Verlag, New York, 1966.

81. A. Maroudas, Studies on the Formation of Hyaluronic Acid Films, in V. Wright (ed.), "Lubrication and Wear in Joints," Sector, London, 1969.

82. V. Dinnar, Two-Porous-Layers Lubrication in Human Synovial Joints, *Ann. Biomed. Eng.,* vol. 4, pp. 91–107, 1976.

83. E. L. Radin and I. L. Paul, A Consolidated Concept of Joint Lubrication, *J. Bone J. Surg.,* vol. 54-A, pp. 607–616, 1972.

84. C. W. McCutchen, Joint Lubrication, in L. Sokoloff (ed.), "The Joints and Synovial Fluid," vol. 11, pp. 437–483, Academic Press, N.Y., 1978.

85. D. Dowson, A. Unsworth, and V. Wright. Analysis of Boosted Lubrication in Human Joints, *J. of Mechanical Eng. Sci.,* vol. 12, no. 5, pp. 364–369, 1970.

86. E. F. Rybicki, W. A. Glaeser, J. S. Strenkowski, and M. A. Tamm, Effects of Cartilage Stiffness and Viscosity on a Nonporous Compliant Bearing Lubrication Model for Living Joints, *J. Biomechanics,* vol. 12, pp. 403–409, 1979.

87. J. M. Zarek and J. Edwards, Dynamic Considerations of the Human Skeletal System, in R. M. Kenedi (ed.), "Biomechanics and Related Bioengineering Topics," pp. 187–204, Pergamon Press, Oxford, 1964.

88. M. A. Biot, General Theory of Three Dimensional Consolidation, *J. Appl. Phys.,* vol. 12, pp. 155–164, 1941.

89. M. A. Biot, Consolidation Settlement under a Rectangular Load, *J. Appl. Phys.,* vol. 12, pp. 426–430, 1941.

90. M. A. Biot, Theory of Elasticity and Consolidation for a Porous Anisotropic Solid, *J. Appl. Phys.,* vol. 26, pp. 182–185, 1955.

91. M. A. Biot, Theory of Propagation of Elastic Waves in Fluid-Saturated Porous Solid. I: Low-Frequency Range. II: Higher-Frequency Range, *J. Acoustical Soc. Am.,* vol. 28, no. 2, pp. 168–191, 1956.

92. M. A. Biot, General Solutions of the Equations of Elasticity and Consolidation for a Porous Material, *J. Appl. Phys.,* vol. 23, pp. 91–96, 1956.

93. M. A. Biot, Mechanics of Deformation and Acoustic Propagation in Porous Media, *J. Appl. Phys.,* vol. 33, no. 4, pp. 1482–1498, 1962.

94. M. C. Mow, Physical Characteristics of a Poroelastic-Elastic Layered System under a Uniformly Moving Load, Ph.D. dissertation, Rensselaer Polytechnic Inst., 1968.

95. M. C. Mow and F. F. Long, On Weeping Lubrication Theory, *Z. Angew. Math. Phys.,* vol. 20, pp. 156–166, 1969.

96. F. F. Ling, A New Model of Articular Cartilage in Human Joints, *J. Lab. Tech. Trans. ASME,* vol. 96F, pp. 449–454, 1974.

97. C. W. McCutchen, Mechanism of Animal Joints: Sponge-Hydrostatic and Weeping Bearings, *Nature,* vol. 18A, pp. 1284–1285, 1959.

98. G. R. Higginson and R. Norman, The Lubrication of Porous Elastic Solids with Reference to the Functioning of Human Joints, *J. Mech. Eng. Sci.,* vol. 16, pp. 250–257, 1974.

99. A. M. Wijesinghe and H. B. Kingsbury, A Poroelastic Analysis of Synovial Joint Lubrication, *Digest 11th Int. Conf. on Med. and Biol. Eng.,* pp. 186–187, Medical Engineering Section, National Research Council, Ottawa, Canada, 1976.

100. P. A. Torzilli and V. C. Mow, On the Fundamental Fluid Transport Mechanisms through Normal and Pathological Articular Cartilage during Function–I. The Formulation, *J. Biomech.,* vol. 9, pp. 541–552, 1976.

101. P. A. Torzilli and V. C. Mow, On the Fundamental Fluid Transport Mechanisms through Normal Pathological Articular Cartilage during Function–II. The Analysis, Solution, and Conclusions, *J. Biomech.,* vol. 9, pp. 587–606, 1976.

102. R. Collins, On the Mechanisms of Joint Lubrication, *Proc. 14th Brit. Theoretical Mechanics Colloq.,* University College, London, 1972.

103. R. Collins, Biological Lubrication, *Proc. 3rd Int. Conf. on Medical Physics including Medical Engineering,* Göteborg, 1972.

104. R. Collins, Une Nouvelle Théorie Globale de la Lubrification des Articulations, *Houille Blanche,* vol. 3, no. 4, pp. 211–218, 1978.

105. R. Collins, The Physics of Human Joint Lubrication, *Proc. 1st Int. Conf. on Mechanics in Medicine and Biology,* pp. 119–123, Witzstrock Publ., Baden-Baden, 1978.

106. R. Collins, A Model of Lubricant Gelling in Synovial Joints, submitted for publication, 1980.

107. J. M. Mansour and V. C. Mow, On the Natural Lubrication of Synovial Joints: Normal and Degenerate, *J. Lubr. Technol.,* vol. 99F, pp. 163–173, 1977.

108. V. C. Mow and J. M. Mansour, The Nonlinear Interaction between Cartilage Deformation and Interstitial Fluid Flow, *J. Biomech.,* vol. 10, pp. 31–39, 1977.

109. S. C. Kuei, V. C. Mow, W. M. Lai, and M. G. Ancona, Biphasic Creep Behavior of Articular Cartilage, *Trans. Orthop. Res. Soc.,* 24th Annual, 3:10, 1978.

110. V. C. Mow, H. Lipshitz, and M. J. Glimcher, Mechanisms for Stress Relaxation in Articular Cartilage, *Trans. Orthop. Res. Soc.,* 23rd Annual, p. 75, 1977.

111. C. W. McCutchen, Comment on Mow et al. (1974 a,b), *J. Biomech.,* vol. 8, p. 261, 1975.

112. S. C. Kuei, Rheological Modeling of Synovial Fluid and Application of the Mixture Theory to Articulate Cartilage, Ph.D. thesis, Rensselaer Polytechnic Institute, Troy, N. Y., 1978.

113. R. M. Bowen, Theory of Mixtures, in A. E. Eringen, III (ed.), "Continuum Physics," pp. 52-76, Academic Press, N.Y., 1976.

114. V. C. Mow and W. M. Lai, Mechanics of Animal Joints: A Review, in M. VanDyke (ed.), "1979 Annual Review of Fluid Mechanics," vol. 11, pp. 247-288, 1979.

115. S. C. Kuei, W. M. Lai, and V. C. Mow, A Biphasic Rheological Model of Articular Cartilage, in R. C. Eberhart (ed.), "1978 Advances in Bioengineering," pp. 17-18, ASME, N.Y., 1978.

116. W. M. Lai and V. C. Mow, Flow Fields in a Single Layer Model of Articular Cartilage Created by a Sliding Load, in M. K. Wells (ed.), "1979 Advances in Bioengineering," pp. 101-104, 1979.

117. V. C. Mow and W. M. Lai, The Optical Sliding Contact Analytical Rheometer (OSCAR) for Flow Visualization at the Articular Surface, in M. K. Wells (ed.), "1979 Advances in Bioengineering," pp. 97-99, 1979.

118. H. Lipschitz, R. Etheredge, and M. J. Glimcher, Changes in the Hexosamine Content and Swelling Ratio of Articular Cartilage as Functions of Depth for Surface, *J. Bone J. Surg.,* vol. 58A, pp. 1149-1153, 1976.

119. A. Maroudas, Balance between Swelling Pressure and Collagen Tension in Normal and Degenerate Articular Cartilage, *Nature,* vol. 260, pp. 808-809, 1972.

120. J. R. Parson and J. Black, Mechanical Behavior of Articular Cartilage: Quantitative Changes with Alteration of Ionic Environment, *J. Biomech.,* vol. 12, pp. 765-773, 1979.

121. L. W. Swenson, R. L. Piziali, and D. J. Schurman, An Electromechanical Model of Human Articular Cartilage, in M. K. Wells (ed.), "1979 Advances in Bioengineering," pp. 105-108, ASME, N.Y., 1979.

122. E. L. Radin, I. L. Paul and D. Pollock. Animal Joint Behavior under Excessive Loading, *Nature,* vol. 226, pp. 554-555, 1970.

123. A. G. Ogston and J. E. Stanier, The Physiological Function of Hyaluronic Acid in Synovial Fluids; Viscous, Elastic and Lubricating Properties, *J. Physiol.,* vol. 119, p. 244, 1953.

124. E. L. Radin, D. A. Swann, and D. A. Weisser, Separation of a Hyaluronic-Free Lubricating Fraction from Synovial Fluid, *Nature,* vol. 228, p. 377, 1970.

125. A. Maroudas, private communication, 1972.

126. R. J. Johns and V. Wright, Relative Importance of Various Tissues in Joint Stiffness, *J. Appl. Physiol.,* vol. 17, pp. 824-828, 1962.

127. A. J. Bollet, Connective Tissue Polysaccharide Metabolism and the Pathogenesis of Osteoarthritis, *Adv. Intern. Med.,* vol. 13, pp. 33-60, 1967.

128. A. J. Bollet, An Essay on the Biology of Osteoarthritis, *Arthritis Rheum.,* vol. 12, no. 2, pp. 152-153, 1969.

129. D. Hamerman, L. C. Rosenberg, and M. Schubert, Diarthrodial Joints Revisited, *J. Bone Jt. Surg.,* vol. 52A, no. 4, pp. 725-768, 1970.

130. E. L. Radin, I. L. Paul, and R. M. Rose, Role of Mechanical Factors in Pathogenesis of Primary Osteoarthritis, *Lancet,* pp. 519-522, March 4, 1972.

131. P. Seller, D. Dowson, M. Longfields, and V. Wright, Requirements of an Artificial Lubricant for Joints, in V. Wright (ed.), "Lubrication and Wear in Joints," Sector, London, 1969.

CHAPTER FOUR

BIOMECHANICAL ASPECTS OF OSTEOARTHRITIC JOINTS: MECHANISMS AND NONINVASIVE DETECTION

James Pugh

The known mechanical changes in osteoarthritic bone, cartilage, and synovial fluid are outlined and related to current observations of subchondral cancellous bone architecture, mechanical properties, and the symbiotic mechanical relationship of the subchondral cancellous bone with the adjacent articular cartilage. The role of dynamic impact loads as a mediator of the osteoarthritic process is emphasized and quantitated in a comparison of the impact response of normal and osteoarthritic knee joints by a noninvasive diagnostic technique. This method of impact testing is discussed in detail and used in an evaluation of the specific modes of shock absorption in the human leg.

1 GENERAL INTRODUCTION

The specific characteristics of osteoarthritis[1] are biochemical, metabolic, histological, and biomechanical in nature and involve the following parts of a typical joint: the

The author gratefully acknowledges the editorial abilities of Susan Rom, the computer and electronics expertise of Alan Streitman, the programming talents of Andrew Miller, and the staff of the Hospital for Joint Diseases and Medical Center for agreeing to constitute our data sets.

[1] The terms osteoarthritis and degenerative joint disease are often used interchangeably. Most authors recognize that they are essentially separate entities [6]. For example, there are

cartilage, the synovial fluid, and the bone [1 to 6]. It is generally accepted [11, 12] that the physical properties of these three entities change during the osteoarthritic process and change the fundamental biomechanical functioning of the joint as the disease progresses. This chapter deals with the biomechanical aspects of osteoarthritis and will only touch on the biochemical and histological aspects of the disease as being supplemental or supporting to the biomechanical characteristics.

Several authors [6, 11, 13] have pointed out that osteoarthritis is essentially a biomechanical phenomenon. Those individuals that tend to develop osteoarthritis generally have joints that are relatively overloaded for a variety of reasons. Nevertheless, there are individuals who seem to be resistant to osteoarthritis although their joint loads are also excessive.

There is considerable controversy over what really is the cause of osteoarthritis. One contention [11, 14] is that a breakdown occurs in the lubrication mechanism in the joint. This could be due to chemical changes in the fluid or cartilage. The central feature here may be an inability of the synovial fluid to provide proper nourishment to the cartilage. It has long been recognized [12] that cartilage itself is avascular and must be nourished indirectly by the synovial membrane. Another contention [15] is that subchondral bone changes are responsible for the disease and that these changes cause the cartilage and fluid to change their role of nutrition and lubrication slightly. The nature of the bone changes was thought to be either chemical or structural, but it is now conceded [16 to 19] that they are structurally induced by a Wolff's-law mechanism that governs the functional adaptation of bone.

The purposes of the present chapter are: (1) to focus on the biomechanical differences between normal and osteoarthritic joints, (2) to consider the effects of these biomechanical differences on the fundamental functioning of the joints, (3) to relate these differences to the observed chemical changes in the joints, and (4) to describe experiments that have been performed in an effort to provide noninvasive detection of osteoarthritis and noninvasive assessment of shock absorption. To do this thoroughly requires a detailed discussion of the cartilage, synovial fluid, bone, lubrication mechanisms, and viscoelastic behavior of the joint.

Many experimental and clinical studies [7 to 10, 20 to 59] have focused on the later stages of osteoarthritis. The gross cartilage fibrillations, bone remodeling, and osteophyte formations occurring in these advanced stages render the joint in a state much different from its original prearthritic condition. Any cartilage and bone studies done on these grossly affected joints really offer only hindsight into the problem. In contrast, the present discussion on grossly normal joints is intended to offer insight into the possibility of determining signs that will allow diagnosis and identification of prearthritic joints before any gross changes occur.

---

degenerative changes associated with senility that are distinct from those degenerative changes associated with osteoarthritis [7 to 10]. Cartilage degeneration in general is usually termed degenerative joint disease. If the characteristics of the cartilage are such that (1) degeneration occurs in weight-bearing areas, (2) a specific proteoglycan depletion, assessable by appropriate staining, is revealed, and (3) there are associated bony changes, then the term osteoarthritis is used to describe this particular type of degenerative joint disease.

2 BIOMECHANICAL FACTORS IN OSTEOARTHRITIS

2.1 Cartilage Changes in Osteoarthritis

Two distinct physical properties are associated with articular cartilage, namely its stiffness and a viscoelastic quantity, the relaxation time [11, 60 to 62]. With advancing osteoarthritis, the cartilage is known to soften; that is, its elastic stiffness decreases and the cartilage becomes more resilient. The changes in relaxation time with osteoarthritis are ill documented, but this parameter probably increases as the resiliency of the cartilage increases.

The effect of this decrease in stiffness is tantamount to a change in the shock-absorbing capacities of the articular cartilage, the more compliant cartilage in osteoarthritis being capable of deflecting more and thus limiting peak loads more effectively. At first consideration this could be advantageous. However, the cartilage in osteoarthritis, being a more effective damper, concurrently becomes a dissipater of greater amounts of impact energy, which ultimately could lead to premature erosion and fibrillation. This is due to the increased magnitude of the deflections osteoarthritic cartilage undergoes in normal activity, relative to the deflections that normal cartilage experiences. In any event, the mechanical changes in the cartilage affect its functioning as a shock absorber. It is clear that the use of impact techniques in diagnosis and the measurement of shock absorption have potential value.

Histologically, cartilage consists of three zones: the superficial tangential zone (STZ), the middle zone, and the deep zone [11]. The change in cartilage stiffness in osteoarthritis is associated with histochemical changes including proteoglycan loss from the superficial tangential zone of the cartilage. The histochemical changes are usually assessed by Safranin-O with methyl-green staining techniques [63]. The initial change in cartilage stiffness also occurs at a stage when the cartilage is increasing its water uptake and when abnormal collagen synthesis is occurring [38, 64]. As the osteoarthritic process advances, the major part of the proteoglycan is washed out of the cartilage, and the chondrocytes begin to clone.

The question as to whether cartilage matrix itself actually carries any load has often been raised [11, 65]. It has been postulated that the water in the cartilage is essentially in a state of hydrostatic pressure, and that load carriage in the cartilage is essentially affected by this water content, the matrix itself carrying minimal load. The finding that osteoarthritic cartilage has a higher water content than normal cartilage is perhaps significant in this regard. If this concept is correct, the matrix bears less inherent load in the degenerative condition than in the normal condition and thus tends to protect itself. Nevertheless, studies of articular cartilage [36, 37, 66, 67] have shown a remarkable similarity between fatigue-produced defects and the osteoarthritic fibrillations. It is possible that the increased water uptake is caused by microscopic fatigue-induced defects in the cartilage. These studies also show that load carriage in cartilage may be significant enough to cause the observed splits. The fact that cartilage matrix does bear some fraction of the load seems to be well established.

Furthermore, another feature that changes subtly with the onset of osteoarthritis is the cartilage surface. Articular cartilage in the normal state is not smooth.[2] There exist three orders of roughness [68], which are termed undulations I, II, and III (see Table 1). These roughnesses have been observed and documented by several investigators [26, 68 to 75] using tracings of replicas and by scanning electron microscopy (SEM). The largest wavelengths, undulations III, are seen to increase in amplitude with degenerative joint disease, and just prior to the occurrence of gross cartilage fibrillation [68]. The undulations II also change their appearance with osteoarthritis, presumably by a chondrocyte "clustering" mechanism [26].

A question to be raised here is the following: Are the roughnesses seen in recent investigations characteristic of cartilage in the "relaxed" state or the "unrelaxed" state? Cartilage has a relaxation time of 10 to 30 min associated with its viscoelastic response. As an example, when we walk at a rate of one step per second, cartilage behaves virtually purely elastically, with negligible viscous behavior, since the loading duration and frequency are much lower than the characteristic relaxation time.

This raises another important question: Is cartilage in joints ever truly in a relaxed state? It is known that the muscles, fascia, and ligaments provide a passive tension that puts cartilage surfaces under load even during so-called resting periods characterized by the lack of physical activity. Even in the swing phase of gait, the hip, for example, is under considerable load [76]. What is not known is whether this load is significant or negligible with regard to the characteristics of the surface of the cartilage. If significant, it could ensure the preservation of an unrelaxed profile of the cartilage *in vivo*, which, in all likelihood, is much different from the relaxed profiles observed in recent SEM studies and intererence contrast microscope studies.

2.2 Synovial Fluid Changes

The changes in synovial fluid at the onset of osteoarthritis are generally ill-documented [77]. The data are inconclusive, owing to the difficulty of obtaining

---

[2] When the cartilage is prepared and examined by conventional techniques involving surgical removal and immediate, direct observation, the roughnesses are evident.

Table 1   Surface roughness features of articular cartilage

Type of undulation	Height (μm)	Wavelength (μm)
I, small ripples	0.2–0.4	0.5
II, depressions	2–4	30–50
III, large waves	10–20	1000

Source: Walker [68].

synovial fluid from normal test subjects as a basis for comparison. It is stated [6] that, at the necropsy table, synovial fluid from patients with degenerative joint disease is more viscous and present in increased quantity relative to that from normal joints. Nevertheless, other authors [77, 78] report a lowering of the amount of the fluid and a decrease in its viscosity. These observations suggest changes in the hyaluronate content of the synovial fluid with osteoarthritis [23, 79, 80].

Synovial fluid provides important lubricating properties to the joint. This has been attributed [81] to the glycoprotein fraction of the mucin. Indeed, digestion of the synovial fluid with hyaluronidase destroys the hyaluronate and consequently the viscosity of the fluid, but does not affect the coefficient of friction of cartilage-on-cartilage interfaces. It has been suggested [82] that the large hyaluronate molecules merely seem to keep the mucin in the joint space.

In view of the histochemical changes occurring in the cartilage with the earliest stages of osteoarthritis, it seems likely that some changes in the synovial fluid also occur. If the properties of the synovial fluid do change, it is also likely that some subtle changes occur in either the lubrication mechanism or the coefficient of friction. Thus a change in the joint fluid is expected to be related somehow to the osteoarthritic process.

Synovial fluid, being non-Newtonian, exhibits an effect known as *shear thinning* [83]. The higher the shear rate in the fluid, the less viscous the fluid is. It is also likely that some change in the shear thinning, or the dependence of the viscosity on shear rate, occurs in osteoarthritis. These effects are also ill documented, since most studies on the viscosity of synovial fluid are taken at one value of shear rate [77].

Current theories for joint lubrication involve the concept of either "boosted" [14] or "weeping" [65] lubrication, both involving the flow of water and small ions through the cartilage surface, out of and into localized "pools" on the cartilage surfaces, respectively. These theories are consistent with the nutritional function that synovial fluid provides for the cartilage. Both these lubrication theories involve pooling on the surface of the cartilage. The locations of the pools are believed to be associated with the undulations III of the cartilage surfaces [68].

In the boosted lubrication theory, the mechanism is a pooling of a concentrated hyaluronate layer on the cartilage surfaces due to water and small ions being forced into the cartilage and away from the contact points during weight bearing. This hyaluronate layer keeps the cartilage surfaces apart as the joint surfaces slide relative to one another. This mechanism allows for nourishment of the chondrocytes, since fluid is forced out of the cartilage and back into it as the contact points change position during normal joint motion. Weeping lubrication, on the other hand, is a postulated mechanism in which water and small ions are forced out of the cartilage into puddles when the cartilage is loaded. Thus, according to this theory, water and small ions tend to collect and form pools under hydrostatic pressure in the depressions on the cartilage surfaces. If either model for the lubrication of cartilage-on-cartilage systems (or even a combination of the two) is correct, there is experimental evidence [84] of the pooling of synovial fluid in the undulations III on the cartilage. Thus, these undulations III play a central role in the cartilage lubrication process [81, 85].

Other investigators have ascribed great importance not to the undulations III, but to the undulations II. Mow and co-workers [72, 86] have postulated that the undulations II in the cartilage could be generated by an elastohydrodynamic interaction between the synovial fluid, the cartilage, and the profile of the moving load, and that these undulations contribute to the lubrication effectiveness. Stable wavelengths are set up on the surface of the cartilage, and these wavelengths may reach an instability leading to cartilage fibrillation under certain conditions if the cartilage stiffness is below a prescribed value. These undulations II have been observed in the SEM by several workers, as noted previously. Again, the question of the relaxed versus unrelaxed state of the cartilage should be brought up. Furthermore, the effect of the removal of the cartilage from the underlying bone leaves open the question of elastic recoil leading to an artifactual ridge pattern [11]. The use of a glutaraldehyde fixation procedure [72, 86, 87] could also be the culprit in producing artifactual profiles.

Interference contrast studies carried out in our laboratories on fresh human condyles did not reveal the ridge pattern corresponding to undulations II, although the features of this pattern are within the limits of resolution of the light microscope (Fig. 1). A collection of localized depressions corresponding to undula-

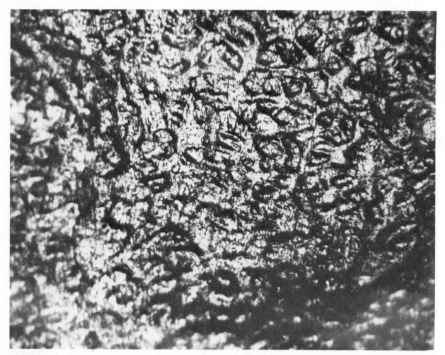

Figure 1 Surface of fresh human medial femoral condyle showing numerous depressions (undulations II) and a contour at the periphery of the field (undulations III). Photomicrograph taken with Leitz orthoplan microscope in the incident-light mode with Smith R interference contrast attachment. 80 ×.

tions II was observed. This has been confirmed by other investigators [69 to 71, 73, 75]. Perhaps significantly, the techniques involving fixation of the cartilage reveal ridges, while the techniques involving replication of fresh cartilage surfaces, freeze drying, or indirect observation of the wet surfaces with the light microscope reveal localized depressions. The undulations II have alternatively been explained as collapsed chondrocyte lacunae [68], an explanation that is supported by the chondrocyte "clustering" effects recently observed on cartilage surfaces [26].

In view of the questions raised as to the existence of ridges having the spacing of the undulations II, the theoretical work of Mow may be irrelevant to the lubrication mechanism and to the biomechanical interactions between the synovial fluid and the cartilage. Our observations of a system of localized depressions corresponding to the undulations II effectively limits the applicability of a theory involving the generation of a set of experimentally observed linear ridges that appear to be artifactual in nature. Furthermore, the effects of pooling in such small-order roughnesses would be minimal. The requirements of fluid interchange and elastohydrodynamic interaction between fluid and cartilage are best satisfied by roughness of the order of undulations III. Thus, a characterization of these undulations III would be expected to give more insight into the problem of osteoarthritis than the minimal insight to be gained in a study relying on the theoretically postulated and unconvincingly exhibited ridge undulations II.

2.3 Subchondral Bone Changes

The effect of the subchondral bone on the functioning of the joints has often been described [72, 86] as passive and minimal. Although numerous authors [33, 88 to 95] have suggested the possible effects of the subchondral bone on the biomechanics of the joint, the diagrams shown often do not recognize the structural inhomogeneity of the subchondral cancellous structure.

An increase in the elastic stiffness of the subchondral bone in a series model for the mechanics of the joint [96] is shown to increase the peak forces experienced by the cartilage in the same manner that a change in the stiffness of the cartilage changes the peak forces in the bone (Chap. 6 of [11]). Cancellous bone is present in the skeleton in regions where an essential shock-absorbing property is required: the diploë layer of the skull, vertebral bodies, and condylar structures. The structure and energy-dissipating effects of cancellous bone have been well documented and are now firmly established [97 to 100].

In view of the effects of the bone on the biomechanical functioning of joints, several investigations have shown differences in the mechanical properties of cancellous bone from joints showing degenerative changes when compared to bone from normal joints. The early work by Radin and Tolkoff ç92´ showed an increase in stiffness and a consequent decrease in the shock-absorbing properties of the bone. The work by Lereim et al. [33] shows an increase in the hardness of bone in osteoarthritics. These differences in mechanical properties are thought to be accompanied by differences in the connectivity and the orientation or spatial arrangement of the trabeculae in the cancellous bone, by a Wolff's-law mechanism [101].

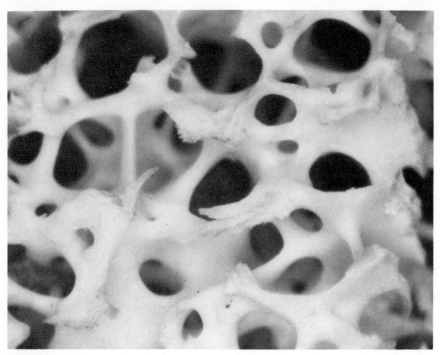

Figure 2 Cancellous bone from human medial femoral condyle. Note the sheet and strut arrangement and the numerous holes penetrating the structure. 20 X.

Cancellous bone is a very complex assemblage of sheets, struts, and rods of bone (Fig. 2). Being a composite, it has often been analyzed using complex and time-consuming stereological techniques [57, 102 to 106]. It is also a very highly loaded system [107]. This precarious combination of high loads and complicated interconnections suggests complex dependencies on spatially oriented stereological parameters.

The assemblage of the trabeculae in the subchondral regions is generally as required by Wolff's law: trabeculae tend to align along directions of maximum stress, with stiffening struts at appropriate intervals [101]. It follows that when the nagnitude and direction of the stresses change in osteoarthritis, considerable rearrangement of the trabeculae in subchondral regions occurs. These changes have been observed experimentally [12], but to quantitate them geometrically requires the use of much more involved techniques than merely density or volume fraction measurements.

The change in the fundamental mechanical property of the cartilage in osteoarthritis, namely a decrease in its stiffness, changes the dynamic stresses in the subchondral cancellous bone. Ultimately, a trabecular remodeling will occur. This is one feedback mechanism that explains the interrelated cartilage and bone changes in osteoarthritis. Conversely, if the bone changes occur in the structure prior to any observable changes in the cartilage, the cartilage itself experiences different dynamic stresses.

One can rationalize a cartilage degeneration model based on either increased or decreased stresses in the cartilage: cartilage erodes if it is either overloaded or underloaded [12]. The gross bony changes could therefore be either sclerosis or atrophy, respectively. To complicate matters further, it is not clear whether the earliest detectable cartilage changes precede or follow the earliest bony changes.

Differences in the bone-mineral contents of the subchondral bone relative to normal bone have also been detected in osteoarthritis [43, 45]. Two geometrically identical pieces of fully calcified bone could have dramatic differences in mechanical properties due to differences in the distribution of mineral at critical sites of stress concentration. The bone-mineral content should also be assessed to fully describe the structure.

2.4 Pathogenesis of Osteoarthritis

Our research to date has consisted of a biomechanical approach to the problem of early primary idiopathic osteoarthritis, with emphasis on delineating the pathogenesis. The possible role of cancellous bone in the etiology has already been discussed and has been alluded to by others as indicated. Preliminary work concerning the interrelations between joint degeneration and the structure and mechanical properties of cancellous bone has already been completed. This involved the use of reflected-light microscopy [108] to quantitate the spatial geometry of the cancellous bone. Special techniques utilizing piezoelectric transducers were developed to measure the mechanical properties [109].

The results were (1) a delineation of the geometric factors governing the mechanical response of cancellous bone [110, 111]; (2) that significant differences in the interconnectivity of the individual trabeculae in the subchondral cancellous region exist between bone from joints exhibiting early osteoarthritic changes (as assessed by Safranin-O stains of sections of the cartilage) and bone from normal joints [112]; (3) the suggestion that microfracture and trabecular collapse play an important role in the remodeling of the trabecular architecture [113, 114]; (4) that cancellous bone exhibits resonant behavior over the range of frequencies 100 to 4000 Hz [115], the resonant behavior apparently being dependent upon the amount of remodeling activity in the cancellous bone [116, 117]; (5) that the properties of the material of individual trabeculae are fundamentally different from the mechanical properties of the material of compact cortical bone [118]; (6) that cancellous bone possesses a directional orientation in the knee in the anterior-posterior direction [119]; (7) that patients with clinically observed osteoarthritis have significantly less shock absorption in the joint than normal patients [120]; and (8) that shock absorption occurring due to tensed muscle per se is not a major mechanism [121].

2.5 Discussion of the Results

In the experimental work done on cancellous bone, the results indicated that the mechanical properties of cancellous bone correlate better with its spatial orientation than with its density or the volume of bone present in the sample [110]. This same concept has been alluded to by others [102]. Thus, subtle differences in the geometry of the trabeculae in the subchondral region have a significant effect on the mechanics of the subchondral bone. Bone remodeling in osteoarthritis by means of trabecular microfracture and collapse in the subchondral region is suggested [113, 114] as a means of obtaining irregular geometries relatively quickly.

The mechanics of individual trabeculae have been delineated by this laboratory [118]. The results fit well with the concept of extensive trabecular buckling and fatigue during normal joint functioning, as put forth by Vernon-Roberts and Pirie [95] in their work on vertebral bodies. This buckling behavior and probable microfracture fit well with current bone remodeling theories [12]. The significant difference in elastic properties of individual trabeculae relative to cortical bone suggests a slightly greater capacity of cancellous bone to limit peak forces than was originally suspected, and consequently a greater importance in its function as a shock absorber in the joint.

The development of piezoelectric techniques for the investigation of bone mechanics is perhaps significant in that samples are now tested immediately upon removal from the cadaver with no damage and high reproducibility [109]. This allows subsequent structural studies on the same bone samples as were tested mechanically, without the disadvantage of artifacts produced during the testing. The testing is carried out at frequencies well away from the resonances previously documented [115], so that the mechanical response is purely elastic at the test frequency selected. The existence of these intrinsic material resonances has been confirmed by two independent investigators [122, 123].

The development of an idealized model for cancellous bone led to the conclusion that the spatial geometry of the trabeculae could have more subtle effects than just merely controlling the overall mechanical properties [111, 124]. The computerized finite-element analyses led to calculations showing the probable effect of bowing of the subchondral bony plate over areas where no supporting trabeculae exist. This bowing, under normal loads, is qualitatively and quantitatively in agreement with the observed cartilage surface undulations III reported by several authors and discussed previously. A high degree of correlation exists for both the amplitude and the wavelength when the theoretical model based on bone deflections is compared to the experimentally obtained data from the cartilage surfaces. Thus, the concept of the underlying bony subchondral plate affecting the microscopic cartilage roughness profile was given at least theoretical justification. The experimental observation that the wavelength of the cartilage undulations III corresponds almost exactly to an intertrabecular spacing is significant.

The concept that the microresponse of the subchondral plate controls the cartilage roughness is not new. Sokoloff [6] reports two suggestions of the probability of the validity of this phenomenon, one as early as 1934. This latter account showed that "bends" in the subchondral bony plate are correlated with cartilage lesions. It seems likely that the concept of focal cartilage degeneration associated with inhomogenous mechanical response of the subchondral bony plate and supporting trabeculae is correct. The recent work of Townsend supports this contention, in experiments on patellar subchondral cancellous bone [142, 143].

The research on cancellous bone and cartilage from cadavers exhibiting early degenerative changes [112] is consistent with these thoughts. Distal ends of human femurs were removed at autopsy from patients having had no history of degenerative joint disease. Safranin-O staining of the cartilage in the weight-bearing areas of the medial condyles enabled characterization of the joints in an expanded Collins classification [92]. All joints were normal or grade I, indicating mucopolysaccharide loss only from the superficial tangential zone of the cartilage. The bone, after preparation and the application of stereological techniques, showed significant differences in the spatial geometry for the two groups, grade 0 (normal) and grade I (early osteoarthritics). In cross section, the bone from the normal joints presents a trabecular arrangement consisting of elongated open spaces running in the direction of the sliding axis of the joint. The bone from the early osteoarthritics shows a more equiaxed distribution of intertrabecular spaces (Fig. 3). "The bone stiffening of 38 per cent from a normal to an early arthritic condition was accompanied by a trabecular contiguity change from 0.7 to 0.8. Since the limits on the contiguity ratio in trabecular bone are one-half and one and the experimentally observed range is 0.6 to 0.9, this increase in contiguity ratio is quite striking" [112].

There was a significant difference in this study in the subchondral cancellous

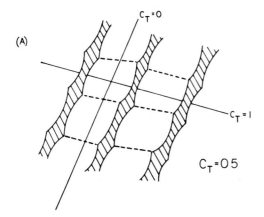

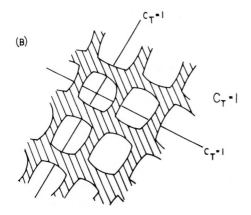

Figure 3 (*A*) Subchondral cancellous bone structure, transverse plane, from joint showing no arthritic change. This shows an average contiguity ratio of 0.5. The articular cartilage surface overlies this structure in the plane of the paper. (*B*) Subchonral cancellous bone structure, transverse plane, from joint showing early arthritic change. This shows an average contiguity ratio of 1.0. The articular cartilage surface in this structure also overlies the structure in the plane of the paper.

bone stiffness, the bone from the arthritic joints being stiffer, and a significant difference in trabecular connectivity (contiguity). No significant difference in amount of bone present was found. In view of the existence of differences in bone pattern between the two groups, instead of between amounts of bone present, the difference in stiffness is postulated to be of less importance than the difference in geometry.

The difference in bone stiffness thus may be a secondary contributor to the decreased proteoglycan content of the cartilage. It would appear that the proteoglycan loss is due to basic differences in the viscoelastic and elastohydrodynamic response of the cartilage brought about by the differences in bone pattern. In essence, the bone "templates" were different in the two groups, leading to differences in possible pooling configurations of fluid on the cartilage surface, and differences in lubrication and fluid flow.

Had there been a simple correlation between bone stiffness and density but not in pattern, the effect of the bone stiffness would have been more directly related to the proteoglycan loss. Whether the "normal" bone remodeled to the arthritic configuration is unclear. It is probably more likely that the bone pattern of the early arthritics was present for quite some time. The time it would take to remodel from a normal pattern to the arthritic pattern, even through a mechanism of trabecular microfracture and rearrangement, would be excessive. Rather, the difference in patterns is suggested to have occurred during the initial ossification.

Thus, the concept of the earliest sign of degenerative change, surface proteoglycan loss from the cartilage, being associated with differences in the subchondral trabecular geometry suggests that the cartilage histochemistry is very sensitive to the micromechanics of the subchondral bony plate. The differences in trabecular geometry suggest differences in the pattern of the undulations III on the cartilage, since the profile of the cartilage surface is sensitive to the subchondral trabecular arrangements.

More recently, Ewald et al. [125] performed hip arthropolasties on dogs and replaced the cancellous bone of the femoral heads with polymethyl methacrylate. The mechanical effect of this procedure is the replacement of the subchondral cancellous bone with a material of identical elasticity but homogeneous geometry. All the dogs subsequently showed osteoarthritis of the hip joint. These experiments are consistent with and support the hypothesis that altered subchondral architecture can be a mediator of osteoarthritis.

3 NONINVASIVE DIAGNOSTIC TECHNIQUES

The only work to date on noninvasive mechanical detection of osteoarthritis has involved either acoustical pattern-recognition techniques [126] or studies of the impact response [127]. The basic principles involved in both these techniques relate to detection of the early arthritic joint, that is, the joint that is not clinically assessable as being arthritic by means of x-ray.

The technique of acoustical pattern recognition involves the measurement of audible sound produced by a moving joint to provide what is referred to as an acoustic signature. A microphone is pressed, for example, on the knee joint of a typical test subject. The joint is moved, and the audible sounds emitted are recorded by means of appropriate electronics. Data reproduction is performed and results are plotted as acoustic output as a function of time, as a frequency spectrum, or as autocorrelation functions. The results of this technique appear to be promising. Unique spectral patterns have been obtained for sounds emitted from normal joints, joints in the rheumatoid arthritic condition, and joints in the osteoarthritic condition. Of course, in the study the patients had radiographically detectable arthritis so it could be established that a joint was indeed arthritic. However, this does not preclude the possible application of these techniques for the identification of prearthritic joints in an effort to subsequently provide rehabilitation to arrest the disease process.

It is evident from the preceding discussion that the mechanical changes associated with osteoarthritic joints result in definite changes in the response of these joints to impact loads and in the fundamental shock-absorbing characteristics of the joint. As was stated, the use of impact techniques appears to have promise in the identification of such changes in shock absorption, especially since the mechanical changes concurrent with osteoarthritis occur early in the disease process and lead to the condition called prearthritic joint. It is appropriate at this time to discuss the use of impact testing to evaluate mechanical properties of bone and joints as well as other techniques that involve the application of a force containing multiple frequencies or high-frequency components.

3.1 Impact Testing

Introduction The orthopedic literature is replete with papers dealing with dynamic measurements on human bodies and on body parts. The present purpose is not to give a review of the literature, but to relate our techniques to the alternative methods. These have utilized a variety of experimental techniques such as ultrasonics, dynamic force plates, and impact loading. Each of these techniques, through the particular nature of the experimental apparatus, is intended to measure a particular mechanical feature of the musculoskeletal system.

Ultrasonics is especially useful in assessing the properties of hard tissue. By its nature, however, the measurements are often invasive. Dynamic force plates are used in assessing the mechanical response of the foot during gait. This equipment is inappropriate for anything but foot-floor reaction forces. Techniques involving impact loading, on the other hand, have the advantage of providing a force similar to that applied to the foot during heel strike as well as the flexibility of applying that force to any part of the body.

The most successful applications of ultrasonics in orthopedics have to date been the assessment of the healing of bone fractures [128] and in the imaging of bone structure [129]. The transducers for such measurements and the associated electronics tend to be costly. The use of mechanical stimulation above 20 kHz is well outside the range of physiologic events, so that the practical use of ultrasonics in the assessment of mechanical response to *in vivo* loads is not feasible.

Several studies using dynamic force plates [130, 131] have shown that during gait the force-time relationship is complex. Such force-time profiles have frequency components centered in the low audio range (DC to 1000 Hz). In comparison, the force-time profile generated in typical impact loading conditions contains much the same frequency components [132]. Thus, a major advantage of the use of impact techniques is the application of loads mechanically similar to the loads the body experiences *in vivo*.

The technique of mechanical impedance[3] measurement involves the assessment of the transmission of a dynamic force from a particular source into or through the body part or tissue being studied [133 to 135]. One method called "swept sine," consists of the application of a sinusoidal mechanical stimulus that is monotonically increasing in frequency, and the determination of the response at each frequency. This is not as physiologically justified as another method: the application of an impact force containing all the frequencies of interest, and the determination of the response as a function of time. The equipment of choice for the latter measurements is a mechanical impedance kit consisting of an instrumented force hammer and an accelerometer (Fig. 4). The force transducer on the hammer allows the determination of the dynamic force input, and the accelerometer allows determination of the response of the body part to that stimulus. The mechanical impedance or mechanical transfer from the hammer to the body part to the accelerometer is taken as the ratio of the response to the stimulus.

A detailed paper [135] has dealt with the electronics necessary to condition the signals generated by the transducers so that reliable recordings can be made. This chapter will be addressed only to the physical basis of the measurements, the interpretation of the results, and the practical advantages to be gained from the interfacing of a computer with the aforementioned electronics. A detailed description of the computer hardware and software can be found elsewhere [121].

Method The accelerometer is placed on the body at a preselected position, a distance away from the point of impaction (Fig. 5). The best choice for points of pickup and impaction tend to be areas of the body with bony prominences close to the skin, i.e., without significant amounts of soft tissue interposed between the bone and the skin. The computer indicates its readiness to accept data by emitting a continuous audible tone. An impact force of short duration is applied at the impaction point. If the level of the force is within a predetermined range, the computer responds by interrupting the tone and printing, on the video display, IMPACT DATA HAS BEEN STORED. If the impact force is too high, the audible tone persists and the computer responds with IMPACT FORCE TOO HIGH, TRY AGAIN. A similar response follows if the impact force is too low. The force and

---

[3]The measurements discussed in the present chapter are not really impedance measurements, but a quantity called inertance, which is defined as acceleration/force. Mechanical impedance is force/velocity. Because of the physical interrelationshps among force, velocity, and acceleration, we chose to use the term mechanical impedance as a generic name for the type of dynamic measurements reported in this chapter.

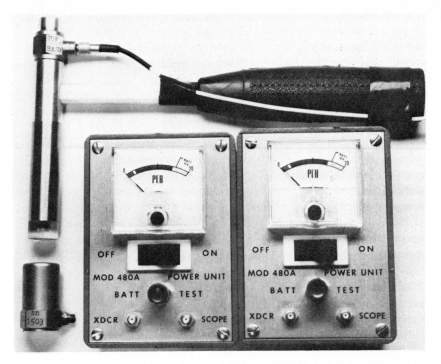

Figure 4 Mechanical impedance kit consisting of instrumented impact hammer, accelerometer, and two power units.

acceleration waveforms are digitized and recorded on a mini-floppy diskette. Only data satisfying the above validity criterion are stored. The data are subsequently analyzed with appropriate software routines.

It is important that the measurements be made by one experimenter, so that the pressure exerted on the transducers tends to be constant [136]. It has been

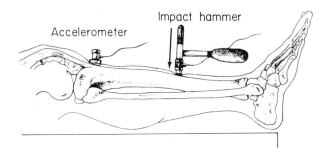

Figure 5 Technique of assessing mechanical impedance of the tibia is to impact the tibia at the midpoint and measure the response at the tibial tubercle. The damped sinusoidal response is controlled by the mass characteristics of the lower leg and the spring constants of the end points of the tibia.

found [137] that humans, with minimal training, are capable of high reproducibility in the application of simple forces requiring finger pressure. It is not important that the impact force be constant, since the data are normalized with regard to this quantity, but data of much higher consistency result when the preload on the accelerometer is maintained constant with hand pressure. In addition, reproducibility is enhanced by care in performing the impaction so that the striker face is parallel to the bone surface and the exact same point is struck in a series of impactions.

The use of a computerized system alleviates several other problems inherent in the measurement of mechanical impedance by a noninvasive technique [137]. Automated data analysis allows more impactions to be performed for each patient, test subject, or test condition, thus assuring a higher level of statistical significance. By providing an interactive mode of testing, spurious impactions and responses are eliminated. These often are caused by slight differences in the positioning of the impact hammer and/or the accelerometer and by slight variations in the pressure of application of either of these devices, as previously mentioned.

Results The previously stored force and acceleration waveforms are analyzed in both the time and frequency domains, using the data-analysis package. This allows the determination of (1) the peak force of impaction F, (2) the magnitude of the maximum peak A_1 of the response, (3) the magnitude of the peak of opposite sign A_2 that follows A_1, (4) the normalized values A_1/F and A_2/F representing the mechanical transfer or inertance, (5) the damping ratio A_2/A_1, and (6) the first 51 Fourier coefficients of the response. Examples of typical results are given in Fig. 6.

The results of all the impactions for a particular test condition can be lumped by the computer, and means and standard deviations automatically printed out. These lumped data can then be automatically tested for significance of difference of the means on either a patient-to-patient basis or a condition-to-condition basis.

Discussion It is instructive to visualize the physical test setup (Fig. 7) as a mass suspended between elastic end points. This reduces to a basic engineering problem, that of forced oscillations of the mass. The mass in this case is the bone onto which

```
AVERAGE IMPACT ANALYSIS PROGRAM

WAVEFORM PEAK VALUES
      -.974 V
      1.248 V
      -.178 V
       .056 V
      -.082 V
       .1  V
      -.04 V

PEAK FORCE INPUT=   .522 V ( 15.1902 LBS.)

    PEAK VALUE (A1)= 1.248 V
    NORMALIZED (A1)= 2.3908

    PEAK VALUE (A2)=-.178 V
    NORMALIZED (A2)=-.340996

  DAMPING RATIO (A2/A1)= .142628

              (a)
```

Figure 6 Typical computer output consisting of the following: (a) peaks of the response, peak force input, normalized values for A_1 and A_2 and the damping ratio, A_2/A_1.

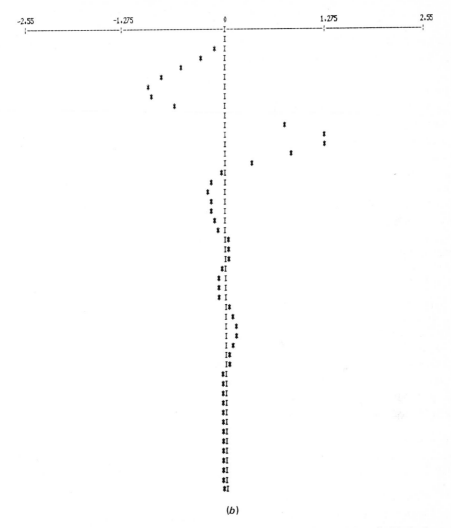

(b)

Figure 6 Typical computer output consisting of the following: (*Continued*) (*b*) Analog reconstruction of the damped sinusoidal response from the digitized data.

the accelerometer is pressed. The elastic end points are the joint surfaces and the associated ligaments and muscle attachments. The response to the impaction is a decaying sinusoid (Fig. 8), which is consistent with such a model. Both the peak normalized force A_1/F and the damping ratio A_2/A_1 are measures of the mechanical transfer during an impaction. Theoretically, differences in the bone mass or in the spring constants of the end points should be reflected in differences in the values of A_1/F and A_2/A_1. Thus, gross bony changes or changes in the joints that alter the spring constants are potentially assessable by the described techniques.

FOURIER SPECTRUM

```
 0  |=================
 1  |=========
 2  |======
 3  |=============
 4  |================
 5  |=====================
 6  |========================
 7  |============================
 8  |============================
 9  |==============================
10  |===================================
11  |==========================================
12  |================================================
13  |=====================================================
14  |======================================================
15  |=======================================================
16  |========================================================
17  |=======================================================
18  |=======================================================
19  |=======================================================
20  |=======================================================
21  |=======================================================
22  |=======================================================
23  |========================================================
24  |=======================================================
25  |=====================================================
26  |===================================================
27  |==============================================
28  |=========================================
29  |======================================
30  |====================================
31  |==================================
32  |================================
33  |=============================
34  |============================
35  |==========================
36  |==========================
37  |=====================
38  |====================
39  |==================
40  |=============
41  |============
42  |==========
43  |=========
44  |========
45  |======
46  |======
47  |=====
48  |====
49  |====
50  |====
```

(c)

Figure 6 Typical computer output consisting of the following: (*Continued*) (*c*) Histogram of the Fourier spectrum.

Furthermore, A_1/F is a measure of the maximum response of the mass under study, or the peak response. Differences in the inherent shock-absorption characteristics of the whole system should be reflected as differences in A_1/F. These peak-response measurements should be relatively independent of the tissue under the point of impaction, since the magnitude of the peak response has been normalized by the impaction force and is thus a measure of the propensity of the system to respond to a unit stimulus. The damping ratio A_2/A_1, in contrast, is a measure of the reduction in

HARMONIC	REAL	IMAGINARY	MAGNITUDE
0	-9.79688E-03	0	9.79688E-03
1	-3.45419E-03	-2.90954E-03	4.51629E-03
2	-5.8239E-04	-3.74321E-03	3.78824E-03
3	-4.26448E-03	-5.41502E-03	6.89263E-03
4	-6.83558E-03	-5.76549E-03	8.94237E-03
5	-8.75917E-03	-5.31829E-03	.0102473
6	-.0113911	-4.36539E-03	.0121989
7	-.0129332	-2.20492E-03	.0131198
8	-.0132484	-1.18414E-03	.0133012
9	-.0152405	-7.94051E-04	.0152611
HARMONIC	REAL	IMAGINARY	MAGNITUDE
10	-.0186813	1.61612E-03	.0187511
11	-.0208855	6.44642E-03	.0218578
12	-.0210072	.0126029	.0244977
13	-.0182187	.0182064	.0257564
14	-.0141915	.0223513	.026476
15	-9.66698E-03	.0251736	.026966
16	-4.16531E-03	.0271206	.0274386
17	1.28629E-03	.0271875	.0272179
18	6.0196E-03	.0263017	.0269818
19	.0108505	.0251523	.0273929
HARMONIC	REAL	IMAGINARY	MAGNITUDE
20	.0155831	.0226752	.0275136
21	.0198322	.019312	.0276816
22	.0235749	.0149016	.0278896
23	.02639	9.10252E-03	.0279157
24	.0272104	2.43565E-03	.0273192
25	.0259419	-4.16076E-03	.0262735
26	.0226195	-.0100992	.0247717
27	.0176105	-.0141475	.0225894
28	.0120787	-.0159093	.019975
29	7.33741E-03	-.015782	.0174043
HARMONIC	REAL	IMAGINARY	MAGNITUDE
30	3.86918E-03	-.01472	.01522
31	1.1303E-03	-.013465	.0135124
32	-9.58678E-04	-.0122413	.0122788
33	-2.76518E-03	-.0109567	.0113003
34	-4.50527E-03	-9.57781E-03	.0105845
35	-6.06556E-03	-7.92993E-03	9.98373E-03
36	-7.17779E-03	-5.93893E-03	9.3162E-03
37	-7.99239E-03	-3.71381E-03	8.8131E-03
38	-8.12465E-03	-1.25416E-03	8.22089E-03
39	-7.44596E-03	1.12427E-03	7.53036E-03
HARMONIC	REAL	IMAGINARY	MAGNITUDE
40	-6.06068E-03	3.10036E-03	6.80765E-03
41	-4.20202E-03	4.32636E-03	6.03112E-03
42	-2.2749E-03	4.74547E-03	5.26258E-03
43	-5.78783E-04	4.54751E-03	4.5842E-03
44	7.14258E-04	3.96181E-03	4.02568E-03
45	1.6581E-03	3.06908E-03	3.48834E-03
46	2.12779E-03	2.18624E-03	3.05076E-03
47	2.30924E-03	1.35911E-03	2.67951E-03
48	2.32219E-03	6.85638E-04	2.42129E-03
49	2.19069E-03	8.07866E-05	2.19218E-03
HARMONIC	REAL	IMAGINARY	MAGNITUDE
50	1.95823E-03	-4.62969E-04	2.01222E-03

(d)

PEAKS (HZ)

233.28
335.34

(e)

Figure 6 Typical computer output consisting of the following: (*Continued*) (*d*) Fourier coefficients of the first 51 components; (*e*) Computer-determined peaks in the Fourier spectrum (this was taken as the center frequency).

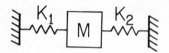

Figure 7 Mass-and-spring model for Fig. 5. The tibia is represented by the mass M. K_1 is the spring constant of the tibio-femoral connection, and K_2 is the spring constant of the connection at the ankle joint.

amplitude of successive oscillations of the mass. High spring constants (stiff cartilage or tense musculature crossing the joint) should result in higher damping ratios. Lower spring constants (softened cartilage) should result in lower damping ratios. Thus, in principle, the peak response and the damping ratio are both measures of the mechanical transfer from the impact hammer into the system and to the accelerometer. The former is a transient response, and the latter is quasi-steady-state.

The data from the Fourier analysis indicate the relative contributions of various frequencies to the response. This is also related to shock absorption in that higher spring constants result in less shock absorption, higher damping ratios, and higher center frequencies of the Fourier series; lower spring constants result in the opposite.

In practice, the measurement of mechanical impedance by the techniques outlined in this chapter has potential value in the noninvasive assessment of the mechanical changes in disease conditions that affect the joints and the bones. The model indicates that the response of the musculoskeletal system to impact forces is damped elastic rebound of the bones between the elastic joints, the constants of which can be varied by muscle tension, bone mass, joint condition, or the physical characteristics of any of the structures spanning a joint.

3.2 Comparison of Impact Responses of Normal and Osteoarthritic Knee Joints

As discussed earlier, the disease process of osteoarthritis is accompanied by clearly delineated physical changes in the afflicted joints. These changes alter the mechanical characteristics of the subchondral bone and the articular cartilage. For example, cartilage softening would result in a predictable change in the force-transmitting properties of the joint. The purpose of this section is to describe the results of experiments designed to characterize the differences in impact response of the lower ex-

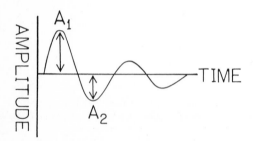

Figure 8 Typical response to impaction showing identification of peaks A_1 and A_2.

tremity in a group of normal test subjects and in a group of patients with varying degrees of osteoarthritis of the knee. Such measurements have potential value in the diagnosis of early changes characteristic of osteoarthritis and in the measurement of changes in shock absorption with osteoarthritis.

The impact force was applied to the heel of supine test subjects. The accelerometer was used to pick up the impact wave at three positions on each test limb: the tibial crest a few centimeters below the tibial tuberosity (shin), over the medial femoral condyle (knee), and on the iliac crest (hip). A total of 19 normal test subjects were impacted on both legs for a total of 38 data points. A total of 17 patients with 33 osteoarthritic knee joints were similarly assessed. The results are shown in Table 2.

Note that a significant difference exists in the amplitude of the impact response for the normals relative to the arthritics at the shin, knee, and hip. The amplitudes are significantly greater for the arthritics. This is consistent with the clinically observed loss of cartilage in the latter group. A reduction in the amount of this shock-absorbing material would be expected to result in higher amplitude of force transmission. Because we are dealing with a series system of mechanical components in the lower extremity, it is not surprising that the amplitudes picked up at the shin and hip are different, although only the knee joint is affected by the disease.

The damping ratio showed a significant difference only at the knee joint. The rebounding of the body parts in the lower extremity exhibits a tendency to damp out at a greater rate for the normals than for the arthritics. This is also consistent with current concepts of shock absorption.

The final part of the study involved a radiographic assessment of the severity of the arthritis of each knee joint. Roentgenograms were distributed in random order to four radiologists. The rating system was from four to zero, with four being the most severe. The main focus of this evaluation was joint space narrowing. However, other features of the disease, such as subchondral sclerosis, cyst formation, periarticular osteophytes, and angulation, were subjectively assessed. The means of the x-ray ratings were then compared with the impact data to find any correlations. No significant correlations were observed. However, for the x-ray ratings versus

**Table 2 Impact data for normals
and osteoarthritics**

Pickup		Normals	Arthritics	Significance
Shin:	A_1	0.74 ± 0.23	1.56 ± 0.62	$p < 0.0005$
	A_2/A_1	0.63 ± 0.23	0.62 ± 0.30	$0.1 < p < 0.25$, NS[*]
Knee:	A_1	0.47 ± 0.20	1.05 ± 0.61	$p < 0.0005$
	A_2/A_2	0.53 ± 0.25	0.69 ± 0.24	$0.005 < p < 0.01$
Hip:	A_1	0.48 ± 0.32	1.07 ± 0.61	$p < 0.0005$
	A_2/A_1	0.48 ± 0.26	0.46 ± 0.21	$0.25 < p$, NS[*]

[*]NS = not significant.

A_2/A_1 at the knee the following data were obtained: $r = 0.239$, $N = 32$, $t = 1.35$, and p was between 0.05 and 0.1. This is just out of the range of significance, and it indicates to us that a functional relationship may exist. We feel that the subjectivity of the x-ray data led to a scatter resulting in a lack of significant p values.

In summary, significant differences were found in the impact responses of a group of normal test subjects and a group of patients with osteoarthritic knees. At the knee, the damping ratio and the amplitude of the impact waves were both significantly higher for the arthritics, consistent with our current understanding of the disease process. The peak-force response of patients with osteoarthritis of the knee joint is shown to be over twice that of patients with normal knee joints. The difference in the response to impact of normal and osteoarthritic knee joints is clearly established. It must be pointed out and emphasized that the patients with osteoarthritis of the knee joint in the present study all had arthritis that was clinically detectable by x-ray, similar to the work on acoustic pattern recognition. However, it can be inferred that this technique also has potential value in assessing the mechanical changes and consequent changes in impact response that exist in prearthritic joints.

3.3 Shock Absorption Due to Musculature in the Constrained Leg

The rigors of the normal daily activity subject the lower extremity to impulsive-type loading. As discussed earlier in this chapter, impact loading has also been related to the propensity for a joint to develop osteoarthritis. It has previously been suggested that bone deformation [97] and the stretching of muscle under tension [138] act to attenuate these potentially destructive dynamic forces. Recent work with rabbits [139] has suggested that these shock-absorbing mechanisms are complementary; i.e., deformation of bone is most effective in reducing higher-frequency peak force components, while muscle contraction under load is more efficient in the attenuation of lower-frequency peak force components. This section presents the results of impact-response studies that have been conducted in an effort to provide further insights into the effect of muscle contraction on the transmission of force in human limbs. This is of value in a description of the precise mechanisms of shock absorption in the musculoskeletal system.

Using an instrumented impact hammer, a force in the range of 9 to 35 lb was applied to the right tibia of 10 grossly normal adult males aged 22 to 49. The midpoint of the distance between the tibial tubercle and malleus was chosen as the tibial impaction point. Transmitted impact-response waveforms were detected by holding a piezoelectric accelerometer firmly against the right tibial tubercle of a supine test subject. The 10 test subjects were impacted under the following conditions: (1) relaxation of the musculature of the right leg prior to and throughout the duration of each impaction, (2) contraction of the quadriceps mechanism of the right leg prior to and throughout the duration of each impaction,

(3) contraction of the quadriceps mechanism of the right leg on command immediately followed by impaction, and (4) relaxation of the quadriceps mechanism of the right leg on command immediately followed by impaction. Thus, the four test conditions were (1) passive relaxed, (2) passive tensed, (3) dynamic tension, and (4) dynamic relaxation. Leg motion occurring during conditions (3) and (4) was limited to 5° or less. The intent of these measurements was to assess the relative shock-absorbing effects of relaxed, tensed, and dynamically tensing and relaxing muscle. Ten impactions per condition were performed, resulting in 40 impactions per subject.

The outputs of the force and acceleration transducers were digitized and recorded on a floppy diskette by a specially designed microcomputer-based impact data acquisition/analysis system [127]. The use of this interactive instrument provided an objective method of recording and analyzing the results of the 400 individual impactions. Stored force and acceleration waveforms were analyzed in the time domain to determine the following waveform characteristics [140]: the peak force of impaction F, the magnitude of the maximum peak A_1 of the transmitted response data and that of the peak of opposite sign A_2 that follows, the normalized values A_1/F and A_2/F, and the damping ratio A_2/A_1. The transmitted response waveforms for each test condition were also averaged in time, and the first 51 Fourier coefficients of the mean data were calculated. The power spectrum was plotted, and the center frequency was determined.

The most consistent results are shown in Tables 3 and 4. No systematic consistencies were noted for the normalized peak responses. There were significant increases in damping ratio for tensed muscle relative to the passive, suggesting reduced shock absorption (1 vs. 2, 1 vs. 3, 1 vs. 4 in Table 3). This is reasonable since tense musculature, whether passive or dynamic, tends to increase the spring constant at the knee joint. It is interesting to note that the greatest increase relative to the passive relaxed muscle was for the passive tensed muscle (65 percent), and

Table 3 Mean A_2/A_1 compared by Student's t-test

| Test subject | Percent difference | | | | | |
	1 vs. 2	1 vs. 3	2 vs. 3	1 vs. 4	2 vs. 4	3 vs. 4
1	↑ 48	↑ 24	↓ 16	↑ 32	NS*	NS*
2	↑ 29	↑ 16	↓ 10	NS	↓ 22	↓ 14
3	↑ 19	NS	↓ 13	NS	↓ 20	↓ 8
4	↑ 25	↑ 67	↑ 33	↑ 38	NS	NS
5	↑ 21	NS	NS	↑ 15	NS	NS
6	NS	NS	↑ 47	NS	↓ 35	↓ 56
7	↑ 43	NS	↓ 24	NS	↓ 39	NS
8	↑ 140	↑ 100	↓ 17	NS	↓ 36	NS
9	NS	↓ 27	↓ 23	↓ 24	↓ 21	NS
10	↑ 194	↑ 67	↓ 43	↑ 44	↓ 51	NS
Mean	↑ 65	↑ 41	↓ 7	↑ 21	↓ 32	↓ 26

*NS = no significant difference.

Table 4 Center frequency compared by Student's *t*-test

Test subjects	Percent difference; change in frequency					
	1 vs. 2	1 vs. 3	2 vs. 3	1 vs. 4	2 vs. 4	3 vs. 4
1	↑ 23; 218→268	NS*	↓ 15; 268→227	NS	NS	NS
2	NS	↓ 11; 226→202	NS	↓ 11; 226→202	NS	NS
3	↓ 19; 259→210	↓ 27; 259→190	↓ 10; 210→190	↓ 14; 259→223	NS	↑ 17; 190→223
4	↑ 21; 174→210	↑ 24; 174→215	NS	↑ 9; 174→190	↓ 10; 210→190	NS
5	↓ 26; 242→178	↓ 22; 242→188	NS	↓ 23; 242→187	NS	NS
6	↑ 47; 158→233	↑ 42; 158→224	NS	NS	↓ 29; 233→166	↓ 26; 224→166
↑7	↑ 108; 149→310	↑ 85; 149→276	NS	↓ 42; 149→212	↓ 32; 310→212	↓ 23; 276→212
8	↑ 28; 172→220	↑ 42; 172→245	NS	NS	↓ 17; 220→182	↓ 26; 245→182
9	↑ 45; 195→282	NS	↓ 27; 282→207	↑ 23; 195→240	↓ 15; 282→240	↑ 16; 207→240
10	↑ 85; 198→366	↑ 41; 198→280	↓ 23; 366→280	↑ 45; 198→288	↓ 21; 366→288	NS
Mean	↑ 35	↑ 22	↓ 19	↓ 10	↓ 21	↓ 8

*NS = no significant difference.

that the increase descended in magnitude in the order dynamic contraction (41 percent) and dynamic relaxation (21 percent).

In comparing passive tensed muscle with the dynamic conditions, the damping ratios both decreased, implying increased shock absorption for dynamic contraction (7 percent) and for dynamic relaxation (32 percent). The 26 percent reduction in damping ratio for dynamic relaxation relative to dynamic contraction further supports the observation of greater shock-absorbing capacity with extension of tensed muscle than with contraction.

The frequency-response measurements showed remarkable consistency with the measurements of damping ratio. With the exception of test condition 1 vs. 4, significant increases or decreases in damping ratio were accompanied by significant increases or decreases, respectively, in center frequency. Shifts to higher frequency are consistent with decreased shock absorption, as are increases in damping ratio.

The finding of significant increases in the damping ratio with passive and dynamic muscle tension relative to the relaxed condition implies a significant shock-absorption contribution of the tensed musculature, consistent with the work of others. However, this study implies, for the constraint of no joint motion, that less shock is absorbed as a result of the tensed musculature. Forced stretching of tensed muscle is generally regarded as a major shock-absorbing mechanism [141]. Furthermore, a tense muscle cannot be forcibly extended except by joint motion. Therefore we conclude that the *major* contributor to dynamic shock absorption is joint motion controlled by tense muscle, rather than shock absorption by tensed muscle per se. There is no apparent shock-absorbing effect due to passively tensed muscle. We did, however, find significant increases in shock absorption for dynamic contraction and relaxation of tensed muscle relative to passively tensed muscle. The fractional change was less than one-third. We take this as further support of our contention that the contribution of muscle to shock absorption is minimal.

We feel that our results confirm the concept that active shock absorption by the musculature must occur concurrently with joint flexion or extension. Furthermore, this implies that the shock absorption occurring in this condition is mainly neuromuscular and dynamic in nature. It is suggested that the actual contribution to shock absorption due to muscle stretching per se without significant joint motion, that is, at heel strike during normal gait, is minimal. This relates to the disease process of osteoarthritis in that more impact energy must be dissipated by the bone and cartilage. Thus, the critical shock-absorbing role of the bone and cartilage in normal joint functioning is further emphasized.

REFERENCES

1. F. T. Hoaglund, Osteoarthritis, *Orthop. Clin. North Am.*, vol. 2, pp. 3–18, 1971.
2. H. J. Mankin and L. Lippiello, Biochemical and Metabolic Abnormalities in Articular Cartilage from Osteo-Arthritic Human Hips, *J. Bone Jt. Surg.*, vol. 52A, pp. 424–434, 1970.
3. H. J. Mankin, Biochemical and Metabolic Aspects of Osteoarthritis, *Orthop. Clin. North Am.*, vol. 2, pp. 19–31, 1971.
4. H. J. Mankin, The Reaction of Articular Cartilage to Injury and Osteoarthritis, part 1, *N. Eng. J. Med.*, vol. 291, pp. 1285–1292, 1974.

5. H. J. Mankin, The Reaction of Articular Cartilage to Injury and Osteoarthritis, part 2, *N. Eng. J. Med.*, vol. 291, pp. 1335–1340, 1974.

6. L. Sokoloff, "The Biology of Degenerative Joint Disease," University of Chicago Press, Chicago, 1969.

7. I. H. Emery and G. Meachin, Surface Morphology and Topography of Patello-Femoral Cartilage Fibrillation in Liverpool Necropsies, *J. Anat.*, vol. 116, pp. 103–120, 1973.

8. P. Ficat, Arthrose et necrose, *Rev. Chir. Orthop.*, vol. 60, pp. 123–133, 1974.

9. E. Vignon, M. Arlot, and G. Vignon, Le Vieillissement de cartilage de la tête fémorale humaine, étude macroscopique de 42 pieces, *Lyon Med.*, vol. 229, pp. 661–669, 1973.

10. G. Vignon, P. Meunier, E. Vignon, and M. Arlot, Le Cartilage fémoral senescent et arthrosique. Données macroscopiques comparatives, *Rev. Rhum.*, vol. 41, pp. 25–27, 1974.

11. M. A. R. Freeman, "Adult Articular Cartilage," Grune & Stratton, New York, 1973.

12. J. Trueta, "Studies of the Development and Decay of the Human Frame," Saunders, Philadelphia, 1968.

13. H. J. Mankin, personal communication, 1973.

14. V. Wright, Tribology and Arthritis, V. Wright (ed.), "Lubrication and Wear in Joints," Lippincott, London, 1969.

15. E. L. Radin, I. L. Paul, and R. M. Rose, Hypothesis: Role of Mechanical Factors in the Pathogenesis of Primary Osteoarthritis, *Lancet*, vol. 1, pp. 519–522, 1972.

16. L. E. Lanyon, Experimental Support for the Trajectorial Theory of Bone Structure, *J. Bone Jt. Surg.*, vol. 56B, pp. 160–166, 1974.

17. K. J. Munzenberg, R. Nienhaus, H. Reischauer, and H. L. Klammer, The Internal Architecture of the Proximal end of Femur as an Indicator of the Loss of Bone Substance Due to Age, *Z. Orthop.*, vol. 111, pp. 874–880, 1973.

18. W. Prager, Optimization of Structural Design, *J. Optim. Theory Appl.*, vol. 6, pp. 1–21, 1970.

19. G. P. Vose, Review of Roentgenographic Bone Demineralization Studies of the Gemini Space Flights, *Am. J. Roentgenol. Radium Ther. Nucl. Med.*, vol. 121, pp. 1–4, 1974.

20. H. Appel and S. Friberg, Effect of Osteotomy on Pain in Idiopathic Osteoarthritis of the Hip, *Acta Orthop. Scand.*, vol. 44, pp. 710–718, 1973.

21. D. R. Bard, M. J. Dickens, J. Edwards, and A. U. Smith, Studies on Slices and Isolated Cells from Fresh Osteoarthritic Human Bone, *J. Bone Jt. Surg.*, vol. 56B, pp. 340–351, 1974.

22. D. R. Bard, M. J. Dickens, J. Edwards, and A. U. Smith, Ultra-Structure, *in Vitro* Cultivation and Metabolism of Cells Isolated from Arthritic Human Bone, *J. Bone Jt. Surg.*, vol. 56B, pp. 352–360, 1974.

23. K. D. Brandt, C. P. Tsiganos, and H. Muir, Immunological Relationships between Proteoglycans of Different Hydrodynamic Size from Articular Cartilage of Foetal and Mature Pigs, *Biochim. Biophys. Acta*, vol. 320, pp. 453–468, 1973.

24. P. D. Byers and M. R. C. Path, The Effect of High Femoral Osteotomy on Osteoarthritis of the Hip, *J. Bone Jt. Surg.*, vol. 56B, pp. 279–290, 1974.

25. P. D. Byers, F. T. Hoaglund, G. W. Purewal, and A. C. M. C. Yau, Articular Cartilage Changes in Caucasian and Asian Hip Joints, *Ann. Rheum. Dis.*, vol. 33, pp. 157–161, 1974.

26. H. O. Dustmann, W. Puhl, and B. Krempien, Phenomenon of Clusters in Arthrotic Articular Cartilage, *Arch. Orthop. Unfall-Chir.*, vol. 79, pp. 321–333, 1974.

27. R. Fridrich and W. Muller, Scanning and Function Studies in Arthritic Disease, *Radiol. Clin. Biol.*, vol. 43, pp. 313–317, 1974.

28. I. Goldie, Erosive Osteoarthritis of the Distal Finger Joints, *Acta Orthop. Scand.*, vol. 43, pp. 469–478, 1972.

29. T. L. Gritzka, L. R. Fry, R. L. Cheesman, and A. LaVigne, Deterioration of Articular Cartilage Caused by Continuous Compression in a Moving Rabbit Joint, *J. Bone Jt. Surg.*, vol. 55A, pp. 1698–1720, 1973.

30. M. Hackenbroch, About Functional Insufficiency, Arthrosis and Prearthrosis, *Z. Orthop.,* vol. 112, pp. 23–27, 1974.

31. F. D. Hart, Pain in Osteoarthrosis, *Practitioner,* vol. 212, pp. 244–250, 1974.

32. R. Lagier, Femoral Cortical Erosions and Osteoarthritis of the Knee with Condrocalcinosis, *Fortschr. Geb. Roentgenstr.,* vol. 120, pp. 460–467, 1974.

33. P. Lereim, I. Goldie, and E. Dahlberg, Hardness of the Subchondral Bone of the Tibial Condyles in the Normal State and in Osteoarthritis and Rheumatoid Arthritis, *Acta Orthop. Scand.,* vol. 45, pp. 614–627, 1974.

34. M. B. Mayor and R. W. Moskowitz, Metabolic Studies in Experimentally Induced Degenerative Joint Disease in the Rabbit, *J. Rheumatol.,* vol. 1, pp. 17–23, 1974.

35. G. Meachim and I. H. Emery, Cartilage Fibrillation in Shoulder and Hip Joints in Liverpool Necropsies, *J. Anat.,* vol. 116, pp. 161–179, 1973.

36. G. Meachim, Articulai Cartilage Lesions in Osteo-Arhtritis of the Femoral Head, *J. Pathol.,* vol. 107, pp. 199–210, 1972.

37. G. Meachim, Light Microscopy of Indian Ink Preparations of Fibrillated Cartilage, *Ann. Rheum. Dis.,* vol. 31, pp. 457–464, 1972.

38. M. Nimni and K. Deshmukh, Differences in Collagen Metabolism between Normal and Osteoarthritic Human Articular Cartilage, *Science,* vol. 181, pp. 751–752, 1973.

39. W. H. Pool, Jr., Cartilage Atrophy, *Radiology,* vol. 112, pp. 47–50, 1974.

40. J. Radke, Autoradiographische Befunde bei degenerativen Huftgel enkserkrankungen, *Z. Orthop.,* vol. 112, pp. 273–282, 1974.

41. U. N. Riede, G. Schweizer, and H. Willenegger, Gelenkmechanische Untersuchungen zum Problem der posttraumatischen Arthrosen im Oberen Sprunggelenk. III, Functional Morphometric Analysis of the Articular Cartilage, *Langenbecks Arch. Chir.,* vol. 333, pp. 91–107, 1973.

42. I. Reimann, Experimental Osteoarthritis of the Knee in Rabbits Induced by Alteration of the Load-Bearing, *Acta Orthop. Scand.,* vol. 44, pp. 496–504, 1973.

43. Y. S. Roh, J. Dequeker, and J. C. Mulier, Cortical Bone Remodeling and Bone Mass in Primary Osteoarthrosis of the Hip, *Invest. Radiol.,* vol. 8, pp. 251–254, 1973.

44. Y. S. Roh, J. Dequeker, and J. C. Mulier, Osteoarthrosis at the Hand Skeleton in Primary Osteoarthrosis of the Hip and in Normal Controls, *Clin. Orthop.,* vol. 90, pp. 90–94, 1973.

45. Y. S. Roh, J. Dequeker, and J. C. Mulier, Bone Mass in Osteoarthrosis, Measured *in Vivo* by Photon Absorption, *J. Bone Jt. Surg.,* vol. 56A, pp. 587–591, 1974.

46. Y. S. Roh, J. Dequeker, and J. C. Mulier, Trabecular Pattern of the Upper End of the Femur in Primary Osteoarthrosis and in Symptomatic Osteoporosis, *J. Belge Radiol.,* vol. 57, pp. 89–94, 1974.

47. J. F. Schweigel, The Rationale for Tibial Osteotomy in the Treatment of Osteoarthritis of the Knee, *Surg. Gynecol. Obstet.,* vol. 138, pp. 533–536, 1974.

48. D. C. Silcox and D. J. McCarthy, Jr., Elevated Inorganic Pyrophosphate Concentrations in Synovial Fluids in Osteoarthritis and Pseudogout, *J. Lab. Clin. Med.,* vol. 83, pp. 518–531, 1974.

49. L. Sokoloff, Cell Biology and the Repair of Articular Cartilage, *J. Rheumatol.,* vol. 1, pp. 9–16, 1974.

50. K. H. Sorensen and H. E. Christensen, Local Amyloid Formation in the Hip Joint Capsule in Osteoarthritis, *Acta Orthop. Scand.,* vol. 44, pp. 460–466, 1973.

51. H. Telhag, Mitosis of Chondrocytes In Experimental "Osteoarthritis" in Rabbits, *Clin. Orthop.,* vol. 86, pp. 224–229, 1972.

52. H. Telhag and L. Lindberg A Method for Inducing Osteoarthritic Changes in Rabbits' Knees, *Clin. Orthop.,* vol. 86, pp. 214–223, 1972.

53. R. C. Thompson, Jr., and C. A. L. Bassett, Histological Observations on Experimentally Induced Degeneration of Articular Cartilage, *J. Bone Jt. Surg.,* vol. 52A, pp. 435–443, 1970.

54. P. A. Toller, Osteoarthrosis of the Mandibular Condyle, *Br. Dent. J.,* vol. 134, pp. 223–231, 1973.

55. R. Ueno, Ergebnisse der Behandlung mit einem Mucopolysaccharidpolyschwefelsaureester bei der experimentallen Arthrose des Kniegelenks, *Z. Orthop.*, vol. 111, pp. 886–892, 1973.

56. E. Vignon, P. Meunier, M. Arlot, J. P. Boissel, L. M. Patricot, and G. Vignon, Données histologiques quantitatives sur les modifications du cartilage de la tête fémorale humaine en fonction des zones de pression, *Pathol. Biol.*, vol. 21, pp. 1057–1061, 1973.

57. V. K. Walcher and P. H. Weitnauer, Quantitative morphometrische Untersuchungen der Sponiosastruktur des Kniegelenkes des Kaninchens nach Immobilization und dosierter Druckbelastung, *Mikrosk. Bull.*, vol 30, pp. 71–79, 1974.

58. C. Weiss and S. Mirow, An Ultrastructural Study of Osteoarthritic Changes in the Articular Cartilage of Human Knees, *J. Bone Jt., Surg.*, vol. 54, pp. 954–972, 1972.

59. C. Weiss, Ultrastructural Characteristics of Osteoarthritis, *Fed. Proc.*, vol. 32, pp. 1459–1466, 1973.

60. G. Arnold and C. Hartung, Histomechanical Behavior of Hyaline Cartilage under Cyclic Deformations, *Z. Anat. Entwicklungsgesch.*, vol. 144, pp. 303–313, 1974.

61. F. Gross, G. Arnold, and C. Hartung, Polorisationsoptische und biomechanische Untersuchungen hyalinen Knorpels, *Z. Orthop.*, vol. 112, pp. 1014–1017, 1974.

62. G. E. Kempson, M. A. R. Freeman, and S. A. V. Swanson, The Determination of a Creep Modulus for Articular Cartilage from Indentation Test on the Human Femoral Head, *J. Biomech.*, vol. 4, pp. 239–250, 1971.

63. L. Rosenberg, Chemical Basis for the Histological Use of Safranin-O in the Study of Articular Cartilage, *J. Bone Jt. Surg.*, vol. 53, pp. 69–82, 1971.

64. H. J. Mankin and A. Zarins, Water Binding in Normal and Osteoarthritic Cartilage, presented at the Annual Meeting of the Orthopaedic Research Society, Dallas, 1974.

65. C. W. McCutchen, Boundary Lubrication by Synovial Fluid: Demonstration and Possible Osmotic Explanation, *Fed. Proc.*, vol. 25, pp. 1061–1068, 1966.

66. G. Meachim, D. Denham, I. H. Emery, and P. H. Wilinson, Collagen Alignments and Artificial Splits at the Surface of Human Articular Cartilage, *J. Anat.*, vol. 118, pp. 101–118, 1974.

67. B. O. Weightman, M. A. R. Freeman, and S. A. V. Swanson, Fatigue of Articular Cartilage, *Nature*, vol. 244, pp. 303–304, 1973.

68. P. Walker, J. Sikorski, D. Dowson, M. Longfield, and V. Wright, Lubrication Mechanism in Human Joints: A Study by Scanning Electron Microscopy, in V. Wright (ed.), "Lubrication and Wear in Joints," pp. 49–56, Lippincott, London, 1969.

69. I. C. Clarke, The Microevaluation of Articular Surface Contours, *Ann. Biomed. Eng.*, vol. 1, pp. 31–43, 1972.

70. D. L. Gardner, The Influence of Microscopic Technology on Knowledge of Cartilage Surface Structure, *Ann. Rheum. Dis.*, vol. 31, pp. 235–258, 1972.

71. F. N. Ghadially, R. L. Ailsby, and A. K. Oryschak, Scanning Electron Microscopy of Superficial Defects in Articular Cartilage, *Ann. Rheum. Dis.*, vol. 33, pp. 327–332, 1974.

72. V. C. Mow, W. M. Lai, and I. Redler, Some Surface Characteristics of Articular Cartilage. I. A Scanning Electron Microscopy Study and a Theoretical Model for the Dynamic Interaction of Synovial Fluid and Articular Cartilage, *J. Biomech.*, vol. 7, pp. 449–456, 1974.

73. W. Puhl, Die Mikromorphologie gesunder Gelenkknorpeloberflachen, *Z. Orthop.*, vol. 112, pp. 262–272, 1974.

74. I. Redler, A Scanning Electron Microscopic Study of Human Normal and Osteoarthritic Articular Cartilage, *Clin. Orthop. Relat. Res.*, vol. 103, pp. 262–268, 1974.

75. H. J. Refior, Vergleichende experimentelle Untersuchen zur Mikromorphologies der Praarthrose zum Beispiel des Kaninchenkniegelenkes, *Z. Orthop.*, vol. 112, pp. 706–709, 1974.

76. N. Rydell, Forces in the Hip-Joint, part II, Intravital Measurements, in R. M. Kenedi (ed.), "Biomechanics and Related Bio-Engineering Topics," pp. 351–357, Pergamon, Oxford, 1965.

77. M. W. Ropes and W. Bauer, "Synovial Fluid Changes in Joint Diseases," Harvard University Press, Cambridge, Mass., 1953.
78. L. Sundblad, Studies on Hyaluronic Acid in Synovial Fluids, *Acta Soc. Med. Ups.*, vol. 58, pp. 113–237, 1953.
79. J. R. E. Fraser, W. K. Foo, and J. S. Maritz, Viscous Interactions of Hyaluronic Acid with Some Proteins and Neutral Saccharides, *Ann. Rheum. Dis.*, vol. 31, pp. 513–520, 1972.
80. D. A. Swann, E. L. Radin, M. Nazimiec, P. A. Weisser, N. Curran, and G. Lewinnek, Role of Hyaluronic Acid in Joint Lubrication, *Ann. Rheum. Dis.*, vol. 33, pp. 318–326, 1974.
81. E. L. Radin and I. L. Paul, A Consolidated Concept of Joint Lubrication, *J. Bone Jt. Surg.*, vol. 54A, pp. 607–616, 1972.
82. C. W. McCutchen, Why Did Nature Make Synovial Fluid Slimy? *Clin. Orthop.*, vol. 64, pp. 18–20, 1969.
83. V. Frankel and A. Burstein, "Orthopaedic Biomechanics," Chap. 6, Lea & Febiger, Philadelphia, 1970.
84. P. S. Walker, The Contact Situation in Joints Shown by Scanning Electron Microscopy, *Rev. Hosp. Spec. Surg.*, vol. 2, pp. 66–76, 1972.
85. R. Kölbel, Current Concepts of Lubrication in Animal Joints, *Arch. Orthop. Unfall-Chir.*, vol. 78, pp. 50–61, 1974.
86. V. C. Mow, W. M. Lai, J. Eisenfeld, and I. Redler, Some Surface Characteristics of Articular Cartilage. II, On the Stability of Articular Surface and a Possible Biomechanical Factor in Etiology of Chondrodegeneration, *J. Biomech.*, vol. 7, pp. 457–468, 1974.
87. M. L. Zimny and I. Redler, Scanning Electron Microscopy of Chondrocytes, *Acta Anat.*, vol. 83, pp. 398–402, 1972.
88. M. A. R. Freeman, W. H. Day, and S. A. V. Swanson, Fatigue Fracture in the Subchondral Bone of the Human Cadaver Femoral Head, *Med. Biol. Eng.*, vol. 9, pp. 619–629, 1971.
89. J. M. Morris and L. D. Blickenstaff, "Fatigue Fractures—A Clinical Study," Thomas, Springfield, Ill., 1967.
90. J. G. Peyron, La Plaque osseuse sous-chondrale, *Rev. Rhum.*, vol. 41, pp. 285–291, 1974.
91. C. J. Pirie, A Technique for Isolating Small Lesions within the Whole Femoral Head, *Med. Lab. Technol.*, vol. 29, pp. 315–318, 1972.
92. E. L. Radin, I. L. Paul, and M. Tolkoff, Subchondral Bone Changes in Patients with Early Degenerative Joint Disease, *Arthritis Rheum.*, vol. 13, pp. 400–405, 1970.
93. S. R. Simon, E. L. Radin, I. L. Paul, and R. M. Rose. The Response of Joints to Impact Loading. II, *in Vivo* Behavior of Subchondral Bone, *J. Biomech.*, vol. 5, pp. 267–272, 1972.
94. R. C. Todd, M. A. R. Freeman, and C. J. Pirie, Isolated Trabecular Fatigue Fractures in the Femoral Head, *J. Bone Jt. Surg.*, vol. 54B, pp. 723–728, 1972.
95. B. Vernon-Roberts and C. J. Pirie, Healing Trabecular Microfractures in the Bodies of Lumbar Vertebrae, *Ann. Rheum. Dis.*, vol. 32, pp. 406–412, 1973.
96. C. E. Crede, "Shock and Vibration Concepts in Engineering Design," p. 128, Prentice-Hall, Englewood Cliffs, N.J., 1965.
97. E. L. Radin and I. L. Paul, Does Cartilage Compliance Reduce Skeletal Impact Loads? The Relative Force-Attenuating Properties of Articular Cartilage, Synovial Fluid, Periarticular Soft Tissues, and Bone, *Arthritis Rheum.* vol. 13, pp. 139–144, 1970.
98. E. L. Radin, I. L. Paul, and M. Lowy, A Comparison of the Dynamic Force-Transmitting Properties of Subchondral Bone and Articular Cartilage, *J. Bone Jt. Surg.*, vol. 52A, pp. 444–456, 1970.
99. S. A. V. Swanson and M. A. R. Freeman, Is Bone Hydraulically Strengthened? *Med. Biol. Eng.*, vol. 4, pp. 433–438, 1966.
100. C. Wistar, "A System of Anatomy," vol. I, p. 2, Carey and Lea, Philadelphia, 1825.
101. J. Wolff, Ueber die innere Architectur der Knochen und ihre Bedeutung fur de Frage vom Knochenwashstum, *Virchows Arch. Pathol. Anat.*, vol. 50, pp. 389–453, 1870.
102. J. C. Behrens, P. S. Walker, and H. Shoji, Variations in Strength and Structure of Cancellous Bone at the Knee, *J. Biomech.*, vol. 7, pp. 201–207, 1974.

103. W. A. Merz and R. K. Schenk, A Quantitative Histological Study on Bone Formation in Human Cancellous Bone, *Acta Anat.*, vol. 76, pp. 1-15, 1970.
104. W. A. Merz and R. K. Schenk, Quantitative Structural Analysis of Human Cancellous Bone, *Acta Anat.*, vol. 75, pp. 54-66, 1970.
105. W. J. Whitehouse, A Stereological Method for Calculating Internal Surface Areas in Structures which Have Become Anisotropic as the Result of Linear Expansions or Contractions, *J. Microsc.*, vol. 101, pp. 169-176, 1974.
106. W. J. Whitehouse, The Quantitative Morphology of Anisotropic Trabecular Bone, *J. Microsc.*, vol. 101, 153-168, 1974.
107. A. H. Burstein, B. W. Shaffer, and V. H. Frankel, Elastic Analysis of Condylar Structures, *ASME Pub.* 70-WA/BHF-1, 1970.
108. J. W. Pugh, R. M. Rose, and E. L. Radin, Techniques for the Study of the Structure of Bone, *Microstructures,* vol. 3, pp. 22-27, 1970.
109. E. L. Radin, H. G. Parker, J. W. Pugh, R. S. Steinberg, I. L. Paul, and R. M. Rose, Response of Joints to Impact Loading. III, Relationship between Trabecular Microfractures and Cartilage Degeneration, *J. Biomech.*, vol. 6, pp. 51-57, 1973.
110. J. W. Pugh, R. M. Rose, and E. L. Radin, Elastic and Viscoelastic Properties of Trabecular Bone, *J. Biomech.*, vol. 6, pp. 475-485, 1973.
111. J. W. Pugh, R. M. Rose, and E. L. Radin, A Structural Model for the Mechanical Behavior of Trabecular Bone, *J. Biomech.,* vol. 6, pp. 657-670, 1973.
112. J. W. Pugh, R. M. Rose, and E. L. Radin, Quantitative Studies of Human Subchondral Cancellous Bone. Its Relationship to the State of Its Overlying Cartilage, *J. Bone Jt. Surg.,* vol. 56, pp. 313-321, 1974.
113. J. W. Pugh, R. M. Rose, and E. L. Radin, A Possible Mechanism of Wolff's Law: Trabecular Microfractures, *Arch. Int. Physiol. Bioch.,* vol. 81, pp. 27-40, 1973.
114. J. W. Pugh, The Micro-Mechanics of Cancellous Bone. I, Microscopic Observations, *Bull. Hosp. Jt. Dis.,* vol. 34, pp. 92-106, 1973.
115. J. W. Pugh, R. M. Rose, E. L. Radin, and I. L. Paul, Mechanical Resonance Spectra in Human Cancellous Bone, *Science,* vol. 181, pp. 271-272, 1973.
116. J. W. Pugh and G. C. Steiner, Relationship between Structure and Mechanical Resonance Spectra in Human Cancellous Bone, Proceedings of the 27th Annual Conference on Engineering in Medicine and Biology, Philadelphia, p. 292, 1974.
117. J. W. Pugh and G. C. Steiner, Relationship between Structure and Mechanical Resonance Spectra in Human Cancellous Bone, *Med. & Biol. Eng.,* vol. 13, pp. 714-716, 1975.
118. J. W. Pugh, J. C. Runkle, R. M. Rose, E. L. Radin, and I. L. Paul, Determination of the Elastic Modulus of Individual Trabeculae by their Buckling Behavior, Proceedings of the 19th Annual Meeting of the Orthopaedic Research Society, Las Vegas, p. 12, 1973; abstracted in *J. Bone Jt. Surg.,* vol. 55, p. 651, 1973.
119. J. W. Pugh, S. P. Lasser, and E. D. Seldman, Preferred Orientations in Cancellous Bone: Techniques for Determination and Possible Biomechanical Significance, Proceedings of the 29th Annual Conference on Engineering in Medicine and Biology, Boston, Massachusetts, p. 110, 1976.
120. R. Israel, A. Streitman and J. Pugh, Impact Response of Normal and Osteoarthritic Knee Joints, *Proc. 30th Annual Conf. Eng. in Med. and Biol.*, p. 85, 1977.
121. A. Streitmen and J. Pugh, Shock Absorption Due to Musculature in the Contrained Leg, *Proc. 32d Annual Conf. Eng. in Med. and Biol.*, p. 68, 1979.
122. J. Black, Comment on Mechanical Resonance Spectra in Human Cancellous Bone, *Science*, vol. 181, p. 273, 1973.
123. E. R. Fitzgerald, personal communication, 1974.
124. J. W. Pugh and R. M. Rose, Mechanical Behavior of Cancellous Bone: A Finite Element Model, Proceedings of the New England Bioengineering Conference, Burlington, Vermont, pp. 46-63, 1973.

125. E. C. Ewald, R. Poss, K. Hirohasi, A. L. Schiller, and C. D. Sledge, Hip Arthroplasty in Dogs Using Normal Articular Cartilage Supported by Methylmethacrylate–An Experimental Model for Osteoarthritis, to be published.

126. M. L. Chu, A. Gradisar, M. R. Railey, and G. F. Bowling, Detection of Knee Joint Diseases Using Acoustical Pattern Recognition Techniques, *J. Biomech.,* vol. 9, pp. 111–114, 1976.

127. A. Streitman, A Microcomputer-Based Data Acquisition/Analysis System for Characterization of the Mechanical Properties of the Lower Extremity, M.S. thesis, Fairleigh-Dickinson University, Teaneck, N.J., 1979.

128. S. A. Brown, Polymeric Fixation and Ultrasonic Assessment of Fractures and Healing, *Bull. Hosp. Jt. Dis.,* vol. 38, pp. 29–30, 1977.

129. R. W. Porter, M. Wicks, and D. Ottewell, Measurement of the Spinal Canal by Diagnostic Ultrasound, *J. Bone Jt. Surg.,* vol. 60B, pp. 481–484, 1978.

130. J. P. Paul, Bio-engineering Studies of the Forces Transmitted by Joints, Part II, Engineering Analysis, in R. M. Kenedi (ed.), "Biomechanics and Related Bioengineering Topics," pp. 369–380, Pergamon, Oxford, 1965.

131. T. P. Andriacchi, J. A. Ogle, and J. O. Galante, Walking Speed as a Basis for Normal and Abnormal Gait Measurements, *J. Biomech.,* vol. 10, pp. 261–268, 1977.

132. J. W. Pugh, A. I. Streitman, and J. F. Stanoch, Studies of the Impact Response of Human Limbs, *Proc.* 28th Annual Conf. *Eng. in Med. and Biol.,* p. 171, 1975.

133. G. F. Lang. Understanding Vibration Measurements, Appl. Note 9, Nicolet Scientific Corp., 245 Livingston St., Northvale, N.J. 07647.

134. G. F. Lang, Shake, Rattle, or Rap? Or How to Conduct Vibration Tests, Appl. Note 10, Nicolet Scientific Corp., 245 Livingston St., Northvale, N.J. 07647, 1975.

135. A. Streitman and J. Pugh, The Response of the Lower Extremity to Impact Forces. I, Design of an Economical Low Frequency Recording System for Physiologic Waveforms, *Bull. Hosp. Jt. Dis.,* vol. 39, pp. 63–73, 1978.

136. S. Saha and R. Lakes, The Effect of Soft Tissue on the Wave-Propagation and Vibration Tests for Determining the *in Vivo* Properties of Bone, *J. Biomech.,* vol. 10, pp. 393–401, 1977.

137. M. Gordon and J. Pugh, Reproducibility of Insertion Torques for a Variety of Bone Screws, to be published.

138. E. L. Radin, I. L. Paul, and R. M. Rose, Hypothesis: Role of Mechanical Factors in the Pathogenesis of Primary Osteoarthritis, *Lancet*, vol. 1, p. 5, 1972.

139. I. L. Paul, M. B. Munro, P. J. Abernethy, S. R. Simon, E. L. Radin, and R. M. Rose, Musculoskeletal Shock Absorption: Relative Contribution of Bone and Soft Tissues at Various Frequencies, *J. Biomech.*, vol. 11, pp. 237–240, 1978.

140. R. M. Israel, A. I. Strictman, and I. W. Pugh, Impact Response of Normal and Osteoarthritic Knee Joints, Proc. 23rd Annual Meeting of the Orthopaedic Research Society, Las Vegas, Nevada, p. 223, 1977.

141. E. L. Radin, "Practical Biomechanics for the Orthopedic Surgeon," pp. 98–99, Wiley, New York, 1979.

142. P. Raux, P. R. Townsend, R. Miegel, R. M. Rose, and E. L. Radin, Trabecular Architecture of the Human Patella, *J. Biomech.*, vol. 8, pp. 1–8, 1975.

143. P. R. Townsend, P. Raux, R. M. Rose, R. E. Miegel, and E. L. Radin, The Distribution and Anisotropy of the Stiffness of Cancellous Bone in the Human Patella, *J. Biomech.*, vol. 8, pp. 363–368, 1975.

FIVE

FINITE-ELEMENT APPLICATIONS IN JOINT-REPLACEMENT DESIGN AND ANALYSIS

Thomas P. Andriacchi and Steven J. Hampton

The formulation of the finite-element method and its application to the stress analysis of total joint implants are presented. Particular attention is given to the analysis of the femoral stem of a total hip prosthesis, its interaction with the cement, its implications in delineating the causes of failure of such prostheses, and suggestions for design improvements.

1 INTRODUCTION

Successful clinical application of total joint replacements is one of the most important recent developments of orthopedic surgery. Indications for their use are, however, still limited, owing to the many unknowns that surround the long-term survival of these devices. At first glance the potential for mechanical failure of these devices seems small. The metal or plastic components have mechanical properties that appear to surpass those of the biological materials being replaced. However, clinical experience has indicated that many of the failures (including component fractures) of these devices can be traced to mechanical causes (Fig. 1). Numerous parameters associated with the design of an implant can be analyzed in purely mechanical terms. Many of these parameters are interrelated, but from a practical viewpoint it is possible to define them as follows: (1) fixation to bone, (2) strength of prosthetic component, (3) wear of articulating surfaces, (4) kinematic requirements, and (5) energy absorption. This overall problem of the mechanical design and analysis of a total joint implant is no doubt multifaceted. However, one of the

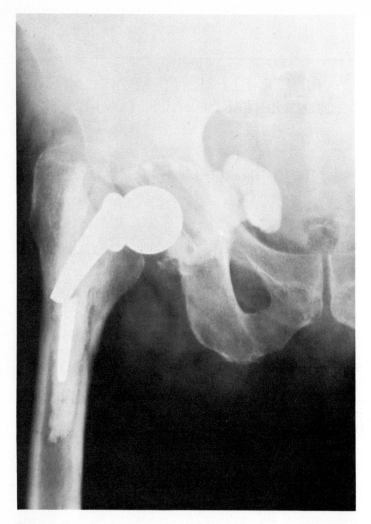

Figure 1 Example of a failure of a total hip replacement resulting from a fatigue fracture of the femoral stem.

chief requirements for design development is the ability to analyze stresses in a bone, implant, and cement system. We shall focus our attention on this aspect in this chapter.

The stress analysis of an implanted total joint replacement represents an exceedingly complex engineering problem. The complexity of the problem in many cases precludes rigorous analysis by classical methods. The finite-element method of analysis is quite applicable to biomechanical studies of this nature. Solids of irregular geometries, composed of several material types and acted on by complex force systems, can be analyzed by using this method. The purpose of this chapter is to summarize the formulation of the finite-element method and describe its application in the stress analysis of total joint implants. In addition, the application of the finite-element method to joint design is illustrated for the femoral stem of a total hip replacement.

2 GENERAL DESCRIPTION OF THE FINITE-ELEMENT METHOD

The finite-element method is a numerical technique used for approximating the solution of the governing differential equation of a continuum. The solution is approximated by subdividing the continuum into a number of simple discrete regions (finite elements). Within each finite element, the approximate solution is expressed in a simple form (usually polynomial). Thus, the overall solution for the continuum is approximated in a piecewise form.

The finite-element formulation of elasticity problems can be derived from a variational principle using an energy approach. Although several energy approaches are available (minimum potential energy, the principle of complementary energy, and the Reissner principle), the most commonly used is the principle of minimum potential energy. When the potential-energy approach is used, the form of the element displacement field must be assumed. In other approaches, the stress field and/or displacement is approximated. For particular problems, one approach may be more suitable than others, but the displacement approach is the simplest to apply and the most commonly used.

Owing to the heuristic nature of this exposition, only the displacement approach using minimum potential energy will be illustrated in the following derivation. The reader is assumed to have a background in solid mechanics.

The strain energy of a linear elastic solid in terms of the displacement field **u** is given as

$$U(\mathbf{u}) = \tfrac{1}{2} \int_{\text{vol}} \epsilon^t \sigma \, dv \tag{1}$$

when ϵ and σ contain the strain components and stress components in matrix form, respectively. By Hooke's law $\sigma = c\epsilon$, with **c** defined as the constitutive matrix, Eq. (1) becomes

$$U(\mathbf{u}) = \tfrac{1}{2} \int \epsilon^T C \epsilon \, dv \tag{2}$$

Substituting the strain displacement relationship $\epsilon = \mathbf{B}\mathbf{u}$ into Eq. (2), we have

$$U(\mathbf{u}) = \tfrac{1}{2} \int \mathbf{u}^t \mathbf{B}^t c \mathbf{B} \mathbf{u} \, dv \tag{3}$$

Thus, the total potential energy can be written in terms of the displacement field **u** as

$$\pi(\mathbf{u}) = \tfrac{1}{2} \int_v \mathbf{u}^t \mathbf{B}^t \mathbf{C} \mathbf{B} \mathbf{U} \, dv - \int_v \mathbf{F}^t \mathbf{u} \, dv - \int_s \mathbf{T}^t \mathbf{u} \, ds \tag{4}$$

where **u** = column matrix of continuous displacement field

B = matrix of differential operators relating strain and displacement

c = constitutive matrix containing material constants

F = body force components (e.g., gravity) acting on volume v

T = surface traction acting on surface s from total displacement

At equilibrium, the displacement field is such that the total potential energy assumes a minimum.

At this point we can develop the general finite-element equations for an elastic continuum. In general, this derivation is independent of the type of element or material constitutive relationships; however, linearity is assumed.

Consider the region in Fig. 2, divided into discrete elements. The potential energy may be written as the sum

$$\pi(\mathbf{u}) = \sum_{i=1}^{M} \pi^i(\mathbf{u}) \tag{5}$$

where M is the number of elements, and π^i is the potential energy of each element. The displacement field within each element must satisfy certain compatibility and completeness conditions to ensure convergence. That is, there must be displacement continuity at element interfaces and at least uniform first derivatives of the displacement within the element. For plane problems, polynomial interpolation functions that contain at least constant and linear terms will satisfy the compatibility and completeness requirements.

To discretize the potential-energy function for one element, the displacement field **u** is expressed in terms of displacements at fixed locations (nodes) within or on the boundary of the element. Thus, the displacement field can be expressed in discrete form as

$$\mathbf{u}^{(e)} = \mathbf{N}\mathbf{d}^{(e)} \tag{6}$$

where $\mathbf{d}^{(e)}$ contains the nodal displacements, and **N** contains the interpolation

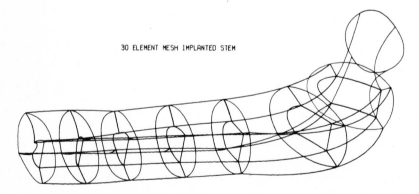

30 ELEMENT MESH IMPLANTED STEM

Figure 2 Illustration of a solid continuum (a femoral stem implanted in a femur) discretized into three-dimensional finite elements.

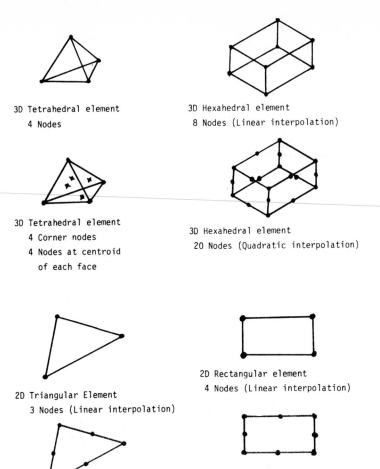

3D Tetrahedral element
    4 Nodes

3D Hexahedral element
    8 Nodes (Linear interpolation)

3D Tetrahedral element
    4 Corner nodes
    4 Nodes at centroid
        of each face

3D Hexahedral element
    20 Nodes (Quadratic interpolation)

2D Triangular Element
    3 Nodes (Linear interpolation)

2D Rectangular element
    4 Nodes (Linear interpolation)

2D Triangular element
    6 Nodes (Quadratic interpolation)

2D Rectangular element
    8 Nodes (Quadratic interpolation)

Figure 3 Examples of two-dimensional and three-dimensional finite elements.

functions. The superscript (e) refers to an element. Similarly, the geometry of the element is determined by the physical arrangement of the nodes and the order of the geometric interpolation function. Elements are classed by their approximate shapes. In two-dimensional analysis triangles and quadrilaterals, and in three dimensions tedrahedrons and hexadrons, are the most common continuum elements (Fig. 3).

Thus the displacement field is expressed in terms of known interpolation functions **N** and unknown nodal displacements **d**. The remainder of the problem involves arranging the equations in a suitable form to solve for the nodal displacements.

The nodal displacements are determined by minimizing the potential-energy function with respect to the nodal displacements, because in this state equilibrium is achieved. Because of the summation principle expressed in Eq. (5), minimization can be achieved element by element.

The potential energy achieves a minimum when the first variation of the functional vanishes, that is,

$$\delta \pi^{(e)}(\mathbf{d}) = 0 \tag{7}$$

where $\mathbf{d}$ is an admissible displacement field. For an element with r degrees of freedom,

$$\delta \pi^{(e)}(d) = \sum_{i=1}^{r} \frac{\partial \pi}{\partial di} \; \delta \; di = 0 \tag{8}$$

But the $\delta \; di$'s are not necessarily zero; thus,

$$\frac{\partial \pi}{\partial di} = 0 \qquad i = 1, \ldots, r \tag{9}$$

must be required for each nodal displacement. Thus the element equations can be written

$$0 = \int_{v} \mathbf{E}^{(e)t} \mathbf{C}^{(e)} \mathbf{E}^{(e)} \mathbf{d}^{(e)} \; dv^{(e)} - \int_{v} \mathbf{E}^{(e)t} \mathbf{F} \; dv - \int_{s} \mathbf{E}^{(e)t} \mathbf{T} \; ds \tag{10}$$

where $\mathbf{E} = \mathbf{BN}$. Eq. (10) is the force displacement relationship for the element. In matrix notation,

$$\mathbf{K}^{(e)} \mathbf{d}^{(e)} = \mathbf{F}_{t}^{(e)} \tag{11}$$

where

$$\mathbf{K}^{(e)} = \int_{v} \mathbf{E}^{(e)t} \mathbf{C}^{(e)} \mathbf{E}^{(e)} \; dv^{(e)}$$

and

$$\mathbf{F}_{T}^{(e)} = \int_{v} \mathbf{E}^{(e)t} \mathbf{F} \; dv + \int_{s} \mathbf{E}^{(e)t} \mathbf{T} \; ds$$

Each element stiffness matrix $\mathbf{K}^{(e)}$ is assembled into an overall force displacement matrix for the entire continuum. The resulting linear system of simultaneous equations is solved for the unknown nodal displacements. The displacements then can be used to compute element strain and stress.

At this point it is useful to review the preceding exposition from a practical viewpoint. The first step in employing the finite-element method consists of discretizing the continuum. Implicit in this step is the goal of adequately representing the physical phenomena under study.

The accuracy of the solution is dependent on the combined choice of element types (i.e., interpolation functions) and the physical arrangement of elements (mesh). There is no firm set of rules for making these choices. However, some helpful guidelines emerge from experience with finite elements, as follows:

1. In regions where the stress gradient is expected to vary rapidly, a finer mesh or elements with higher-order interpolation functions should be used.
2. Elements should be given a well-proportioned shape, that is, the ratio of an element's smallest dimension to its largest dimension (aspect ratio) should be near unity where possible. Long, narrow elements should be avoided because they lead to a solution with directional bias.
3. If possible, nodes should be placed where external forces are applied.
4. Element density should be increased in regions of abrupt changes in geometry. In general, increased accuracy can be expected from an increase in the number of elements used to model a particular problem. Increasing the number of elements (mesh refinement) usually represents a compromise between computational expense and accuracy. However, there will be a point where further mesh refinement may cause loss of accuracy because of computational round-off errors.
5. Large differences in the stiffnesses of different elements can lead to an ill-conditioned stiffness matrix and thus solution errors. This situation may occur in the analysis of total joint replacements where a large difference in elastic modulus between cement and steel exists.

It should again be noted that linearity was assumed in the preceding derivation. If the finite-element approach is to be used for problems where material non-linearities (e.g., biological tissue) or geometric nonlinearities are important, then a nonlinear formulation should be used. A common method of handling nonlinearities is an incremental linearization scheme. Finite-element codes are available (Table 1) to handle nonlinearities and/or dynamic problems. In the study of joint replacement design, many problems may require both time-dependent as well as nonlinear formulations. The reader is referred to Zienkiewicz [1], Przemieniecki [2], and

Table 1 Finite-element stress analysis computer codes

Program name	Class of problems	Element types	Source
SAP IV	Static, dynamic, linear, 2-D and 3-D analysis	Truss, beam, plane stress, plane strain, membrane, 3-D solid, axisymmetric	NISEE, 729 Davis Hall, Univ. of Calif., Berkeley, CA
NON SAP	Static, dynamic, 2-D and 3-D linear and nonlinear analysis	Truss, beam, plane stress, plane strain, 3-D solid, axisymmetric	NISEE, 729 Davis Hall, Univ. of Calif., Berkeley, CA
NASTRAN	Static and dynamic 2-D and 3-D linear elastic analysis	Beam, membrane, plane strain, plane stress, 3-D solid	COSMIC

Huebner [3], which describe the development and application of finite elements in more detail than is possible in this chapter.

3 GENERAL ORTHOPEDIC APPLICATIONS
OF FINITE–ELEMENT METHODS

Finite-element methods have been used in several general areas of orthopedic applications: (1) basic studies of stress distribution in bone and soft tissue structures; (2) studies of the stress distribution resulting from internal fracture fixation; and (3) studies of internal prosthetic joint replacement, stress analysis, and design. An examination of the methodology used by some of the investigators in these studies is a helpful first step toward understanding the application and limitations of the use of finite-element methods in orthopedic problems.

Rybicki et al. [4] were among the first to use a two-dimensional finite-element analysis to study stress distributions in a normal human femur. Woo et al. [5] and Simon et al. [6] used a combined finite-element and experimental approach to study internal fracture fixation. Hayes et al. [7] used a three-dimensional finite-element analysis to examine the functional structure of the human patella. Kulak et al. [8] and Belytschko et al. [9] used an axisymmetric finite-element model to study stresses in the human intervertebral disk. Piziali et al. [10] and Hayes et al. [11] used finite-element models to study stresses leading to fractures in the human tibia. The femoral stem of the total hip replacement has been the focus of a number of finite-element studies. Among investigators who studied this problem are Bartel and Samehyeh [12], McNeice et al. [13], Andriacchi et al. [14], and Hampton et al. [15]. Lewis et al. [16] reported a two-dimensional and three-dimensional analysis of a geomedic total knee replacement using finite-element methods.

4 PROSTHESIS ANALYSIS AND DESIGN

As indicated by the studies described above, stress-analysis problems associated with total joint replacement have been analyzed using the finite-element method. However, even with powerful methods such as the finite-element technique, the stress analysis of a metallic or polyethylene prosthesis cemented into human bone will require a number of simplifications. Within the scope of the available finite-element techniques (Table 1), the investigator is faced with a number of decisions. Should a two-dimensional or three-dimensional method of analysis be used for a specific problem? What type of element would be most applicable and provide an accurate solution? What are the limitations of the results using such techniques? How should alternative methods of analysis, either experimental or analytical, be used to test the validity of the finite-element results? Finally, there is the question of the application of finite-element methods to the design of total joint replacements. Many of these questions will be addressed in the remainder of this chapter.

In attempting to select the appropriate simplifications and assumptions necessary to model a bone implant system, it is useful first to examine the mechanical characteristics of each of these components. The most complex of the components is living human bone. Human bone is neither isotropic nor homogeneous; it exhibits material nonlinearities as well as time-dependent material behavior. In addition, its geometry is complex and irregular. Although it is within the capacity of the finite-element method to incorporate many of these features into a model, the lack of appropriate physical property data and/or computational costs may preclude the use of such sophisticated analytical approaches. The mechanical characteristics of cement are nearly as difficult to characterize as those of bone. Although, in the laboratory, cement can be considered isotropic and homogeneous, the *in vivo* situation of a cemented prosthesis may be considerably different. The easiest component of the system to model is the prosthesis itself. It is composed of metallic or plastic material with clearly delineated mechanical properties and geometries. A difficulty that may arise is modeling the three-dimensional geometric characteristics of the component.

The most difficult aspects in the analysis of the joint replacement problem are the cement-bone and prosthesis-bone interfaces. These interfaces are not perfect bonds. The interface between prosthesis and cement can be described as a mechanical interlock that breaks down under low tensile or shear stresses. An appropriate analysis of both prosthesis loosening and postprosthesis loosening failure should incorporate this concept. Analytical capabilities for these types of interface elements exist; however, the paucity of appropriate experimental data on interface characteristics again seems to be the limitation. It is at this point that the investigator must decide what simplifications can be used to solve the problem. A review of the current state of the art is useful at this point.

4.1 Analysis of Currently Employed Prostheses

Bartel and Semehyeh [12] used an idealized model of a bone-cement-stem system to analyze the effect of cement modulus and thickness on stresses in the bone, cement, and prosthesis system. The bone and prosthesis stem were considered to be circular and concentric and subject to compressive, bending, and transverse loads. It was assumed that the bone, cement, and prosthesis were linear, homogeneous, and isotropic materials. Stresses were computed in two ways. A three-dimensional solution from the theory of elasticity and a three-dimensional finite-element model were used. The finite-element model was used in regions where abrupt changes in geometry would produce stress concentrations. The results indicated reasonable agreement between the theory-of-elasticity solution and the finite-element method in this idealized model, except in the regions where stress concentration may exist. In this application the investigators significantly simplified both the geometry and the material characteristics to examine the relative effects of the cement modulus and thickness of the components in this composite system.

McNeice et al. [13] used a two-dimensional model of the femoral component of a total hip prosthesis cemented into bone to study stresses in the bone, cement, and prosthesis. They chose the frontal plane for the analysis; however, they attempted to account for the full three-dimensional geometry of the stem, cement, and bone by using a method of composite materials. The three-dimensional stiffness characteristics of the entire cross section of the composite prosthesis, cement, and bone were lumped into the plane of the prosthesis. Each of the components was assumed to be linear, homogeneous, and isotropic. They analyzed three types of prostheses: the McKee-Farrar, Moore, and Trapazoidal 28. Their model also assumed a continuous interface between prosthesis and cement and cement and bone. They studied the stresses in bone, cement, and stem.

A two-dimensional finite-element model was used by Andriacchi et al. [14] to examine the stresses in the femoral stem of a total hip replacement. The model included a representation of an implanted stem in cement surrounded by the proximal portion of the femur (Fig. 4). Linear displacement elements (triangle and quadrilateral) were used to discretize the continuum. The number and arrangement of elements were selected on the basis of anticipated stress distributions and the goal of analyzing stresses in the implant. This model differed from the one described by McNeice et al. in that only the cement and bone lying in the plane of the stem were included in the model. It was also assumed that the material components behaved linearly and that each component was isotropic (Table 2). The primary purpose of this model was to analyze factors that influence stresses in the

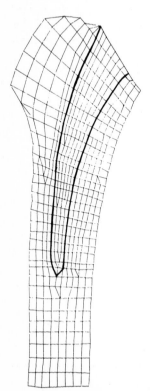

Figure 4 Two-dimensional continuum finite-element model of an implanted Mueller femoral stem.

Table 2 Material property data

Material type	Young's modulus E (N/cm²)	Poisson's ratio v
Stainless 316	1.96×10^7	0.29
Cortical bone	1.76×10^5	0.30
Trabecular	2.8×10^4	0.30
Bone cement	2.3×10^5	0.23

femoral stem. A summary of the types and numbers of elements used in several studies is given in Table 3.

Femoral-stem stress distribution The stress distribution throughout the stem, bone, and cement was computed via the model for each case. However, only stresses in the femoral stem were analyzed, owing to the lack of adequate validation of the stresses computed in the other components. Shown in Fig. 5 is a typical distribution of longitudinal stresses occurring along the lateral and medial edges of the femoral stem and resulting from a load of 1 N applied at $0°$. Tensile stresses are distributed along the lateral edge, and compressive stresses along the medial edge. The stresses reach a peak magnitude at midstem and decrease to approximately 0 at the distal tip. Note that the region of maximum stress occurs in approximately the middle third of the stem, the region where fractures are reported clinically. Stress distributions similar to that shown in Fig. 5 were found for every stem configuration studied, although the magnitudes of the stresses were different. The stress distribution shown in Fig. 5 is indicative of a bending deformation. Although the

Table 3 Finite-element model parameters and maximum tensile stress predictions

	Element types	Number of elements	Normalized maximum femoral-stem stress (N/cm²/N)	
			Fully supported	Partially supported
Charnley	Linear displacement triangles	683	4.8	7.9
Mueller	Linear displacement triangles, quadrilaterals	473	6.21	7.11
CAD	Linear displacement triangles and quadrilaterals	236	5.080	5.676
T28*	Four-node quadrilateral	897	6.4	12.8

*From McNiece et al. [13].

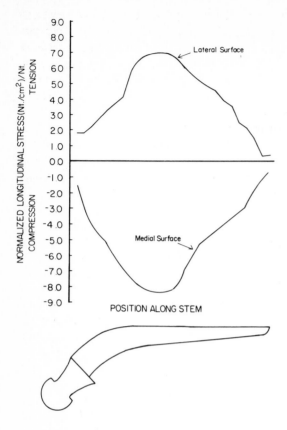

Figure 5 Typical stress distribution in the femoral stem.

stem sustains both bending and compressive stresses, the bending stresses appear to be dominant. A summary of maximum tensile stresses along the lateral surface of the stem for various stem designs is given in Table 3.

4.2 Validation and Clinical Correlation

Hampton et al. [15] examined the validity of several assumptions used in the technique described above. This study provided both analytical and experimental justification for the assumptions in the two-dimensional analysis described by Andriacchi et al. The validation study included a comparison of two-dimensional and three-dimensional finite-element models with experimental results obtained from two femoral stems instrumented with foil strain gauges on the lateral surface and implanted in wet cadaver femurs. Loads were applied in the frontal plane to the femoral head, and longitudinal stresses were recorded. The results of this study (Fig. 6) indicated that the effects of loads lying in the frontal plane of the prosthesis can be analyzed using the two-dimensional representation of the stem implanted in the femur. It was concluded that the portion of the femur and cement not included in the two-dimensional model have a secondary effect on stem stresses. The response of the system to the critical loadings can be efficiently studied via the two-dimensional finite-element representation of the frontal plane.

On the basis of these findings it appears that support at the boundaries along the lateral and medial surfaces of the femoral stem is dominant, in the sense that any support derived from cemented bone not in the plane of the prosthesis probably will play a secondary role for the types of loads assumed to produce the maximum tensile stresses on the femoral stem. Although the validity of the model for computing stresses in the stem seems to be adequate, the stresses in the cement and bone computed with finite-element methods remain unchecked.

A summary of data for 11 failed femoral stems is given in Table 4. Six of these failures were reported by Galante et al. [17]. An additional five were observed subsequently. Fatigue failure, occurring an average of 35 mo after implantation, was the cause of stem fracture in all 11 cases. The average failure location site was 68.4 mm from the proximal lateral shoulder, measured along the lateral surface. The range was from 56 to 80 mm. Thus, all failures occurred in the middle third of the stem. Although these data are not yet statistically significant, they appear to indicate that the mean failure location for the Charnley stem design was more proximal (65 mm) than for the Mueller stem (70.3 mm).

Note that the region of maximum tensile stresses predicted by the finite-element models (Fig. 5) occurs in the region where stem fractures are observed clinically. In addition, it was predicted that the Mueller stem sustains maximum tensile stresses slightly more distal than the Charnley stem. Thus, there appears to be a positive qualitative correlation between clinical observation and model prediction.

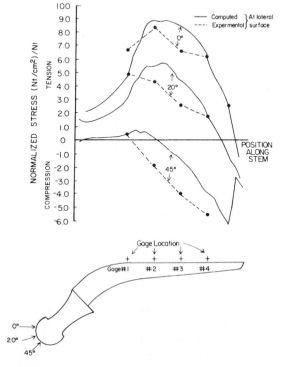

Figure 6 Example of the results of an experimental validation of predicted finite-element results. Tensile stresses along the lateral surface of the stem are shown.

Table 4 Summary of 11 femoral-stem failures

Prosthesis stem design	Fracture location[*]	Time to failure postoperatively (mo)	Patient age (yr)
Charnley, standard	66	19	58
Charnley, standard	65	40	70
Charnley, standard	73	29	63
Charnley, straight stem	56	61	67
Mueller, short neck	56	10	80
Mueller, short neck	68	24	61
Mueller, standard neck	80	27	61
Mueller, standard neck	56	48	56
Mueller, long neck	69	4	72
Mueller, long neck	86	50	71
Mueller, long neck	77	36	67

[*]Distance measured from shoulder along the lateral stem curvature.

4.3 Failure Analysis—Current Design

To illustrate the manner in which the magnitude of the maximum tensile stress, the number of cycles, and the range of stress fluctuations combine to produce fatigue failure, times were predicted for subjects weighing between 60 and 90 kg (Table 5). Maximum tensile stresses were determined as already described. The number of

Table 5 Relative effects of body weight, number of cyles, and range of stress fluctuations on stem fatigue life under maximum stress conditions

Body weight (kg)	Maximum tensile stress (N/cm^2)	Stem fatigue life[*]	
		Stress range $R = 0$ (no. of cycles)	Stress range $R = -0.5$ (no. of cycles)
90	4.5×10^4 (6.3×10^4 lb/in^2)	4×10^4 (1 yr)[†]	0.25×10 (3 mo)
80	4.0×10^4 (5.75×10^4 lb/in^2)	1.25×10^6 (3 yr)	0.25×10^6 (7 mo)
70	3.5×10^4 (5.2×10^4 lb/in^2)	4.25×10^6 (10 yr)	6×10^6 (1.5 yr)
60	3.0×10^4 (4.3×10^4 lb/in^2)	5×10^7 (30 yr)	1.25×10^6 (3 yr)

[*]Fatigue data derived from Miller et al. [18] on cobalt-chromium-molybdenum prosthesis alloy.

[†]Time estimates determined by assuming 4×10^5 walking cycles per year.

cycles to failure, derived from data reported by Miller et al. [18] on cast cobalt-chrome alloy, were determined for two different ranges of stress fluctuations. In the first case ($R = 0$), stresses cycled from the maximum tensile stress to zero. In the second case ($R = -0.5$), stresses cycled from the maximum tensile stress to a compressive stress equal to 50 percent of the maximum tensile stress. *In vivo* conditions probably fall between these two extremes. The number of years to failure was computed by assuming 4×10^5 walking cycles per year based on walking approximately 1 km/day with a stride length of 1 m.

These results indicate the importance of the effects of the range of stress fluctuations on fatigue life. For example, a stem implanted in a 60-kg subject will fail in 30 yr at stresses cycled from zero to the maximum tensile stresses, and will fail in 3 yr at stresses cycled from the same maximum tensile stress to a compressive stress equal in magnitude to 50 percent of the maximum tensile stress.

Body weight, because it is proportional to the magnitude of the maximum tensile stress, is also an important parameter to the fatigue life of the femoral stem. A stem in a 90-kg subject for the stress conditions $R = 0$ would experience fatigue failure at 1 yr. A 60-kg subject with the same stem conditions will not sustain fatigue failure until 30 yr of service. It should be emphasized that the data illustrated in Table 5 represent the highest stress conditions computed for this study and may only result *in vivo* following lack of proximal support at the level of the calcar femorale and failure at the cement-bone interface.

4.4 Suggested Improvements—Current Design

The maintenance of low stresses in the femoral stem is dependent on maintaining a stiff medium supporting the proximal medial portion of the stem. Because an equal volume of cortical bone is stiffer than either cement or trabecular bone, a stem supported by cortical bone will sustain lower maximum tensile stresses than one supported by either cement or trabecular bone. Given the constraints of the current stem designs, it may not be possible to place the proximal medial portion of the stem directly on cortical bone. In this case, a reasonably stiff support could be achieved by a layer of cement between cortical bone and the stem. Cement should be used to provide the largest possible contact area for the stem, and the thickness of the cement layer in this region should be minimized.

Results of these studies indicate that adequate stem support is most important in preventing excessive stresses in the femoral stem (Table 3). Although stem orientation plays a role in reducing tensile stresses in the stem, surgeons should not neglect the need for adequate stem support at the calcar in attempting to achieve proper orientation.

These stress-analysis studies indicate that future stem designs should incorporate some means of assuring adequate support at the calcar throughout the life of the prosthesis. In addition, stem cross sections should be designed to achieve maximum bending stiffness in the middle one-third of the stem, where the maximum tensile stresses occur. Although design was not the specific objective of the above-mentioned studies, the results are directly applicable to future design improvements for the femoral stem.

It is important to examine the assumptions used in applying the finite-element methods in the studies mentioned above. In each study, all the materials including bone were approximated as isotropic, elastic, and homogeneous materials. It is difficult to argue the validity of any approach on an intuitive basis. In bio-mechanical studies, where significant simplifications are made, there is an implicit need to test the validity of these assumptions using alternative approaches.

All the currently reported models of bone-cement-implant systems assume the interfaces are perfect bonds. Thus, linear stress-analysis programs have been suffi-cient. The work described by Andriacchi et al. [14] and Hampton et al. [15] has shown through experimental validation that this assumption is appropriate if only stresses in the prosthesis are analyzed. However, no study currently available has shown that the stresses predicted by the linear models at the cement-bone and prosthesis-bone interfaces are valid. It should be noted that component loosening resulting from interface breakdown is a common failure model of total joint implants that requires further study. However, the state of the art described here (i.e., component failure analysis) should be considered as only a first step toward an optimal design.

4.5 Design Development Approaches

The question of the usefulness of finite-element analysis for joint replacement design can be answered only after appropriate decisions regarding design variables have been made. An analysis of the femoral stem of a total hip replacement provides a useful illustration of the use of finite-element methods in joint replacements.

After examining the difficulties and potential pitfalls associated with the analysis of total joint replacement, it is not unreasonable to suggest that establishing an optimal joint design using a single finite-element model is unrealistic at this time. The difficulty arises in part from a multiplicity of rather ill-defined factors that must be considered before appropriate optimization criteria can be established. In addition, it may not be feasible or wise to incorporate all the possible design criteria into a single finite-element model. An approach to joint design, which may be feasible based on the current state of the art, is indicated in the following steps.

1. Form hypotheses, based on experience with joint replacements, regarding the potential critical design criteria in the bone-cement-prosthesis system, determine which parameters affect the selected design criteria, and place appropriate anatomic, surgical, and biological constraints on these parameters.
2. Develop a finite-element model or models to evaluate the parameters selected for implants currently used.
3. Test the validity of the finite-element model or models in accurately predicting the influence of the selected parameters. (Note that the model need not necessarily be a valid representation of the entire solid, so long as the selected design parameters can be accurately evaluated).
4. Select design parameters, on the basis of an analysis of current designs, that can

be modified (within appropriate constraints) to converge to the chosen criteria. Formulate a design that incorporates selected modifications.

5. Evaluate the modified design using the model developed in step 2 against chosen criteria. If the criteria are not satisfied, reevaluate the choice of selected parameters in step 4 and make alternative design modifications.

The analysis of stresses in the femoral stem provides a useful illustration of the application of the approach described above to the design of joint replacements. There are many possible failure modes of a total hip replacement, including component loosening, component fracture, and dislocation. The objective of this study was to isolate the problem of stem fractures as a first step toward the design modification of the total hip replacement.

The first step involved observations of femoral stem fractures. These observations indicated that failures originated along the lateral surface of the stem approximately in the middle one-third of the length of the stem. Available design parameters included stem orientation, cross-sectional design, stem profile, and stem material properties. A set of rather obvious physical constraints was imposed by the anatomy of the proximal femur.

The second step was to develop a finite-element model of a femoral stem implanted in the proximal femur with cement. The model was designed to analyze the parameters described above. Modeling assumptions included load direction, material property representation, and two-dimensional analysis.

The next step involved model validation. The validity of this model was examined by two methods, an analytical three-dimensional finite-element model and an experimental study. Because many of the same assumptions were used in the construction of the three-dimensional model as were used in the two-dimensional model, it was necessary to validate the results experimentally.

Design-parameter modification involved changing the design parameters described above, with the goal of reducing the maximum tensile stress in the stem. It was found that reducing the stiffness of the implanted stem produced lower maximum stresses in the stem. In addition, stem length was studied by varying the length of stems of current design. The effect of shortening stem length was to reduce stresses in the stem. Study of stem orientation indicated that valgus positioning and proximal-lateral cortical support resulted in lower stresses in the stem. Proximal medial support in the stem was also found to be a significant factor in determining the level of maximum stress in the stem. Through constantly modifying these design parameters with the goal of reducing stresses, a design modification of the stem was accomplished. It should be noted that at all times design alterations to the stem must be weighed against given anatomical constraints of the proximal femur, biocompatibility of implant materials, and the mechanics of implantation.

The convergence of this approach to design improvement is dependent on a number of factors: First, and probably most important, is the appropriate selection of attainable design criteria. Second is the intuitive ability of the investigator to select the appropriate design modifications that will satisfy the selected criteria.

Third, convergence is dependent on the ability of the analytical and experimental models to predict and evaluate the response caused by variation of the selected design parameters.

5 CONCLUDING REMARKS

The need for improved analysis and design of total joint replacements is unquestioned. Finite-element methods represent a powerful tool for problems of implant designs when properly used. The user in this area should have an understanding of the mathematical and conceptual basis for finite elements as well as the potential pitfalls associated with their use. The following factors have been shown to be important considerations in using finite elements: (1) mesh construction, (2) element interpolation functions, (3) element aspect ratio, (4) accuracy of solution, and (5) numerical conditioning.

The methods and assumptions used to model bone, cement, and implant systems using finite elements comprise an important consideration. The choice of appropriate simplifications as well as the implication of these simplifications should be examined. The limitations of solutions and the necessity for validity confirmation in such problems are important considerations. Finite-element methods represent an important and useful tool when used with appropriate simplifications, insight, and care. The finite-element method, used as an analytical tool in the design procedure, can lead to significant improvement in the field of total joint replacement.

REFERENCES

1. O. C. Zienkiewicz, "The Finite Element Method in Engineering Science," McGraw-Hill, New York, 1971.
2. J. S. Przemieniecki, "Theory of Matrix Structural Analysis," McGraw-Hill, New York, 1968.
3. K. H. Huebner, "The Finite Element Method for Engineers," Wiley, New York, 1975.
4. E. F. Rybicki, F. A. Simonen, and E. B. Weis, On the Mathematical Analysis of Stress in the Human Femur, *J. Biomech.*, vol. 5, pp. 203–215, 1972.
5. S. L-Y Woo, B. R. Simon, and W. H. Akeson, An Interdisciplinary Approach to Evaluate the Rigidity of Internal Fixation Plate on Long Bone Remodeling, *Proc. 28th Ann. Conf. Eng. in Medicine and Biology, New Orleans, La.*, vol. 17, paper C1.10, Alliance for Engineering in Medicine and Biology, September, 1975.
6. B. R. Simon, S. L-Y. Woo, S. R. Olmstead, and W. H. Akeson, Parametric Stress Analysis of Internal Fixation Plating, *Trans. 22d Ann. Orthop. Res. Soc., New Orleans, La.*, vol. 1, paper 2, January, 1976.
7. W. C. Hayes, D. J. Boyle, and A. Velez, Functional Adaptation in the Trabecular Architecture of the Human Patella, *23rd Ann. Orthop. Res. Soc., Las Vegas, Nev.*, paper 110, February, 1977.
8. R. F. Kulak, T. B. Belytschko, A. B. Schultz, and J. O. Galante, Nonlinear Behavior of the Human Intervertebral Disc under Axial Load, *J. Biomech.*, vol. 9, pp. 377–386, 1976.
9. T. Belytschko, R. F. Kulak, A. B. Schultz, and J. O. Galante, Finite Element Stress Analysis of an Intervertebral Disc, *J. Biomech.*, vol. 7, pp. 277–285, 1974.
10. R. L. Piziali, T. K. Hight, and D. A. Nagel, An Extended Structural Analysis of Long Bones—Application to the Human Tibia, *J. Biomech.*, vol. 9, pp. 695–701, 1976.

11. W. C. Hayes, L. W. Swenson, and D. J. Schurman, Mechanics of Tibial Plateau Fractures, *Trans. 22d Ann. Orthop. Res. Soc., New Orleans, La.,* vol. 1, paper 9, January, 1976.
12. D. L. Bartel and E. Samehyeh, The Effect of Cement Modulus and Thickness on Stresses in Bone-Prosthesis Systems, *Trans. 22d Ann. Orthop. Res. Soc., New Orleans, La.,* vol. 1, paper 3, January, 1976.
13. G. M. McNeice, P. Eng, and H. C. Amstutz, Finite Element Studies in the Hip Reconstruction, *Int. Ser. Biomech.,* vol. V-A, pp. 399–405, P. V. Komi (ed.), Baltimore: University Park Press, 1976.
14. T. P. Andriacchi, J. O. Galante, T. Belytschko, and S. Hampton, A Stress Analysis of the Femoral Stem in Total Hip Prosthesis, *J. Bone Jt. Surg.,* vol. 58A, pp. 618–624, 1976.
15. S. J. Hampton, T. P. Andriacchi, J. O. Galante, and T. B. Belytschko, Analytical Approaches to the Study of Stresses in the Femoral Stem of Total Hip Prostheses, *29 Ann. Conf. Eng. in Medicine and Biology, Boston, Mass.,* paper 32.1, November, 1976.
16. J. L. Lewis, D. Jaycox, and O. Wang, Stress Analysis of Some Features of Knee Prostheses by Finite Element, *Trans. 23rd Ann. Orthop. Res. Soc., Las Vegas, Nev.,* vol. 2, paper 53, February, 1977.
17. J. O. Galante, W. Rostoker, and J. M. Doyle, Failed Femoral Stems in Total Hip Prostheses: A Report of Six Cases, *J. Bone Jt. Surg.,* vol. 57A, pp. 230–236, 1975.
18. H. Miller, W. Rostoker, and J. O. Galante, A Statistical Treatment of Fatigue on the Cast Co-Cr-Mo Prosthesis, *J. Biomed. Mater. Res.,* vol. 10, pp. 399–412, 1976.

BIOMECHANICAL ASPECTS
OF ARTIFICIAL JOINTS

Peter S. Walker

This chapter provides the biomechanical perspectives of artificial joints. It consists of three sections. The first is a historical tracking of the evolution of artificial joints. The second clarifies the kinematics, kinetics, morphology and properties, and biomaterials criteria of artificial joints. The third section not only treats the approaches to design analysis and evaluations of the various types of artificial joints, but attempts to provide insight into the basis of their performance characteristics.

1 HISTORICAL INTRODUCTION

Artificial joints were developed in an effort to satisfactorily treat arthritis or posttraumatic conditions. In the 1890s Theophilus Gluck treated wartime injuries with components machined from ivory as well as from other materials. He implanted joints in the hip, finger, and thumb, and probably elsewhere as the need arose. Noting the subsequent loosening that sometimes occurred, he made components with intramedullary stems and cemented them in place. Around the turn of the century, Jones tried the interposition of gold foil in arthritic joints, and later, in the 1920s, rigid materials were used. The rationale was that if the roughened surfaces were reamed so that the interpositional component were a close fit, the motion at the bone surfaces would lead to the formation of cartilage. The materials

Mr. William Thackeray is thanked for his excellent drawings. The author is grateful to Howmedica, Inc., for permission to publish this chapter.

chosen were believed to be biocompatible and able to withstand the joint forces, even though there was little information on the latter.

After Smith-Peterson had tried glass and other materials in the hip, cobalt-chrome alloy was used from about 1937. This was the cup arthroplasty that was used in thousands of cases up to the mid-1960s, with good results for the most part. From about 1926 onward, several surgeons experimented with complete femoral head replacements with straight stems for attaching through the neck. Hey Groves used ivory, whereas Bohlman tried metal and extended the stems through the lateral wall of the femur for extra fixation. In 1941, Moore and Bohlman designed a complete upper femur, the forerunner of the Moore hip (Fig. 1). The Judet femoral head prosthesis made from acrylic, and sometimes with a metal stem, was used in hundreds of cases from 1947 onward. They loosened or broke in large numbers, the former complication persisting even after a change to metal.

The first "total hip replacement," where components were provided for both articulating surfaces, was developed by Philip Wiles in 1938. An improved design was introduced in the 1950s. Most of these prostheses, which used bolts and screws for attachment to the bone, suffered loosening or component breakage. In 1951, femoral head prostheses with intramedullary stems were first developed. The usual indications were nonunited femoral neck fractures and avascular necrosis of the femoral head. The stems were press-fitted for good initial fixation. These prostheses, particularly the Moore, have been widely used and still have an important place today, more especially when the acetabulum is well preserved.

McKee and Watson-Farrar from Norwich, England, pursued the idea of a total hip by using a modified Thompson femoral component with a metallic acetabular cup. In the cases performed during the 1950s, screws were used for fixation, giving the inevitable loosening problems. The first recorded total hip replacement where

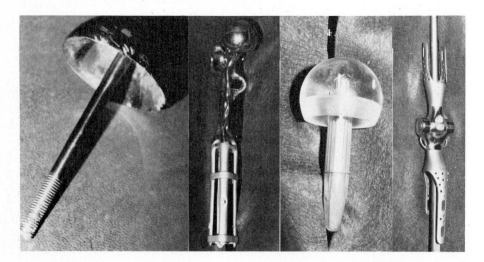

Figure 1 Historical items. Left to right: part of a Wiles total hip; Moore and Bohlman proximal femur; Judet femoral head (note metal rod embedded in acrylic); mechanical elbow hinge.

the components were cemented in place was by Edward Haboush [1] in 1951. Unfortunately, the hip dislocated shortly after surgery, and the technique was never pursued. It was not until 1960 that cemented components were tried again, this time by Charnley [2], using a self-curing methyl methacrylate suggested by Dennis Smith. Charnley used a surface replacement design initially, but soon moved to a cemented femoral stem with a 22-mm-diameter ball to reduce friction, working in a press-fitted socket made from polytetrafluoroethylene (PTFE). In 1963, Charnley switched to cemented sockets made from high-molecular-weight polyethylene, having experienced severe wear of PTFE as well as loosening of uncemented components. The all-metal McKee-Farrar design was also being cemented in place by this time.

Components for the knee appeared about 1940, with Campbell's femoral mold, Aufranc and Smith-Peterson's center-board insert, and Virgin and Carrell's metallic tibial plateau. McKeever's metallic patella replacement was introduced in 1949 and still finds use today in selected indications. With severe knee arthritis in mind, knee hinges were worked on from about 1950.

The Walldius hinge, which is used to this day, was first constructed in 1951 in acrylic and was changed to cobalt-chrome alloy in 1958 [3]. The Shiers stainless steel hinge was designed in 1953. While serving usefully in many patients, these and similar hinges suffered from the large amount of bone removal necessary for insertion, loosening and settling in the bone, skin irritation, and infection. McKeever developed a conservative approach to the knee in 1952 with unicompartmental metallic tibial replacements. The MacIntosh plateaus [4] were similar but without fixation keels. This prosthesis relied on tightening and realignment of the joint and was widely and successfully used until about 1970. The Massachusetts General Hospital and the Sbarboro femoral molds, although not widely used, gave successful results in many cases [5]. In 1969, about 10 yr after Charnley's cemented total hips, a cemented metal-plastic "polycentric" knee prosthesis [6] was designed at Charnley's hip center in Wrightington.

Except for scattered instances, developments for other joints postdated those of the hip and the knee. Metallic hinges for the elbow were used from the early 1950s by surgeons including Buckman, Dugdale, and Bateman. F. R. Thompson's metal hinges for the metacarpophalangeal (MCP) and proximal interphalangeal (PIP) joints were of the same vintage. Most of these noncemented hinges apparently suffered from loosening, and in some cases the stems penetrated the cortices of the bone. Dee's cemented elbow hinge was introduced in the early 1970s, but it too suffered loosening and extrusion after a few years of use. Neer's humeral head replacement dates back to about 1953 and is still used today. Flatt's modification of Thompson's finger prosthesis, although having some advantages, did not solve the problems. In the mid 1960s, Niebauer and Swanson independently developed silastic spacers for the MCP joint. These joints combine simplicity of design and insertion with satisfactory results, and up to the time of this writing, despite the residual problems, remain unsurpassed. This is so despite the development of cemented metal-plastic designs such as that of Steffee, who began experimentally with animals in 1964.

The early to mid-1970s saw a rash of developments of cemented metal-plastic designs for the less used joints such as the wrist, ankle, and shoulder, as well as many variations of prostheses for the hip and the knee. The field is anything but stagnant. Not only are improved mechanical configurations for the bearings being designed, but so are new methods of fixation, and alternative materials to metal on plastic. The next decade will undoubtedly bring benefits from an exploitation of these new possibilities, as well as from increased knowledge of joint biomechanics.

2 CONSIDERATIONS FOR DESIGN

Three primary factors must be considered in the design of artificial joints:

1. Motion and restraint requirements
2. Forces and moments that will be sustained
3. The morphology and properties of the anatomic joint

Other considerations are the materials to be used, ease of manufacture and cost, ease of surgery, instrumentation and technique, and life requirements. These will not be discussed in detail here.

2.1 Motion and Restraints

To relieve the pain and instability of arthritic joints, there are several options. Fusion is often possible and is often preferred to artificial replacement when adjacent joints can compensate. Examples are the tibiotalar, the wrist, and the glenohumeral joints. On the other hand, it would be considered undesirable to fuse the hip, knee, elbow, or the MCP joints. Osteotomy is an attempt to realign the joint and to redistribute the stresses. In selected cases and when performed correctly, successful results can be achieved, particularly for the hip and knee [7].

Joint motion has been the subject of many studies, dating back to the classical studies in the last century of the Weber brothers, Braune and Fischer, and Marey [8]. For studying the motion of joint specimens, the globe excursion method of Albert, Strasser, and Dann is worthy of particular note.

Some of the recent methods that have been used to quantitate joint motion are

1. Still photographs
2. Stroboscopic photography
3. Optical scanning using the Selspot system or the EMR optical image digitizer
4. Television videotape-computer system
5. Electromechanical goniometer
6. Bioplanar x-rays or cineradiography
7. Accelerometry

A method used for many years, primarily applicable to the lower limb in gait, was to take cinephotographs of the limb, with markers attached at points on the limb segments. Stick patterns depicting the motion were obtained. Motion in other planes can be seen by taking overhead views using mirrors [9]. In a recent study of the upper extremity, markers were fixed externally to the limb segments, related to bony coordinates by radiographs, and then filmed by two cameras during desired activities [10]. Other recent methods have used two cameras for obtaining three-dimensional data, light-emitting diodes as reference points, and automatic data storage for subsequently obtaining television or printed displays [11, 12, 13]. Electrogoniometry has been used extensively for obtaining on-line simultaneous data on joint segment motion [14]. So far, this method has been applied mainly to gait analysis. Another approach under development is the use of accelerometers [15] from which motion data can be obtained. The greatest drawback of all these systems involving external markers is the movement of the marker relative to the bone, but in certain cases this can be measured on specimens and then factored into the computations.

Motion provided by the prosthesis Motion is an essential characteristic of a joint, and the artificial joint must provide sufficient motion for the functional requirements of the patient. There is a question as to whether the required motion should be defined in terms of the passive motions possible at the joint, or as a summation of the active motions used in various activities. The preferred solution is that the prosthesis permit motions in all planes in excess of normal physiological motions, for three reasons. First, it is important that impingements do not occur that might cause loosening; second, there are insufficient data on the ranges in different activities; third, if a prosthesis permits only functional motion, inaccurate placement at surgery will lead to impingements. However, if there are instabilities in certain planes because of soft-tissue deficiency or muscle weakness, certain restraints in the prosthesis may be necessary. Based on these considerations, there are several possibillities:

1. The prosthesis permits motion beyond all the normal passive range with no restrictions.
2. The prosthesis allows most of the normal passive ranges of motion but has guides or nonrigid restraints to motion in certain planes.
3. The prosthesis allows motion in selected planes only and prevents motion in other planes.

Which is applicable depends largely on the severity of the arthritis. The following examples illustrate these three cases.

The conventional ball-in-socket total hip is an example of the first case, in that the motion is unrestricted and there is seldom a reason for any restraint. An important parameter in defining motion before neck impingement is the neck/head diameter ratio, which is about 0.7 in the normal hip (Fig. 2). Assuming an anatomically oriented socket, an artificial hip would provide the same motion as normal with a neck/head ratio of 0.7 or less. For an endoprosthesis, greater than normal range is achieved by making the neck diameter smaller than that of the

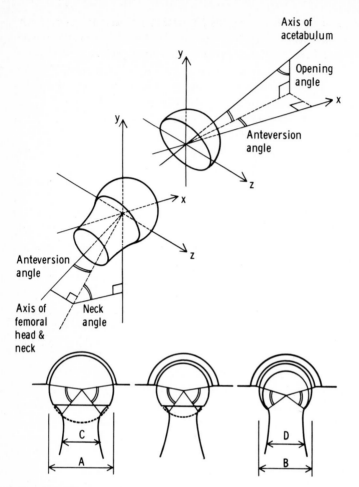

Figure 2 Definitions of angles in the hip. Range of motion is a function of C/A or D/B. Left, normal hip; center, total hip; right, surface replacement.

normal femoral neck. On the hypothesis that reducing the relative sliding between the metal ball and the cartilage will reduce erosion, a new type of endoprosthesis has been introduced, the floating cup originated by Bateman [16]. This uses the fact that in walking the motion is principally rotation about a horizontal transverse axis. The femoral ball is snapped into a plastic socket that is, in turn, fixed into a metal housing. Long-term results are awaited to assess the value of the device.

In the all-metal McKee-Farrar prosthesis, impingement occurred in many cases between the neck of the femoral component and the rim of the acetabulum, with a likely adverse effect on the fixation. In metal-plastic total hips, using the current Charnley and Charnley-Müller designs as examples, the head/neck ratios are 0.6 and 0.5, respectively. Even so, owing to surgical variations in component placement, they are known to sublux temporarily or even dislocate during certain activities. On the basis of motion alone, there seems to be no justification for a snap-in socket, where the socket is cemented in place. One of the design problems of "surface replacement" hip prostheses, such as the Wagner and Tharies designs [17], is to provide sufficient range of motion. Theoretically, so long as the diameter of the femoral cap is not less than the original, and the acetabular component does not protrude beyond the normal periphery, the motion will be at least normal, but these criteria are not easy to meet in practice.

Another example of an unconstrained prosthesis is the modular type of knee, where the femoral components are anatomically shaped metal runners, and the tibial components are close to flat surfaces, examples being the Marmor, Sledge, and Charnley Load Angle Inlay (Fig. 3). This arrangement allows more freedom of motion than normal in that the dishing of the medial compartment of the tibia and the menisci themselves are not mechanically reproduced. A recent entry into the unrestricted type is that in which the femoral components are doubly convex runners, locating into wedge-shaped plastic washers that are free to slide on flat metal plates on the upper tibia [18].

When the arthritic knee is too unstable to accept an unconstrained prosthesis, a partially constrained type is required—an example of case 2. In the condylar replacement type of prosthesis, the constraint is usually provided by some degree of conformity between the femoral and tibial components. The degree can vary

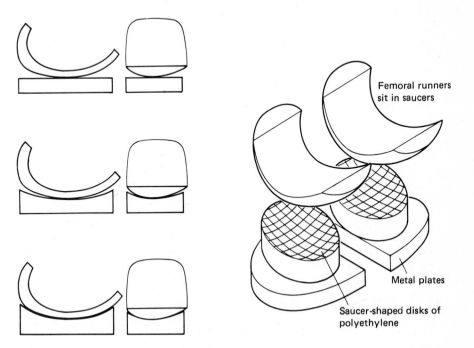

Femoral runners
sit in saucers

Metal plates

Saucer-shaped disks of
polyethylene

Figure 3 Conformity in knee prostheses. Top, nonconforming; center, partially conforming; bottom, fully conforming (in extension); right, fully conforming, nonconstrained design.

considerably, from the low conformity of, say, the Townley and Anametric prostheses, to the moderate conformity of the total condylar and Duopatella, and to the almost complete conformity of the early Geomedic. The limits of motion in the MCP joint are determined by the ligaments and the passive restraints of the muscles, rather than by the spherical surfaces. The Swanson Silastic spacers are partially constrained in the sense that the elasticity of the material provides progressive restriction to radial and ulnar deviation, but the hinge arrangement permits the flexion-extension range with relatively little resistance. The metal-plastic designs provide various degrees of mechanical restriction to radial and ulnar motion (Fig. 4).

The earliest finger designs are uniaxial hinges, examples of the third type of

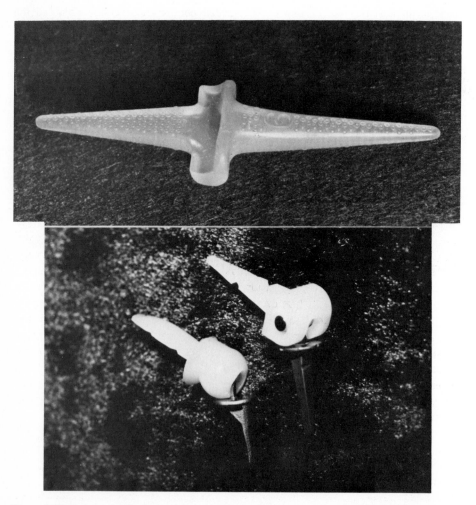

Figure 4 Finger prosthesis. Top, Swanson Silastic spacer; center, Strickland (now obsolete); bottom, Steffee.

prosthesis, where motion is restricted to a particular plane. All fixed hinges are also examples: for the knee, the Shiers, Walldius, and Guépar; for the elbow, the Dee (now obsolete), the Coonrad, and the Stanmore. Some of the more recent knee "hinges," while allowing unrestricted flexion-extension, allow constrained or partially constrained motion in other planes. Thus the Attenborough and the Spherocentric partially constrain transverse rotation, but fully constrain linear motions in the anterior-posterior (a-p) and medial-lateral (m-l) directions.

The above shows how difficult it is to define a prosthesis as nonconstrained, partially constrained, or fully constrained. The only methodical way of doing this is to consider three fixed orthogonal axes on one of the bones (e.g., the ulna for the elbow, the tibia for the knee, the phalanx for the MCP) and to examine the motions in the six degrees of freedom, three rotational and three linear. Questions of constrainment, laxity, and stability will be dealt with in more detail in a later section of this chapter.

Definition of motion and mechanical analogs To define the range of motion in a joint, clinical terms such as flexion-extension, abduction-adduction, and internal-external rotation are used. Generally speaking, these motions are readily understood and can be measured by external goniometry, from radiographs, or by more sophisticated methods. When flexion-extension is the primary motion of a joint, the other motions should be specified with reference to a particular flexion-extension angle. For example, at $0°$ flexion, the internal-external rotation of the knee joint is only a few degrees, but at $30°$ flexion and beyond, the rotation is about $20°$.

A rigorous method of defining the position of a joint is to use Eulerian angles [19]. One bone is regarded as fixed, and X, Y, Z axes are set in this bone (Fig. 5). Then x, y, z axes are set in the moving bone such that in the zero position of the joint (e.g., extended), the two sets of axes are in register. Any new joint position can be uniquely described as the result of three angular rotations: (1) flexion-extension, rotation about the fixed Z axis; (2) abduction-adduction, rotation about the moving y axis; and (3) axial rotation, rotation about the moving x axis.

These three angles cannot be determined directly using simple measurements on a patient or from radiographs. However, such a measurement system is necessary when the motions of joints need to be scientifically described. A typical method of determining Eulerian angles is to consider three points fixed in each bone. These points can be small pellets, the tips of pins, or well-identified bony landmarks. In successive positions the X, Y, Z coordinates of each point are measured, and hence the relative motion from one position to the next can be computed. This method has been applied to studies of the elbow, finger, and spine.

To conceptualize a six-degree-of-freedom system, with three rotational and three linear movements, mechanical analogs can be useful. This is particularly so in this case, where the analogs represent current and possible configurations of artificial joints. In Fig. 6 it is assumed that there is sufficient force to keep the surfaces in contact. The fixed axes are in the lower component. The difference between analogs a and b is that the former allows translation along all three axes, whereas the latter allows no translation. Analog c is the same as b, except that

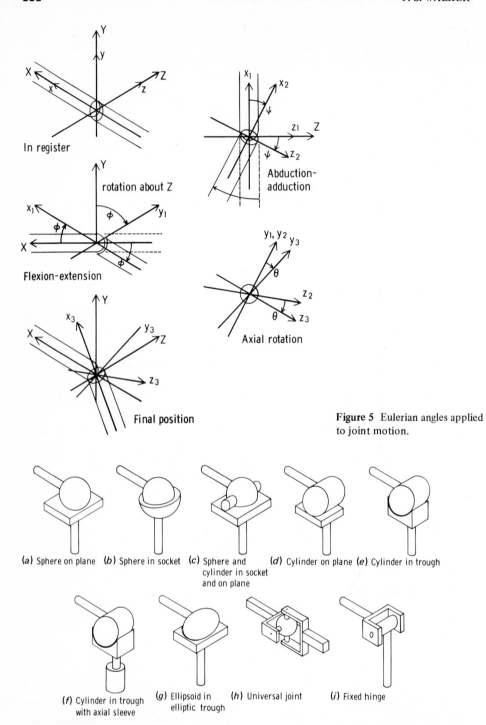

In register

rotation about Z

Flexion-extension

Final position

Abduction-adduction

Axial rotation

Figure 5 Eulerian angles applied to joint motion.

(a) Sphere on plane   (b) Sphere in socket   (c) Sphere and cylinder in socket and on plane   (d) Cylinder on plane   (e) Cylinder in trough

(f) Cylinder in trough with axial sleeve   (g) Ellipsoid in elliptic trough   (h) Universal joint   (i) Fixed hinge

Figure 6 Mechanical analogs to describe configurations of prostheses and the motions they allow.

rotation about the Z axis is prevented. Were analog e to be restricted along x, it would be equivalent to i. So long as there is no tilting or subluxation, g is equivalent to analog i. In the universal joint, relative rotation about the Y axis is prevented.

Summary In the design and selection of prostheses, the following considerations apply:

1. Motions that the normal intact joint provides
2. Which of the motions are restricted primarily by soft tissues, and which by the surfaces, with recognition of their interplay
3. Whether the prosthesis should replace the surfaces only, or whether restraints should be designed that effectively replace soft tissues
4. The ranges of motion and translations required of the prosthesis with respect to orthogonal axes

2.2 Forces and Moments

As implied, one of the main purposes of a joint is to enable the body to change its position, or to move an extremity to a required position. A second purpose is to transmit forces and moments across adjacent segments, under stationary and moving conditions. A simplified two-dimensional quasi-static representation of a limb segment is shown in Fig. 7. If the resultant foot-to-ground force passes anteriorly to the knee, the hamstrings are required to balance the extending moment on the leg. It is easy to see that the muscle force may be two to three times the ground reaction force because of the lever arm requirements, giving a resultant joint force of three to four times body weight. Furthermore, owing to foot-to-ground shearing forces and to the angulation of the joint and the musculature, shear forces are developed across the joint surfaces. Three-dimensional considerations indicate that moments are also transmitted to the joint. As for analyzing motion, it is useful for force analysis to set orthogonal axes in the reference bone and to define three components of force and three of motion.

In a complete force analysis, a considerable amount of data is needed:

1. Positions of the limb segments
2. Velocities and accelerations of the limb segments
3. External forces and moments
4. Geometry in and around the joint
5. Forces acting in individual muscles

The determination of the segment positions, velocities, and acceleration positions was described in Sec. 2.1. The average masses and centers of gravity of bone segment have been reviewed recently by Contini [20]. External forces and moments have been determined by force plates for the lower extremity during ambulation, by simple force transducers in studying knee or elbow extension strength, and by

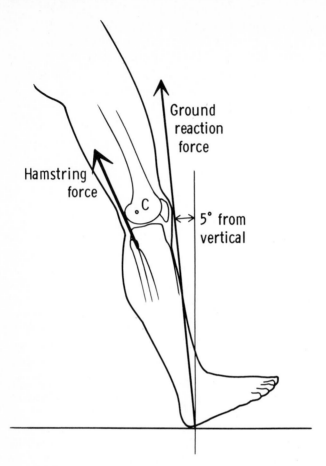

Figure 7 Simplified representation of the lower limb in walking.

strain-gauged grips for studying pinch or grip strength [21]. The internal geometry of joints is an imprecise subject, and in any case it varies from joint to joint. The lines of action of muscles are difficult to define precisely, because the center of force across a given section may not be at the centrode, and the muscles do not appear to act in straight lines because of sheaths, soft tissue, and bony and other interventions.

One approach to the problem has been to cut sections of a specimen embedded at the required position [22]. Another technique for analysis in multiple positions is to determine the coordinates of insertions and attachments and to assume straight-line action, allowing for bony intervention [23]. Muscle activity is determined by electromyographic (EMG) techniques, but it is not yet possible to accurately specify the force, although relations have been proposed among integrated EMG signal, the area of the muscle, and the force. The redundancy problem in joint force analysis has been dealt with by ignoring antagonistic muscle action; by grouping muscles; or by assuming that the total joint force, the shearing force, the joint moments, or weighted combinations, are minimized [24].

The following examples will serve to illustrate the effects of forces and moments on artificial joints.

Upper extremity Although the joints of the upper extremity are not subjected to the frequent and repetitive forces of ambulation, the forces can be of considerable magnitude, and the range of activities is great. In the simple activity of elevating the arm to 90°, the force in the glenohumeral joint reaches about 0.9 times body weight, while the shearing force reaches 0.4 times body weight. With a 1-kg weight in the hand, the forces are increased 60 percent. With the arm elevated to 90° and the elbow flexed to 90°, the forces are reduced by 30 percent [25]. The vectors are shown in Fig. 8 in relation to average relative positions of the humerus and the scapula.

The simplest type of shoulder prosthesis is the Neer humeral head replacement. When a plastic glenoid resurfacing is used, the amount of conformity and the degree of enclosure around the humeral head determine the shearing component that can be transmitted. It is significant that the direction of the shear force changes from downward to upward as the arm is elevated, which rocks the glenoid component back and forth. This effect is more serious in those prostheses that rely on a ball-in-socket configuration for increased stability, where the ball protrudes from the socket (Fig. 8).

On lifting a weight in the hand with the elbow flexed and the arm in a vertical plane, the brachialis is the major muscle acting in the elbow, with assistance from the biceps and brachioradialis at higher loads. In supporting a weight of 1 kg, the joint force is estimated to be 216 N at 90° of flexion, and 431 N at 45° of flexion. The resultant has a component passing anteriorly on the distal humerus at small flexion angles, and posteriorly after, say, 30° of flexion [22]. Toggling of the humeral component will occur and will be deleterious to fixation. At maximum isometric contraction in extension, the joint force is twice the body weight. The biceps will apply a moment in relation to the humerus, which in extension and pronation can reach 9.8 N m, and in flexion 3 N m.

A detailed study of elbow function was carried out by Nicol for the activities of eating, reaching, table pull, and seat rise. The force and moment vectors acting in and around the radioulnar and humeroulnar joints were calculated. In eating, the humeroulnar force was only 400 N, equally disposed on the medial and lateral sides of the joint. There was a radial head force of 200 N when the hand was near the table. The forces in reaching were of about the same magnitude. In seat rise, however, using the hands and arms for assistance with the legs stretched outward, the humeroulnar force was initially 500 N, rising to 1800 N at the end of the activity, the medial force rising steadily during the activity. The tension in the lateral ligament was about 600 N throughout the activity (Fig. 9). Note that if the ligaments are not present, the force that would otherwise be acting will be translated as a moment on a prosthesis.

The multitude of force and moment patterns has a wide-ranging effect on prosthetic components (Fig. 10). Whether the prosthesis is a surface replacement, is partially constrained, or is a hinged type is also important. The first type can be

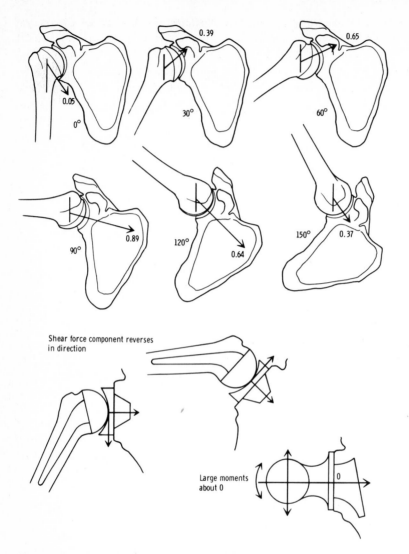

Figure 8 The force vectors at the glenohumeral joint in isometric abduction.

stiff in rotation when there is a compressive force, while the hinges are stiff to all forces and moments except flexion-extension moments. The major force will act approximately in line with the distal humerus, regardless of flexion angle. Forces normally carried by ligaments are of particular significance with hinged prostheses. Here, all of the moment will be carried by the prosthesis, amounting in seat rise to 600 N × 28 mm (average lever arm), a considerable moment. Another factor to consider is the presence or absence of the radial head. In the latter case, there will be a resulting moment about the ulna axis as well as increased humeroulnar forces.

The MCP joint is commonly replaced in rheumatoid arthritis, and with lesser frequency in osteoarthritis and posttraumatic conditions. Walker and Davidson [21] measured the external forces applied during various forms of pinch and grip. Pinch forces averaged 57 and 75 N in females and males, respectively, whereas arthritic patients averaged only 13 N. Grip strength was 153 N in males, and half that in females. Chao et al. [26] calculated the joint forces in normal hands for pinch and grasp activities. Relative to axes in the index metacarpal, for a unit tip pinch force,

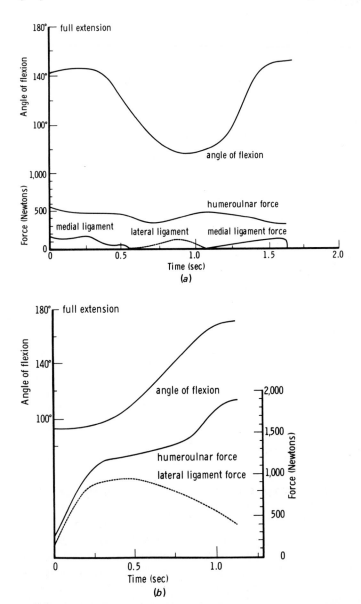

Figure 9 Forces at the elbow joint in (*a*) eating and (*b*) seat-rise activities. (*After Nicol [10].*)

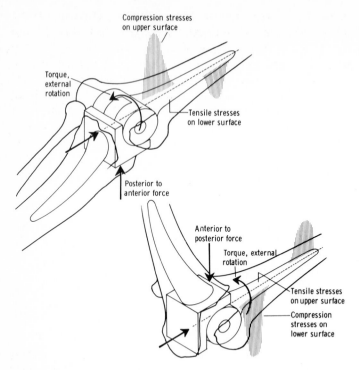

Figure 10 Indication of the shifting forces and stresses on a linked type of elbow prosthesis.

the compressive force was 8 times, the volar shear on the phalanx was 2.7 times, and the lateral shear 2.4 times. In grasp, the compressive force was 11.4 times, and the shearing forces were 1 to 2 times the above. Therefore, in pinch, the joint force would be 450 N and the shear force 150 N, in females. An analysis of the turning of a tap and pinching a 45-mm cylinder was made by Berme et al. [27]. In turning, the compressive and shear forces were about 170 and 50 N, respectively. In pinching, the corresponding forces were about 100 and 30 N. The discrepancy in the external forces between this study and that of Walker and Davidson [21] probably results from the 45-mm span compared with the tip-to-tip pinch. Some of the forces described above, together with moments in other actions such as lateral pinch, are shown in relation to a mechanical type of prosthesis in Fig. 11. The Silastic type of prosthesis would be unable to sustain these average "normal" forces, but even after prosthetic replacement in an arthritic hand, the forces applied have been found to be much smaller than normal [28].

Lower extremity Most of the force studies have been of level walking and stair and ramp activities, but there has been one study of squatting and stooping. The landmark reports for the hip joint are those of Rydell [29] and Paul [30]. During the stance phase of walking, there were found to be two force peaks, occurring at heel strike and at toe-off, of the order of 3 times and 4.5 times body weight, respectively. In fast walking, or in walking up and down stairs, the peaks reached about seven times body weight. The vectors for level walking are shown in Fig. 12.

For an appreciation of the stresses on the upper femur as a whole, the abductor force must be accounted for. The force on the femoral head results in a compressive force down the femoral axis and a bending moment, in the frontal plane, that diminishes steadily to zero where the force line crosses the neutral axis of the femur. Secondarily, there is a bending moment in the sagittal plane at heel strike and at toe-off, as well as a moment about the long axis of the femur. In squatting and stooping, large sagittal moments and torques about the long axis are developed [31] because the femur is now inclined to the horizontal by only about 30°. In relation to a prosthesis, the forces during one-legged stance are of interest. The line of action and the magnitude were found to vary considerably [32], depending on whether the pelvis was erect or sagging.

For the knee joint, the important forces are the compressive femorotibial force and its distribution between the medial and lateral condyles, the varus and valgus moments (particularly if toppling occurs), the a-p shearing forces, and the moments about the tibial axis. The work of Morrison [33, 34] provides these data for walking, ramp, and stair activities. In level walking, the compressive force had three peaks. The first two peaks, of two to three times body weight, corresponded with activity in the hamstrings and quadriceps; the third peak, of three to four times body weight, occurred at push-off as the gastrocnemius was active.

The line of the resultant seen in the frontal plane was central on heel strike but quickly moved 20 mm to the medial side for the rest of the stance phase. Walking up and down a ramp or stairs did not affect the basic force patterns but increased the peak force to about five times body weight. The shearing forces during walking

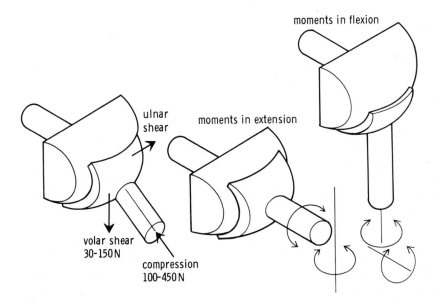

Figure 11 Some of the forces and moments acting on an MCP finger prosthesis.

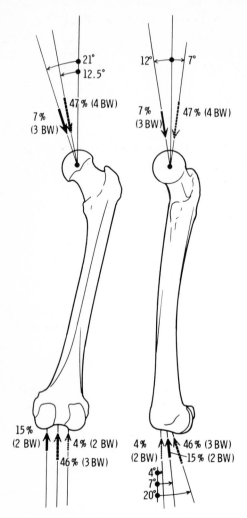

Figure 12 Force vectors at the hip and the knee for level walking. (*After Paul [82].*)

were translated into cruciate ligament forces, which amounted to two 250-N peaks in early and late stance for the posterior cruciate, and a peak of 100 N in midstance for the anterior. In walking up stairs, the posterior cruciate force peaked at 1240 N, whereas in walking down a ramp there was a 450-N peak in the anterior cruciate. The external torque on the tibia peaked at 11.5 N m in late stance. The forces and moments transmitted to a prosthesis will depend on the type of prosthesis. For an unconstrained condylar replacement, only the compressive forces will be transmitted (ignoring friction); for a conforming condylar replacement, the axial torques and a-p forces will be additionally carried; for a fixed-axis hinge, all the forces and moments will be carried except in the flexion-extension plane. The patellofemoral force reaches nearly three times body weight in ascending stairs, but only one body weight in level walking. The resultant force moves from the lower to the upper aspect of the patella with flexion, and the contact splits into two separate areas past about

$90°$ of flexion. These data are relevant to the design of plastic patella "buttons."

The ankle joint, even in level walking, sustains about five times body weight, because of the long lever arm of the foot-to-ground force about the center of the ankle at toe-off. The a-p shearing force of up to 0.7 times body weight was biphasic, acting in the aft direction on the foot in early stance, and the reverse in late stance [35]. Because of the small area of the ankle, such forces exert considerable stresses at the implant-bone interface in a prosthesis.

Summary Although the force and motion patterns for each joint vary in multitudes of ways depending on the activity, certain features are common to all joints, whether in the upper or lower extremity:

1. The internal forces in the joints are usually several times larger than the external forces, because of the muscle forces needed to maintain equilibrium.
2. With respect to axes in a bone with a concave joint surface (glenoid, ulna, radial head, phalanx, acetabulum, tibia), the longitudinal force is dominant, there is a significant shear force in the flexion-extension plane, and a less significant shear force in the third direction.
3. With respect to a bone with a convex bearing surface (humerus, femur, metacarpal), the long axis of the bone can change its orientation significantly with respect to the long axis of the concave surface, such that the dominant force component can exert a sizable shearing force or bending moment on an affixed prosthetic component.
4. Moments in the principal plane of motion are not normally carried by the joint; moments about the other two axes may be significant and will be carried by the joint complex.
5. Forces and moments are repetitive such that fatigue becomes an important question, more especially in the lower extremity.
6. Certain forces and moments cycle in direction, producing "reverse bending."

2.3 Morphology and Material Properties

The most basic information needed in prosthesis design is the dimensions. This information is by no means extensive, but data have been provided for the hip by Oh and Harris [36], for the knee by Mensch and Amstutz [37], and for the elbow by Amis et al. [38].

Configuration of a prosthesis It seems self-evident that a prosthesis should be compatible with the geometry of the bones to which it is fitted, but it is surprising how frequently the fit is not ideal. However, it is not an easy problem to define the shape of the joint, because of the irregular geometry and the variations among different specimens. The geometric differences between arthritic and normal joints must also be taken into consideration. The ligaments and muscles must be regarded as part of the joint, because these will place limitations on the shape of a particular design. There are also surgical considerations, in terms of the available space for inserting the components, placing fixation spikes, inserting axles, and so on. All these factors impose an "acceptable envelope" within which the prosthetic components must fall.

These points can be illustrated in relation to the design of hip prostheses (Fig. 13). Under the assumption that the major problem is erosion of the joint surfaces, a simple solution was to rasp the surfaces to spherical shapes, and to insert a spacer of polished metal. This is equivalent to cup arthroplasty. Although the stresses across the bone may be close to physiological, a clinical drawback appeared to be that sliding between metal and cartilage was not fully tolerated. The basic idea has been revived in the past few years by using a cup in a cup, the components being cemented to the femoral head and to the acetabulum. The sliding now occurs between metal and plastic, and the overall clinical result is better than for a cup.

When the femoral head is too misshapen or is osteoporotic, a cup cannot be used. One option, popularized in the Judet type of prosthesis, is a metal tack. However, the stresses on the bone will now be completely different from normal, and in this case the high stresses beneath the proximal stem led to loosening and eventual failure. The femoral head replacement, such as the Moore, uses an intramedullary stem to fit down the femoral canal and a collar for location against

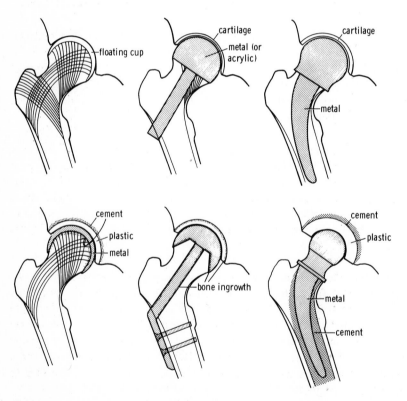

Figure 13 Some of the configurations that have been used, or are under experimentation, for a hip prosthesis.

the calcar. The size and orientation of the collar and the broad metal surfaces against the endosteum produce tolerable stresses, accounting for the ongoing success of this design. However, in some cases there is a certain amount of bone resorption of the neck and calcar because of stress and micromovement.

Cementing the component and articulating with a cemented plastic socket give the familiar and widely used total hip replacement. By their nature, such total hips lead to an abnormal stress pattern in the femur. The bending stresses in the bone are reduced, owing to the portion of bending carried by the stem. There are other alternative forms, using mechanical fixation, cement, or porous bone ingrowth for fixation. For example, the metal tack could be supported by a plate on the lateral cortex, such as the form originated by Wiles and by Coonse. For further support of the component of force perpendicular to the neck, the femoral head portion can enclose a preserved portion of the femoral head.

The different forms, applicable to other joints, can be summarized as follows:

1. Interposition surface replacement not attached to bone (e.g., Smith-Peterson cup)
2. Surface replacement attached to bone (surface-replacement hips, modular-knee tibial components)
3. Surface replacement supplemented by external "cuffs" (early Haboush femoral component)
4. Surface replacement supplemented by short studs or blades (ankle prostheses, condylar replacement knees)
5. Condylar replacement supplemented by intracancellous pegs (total condylar tibial components, Spherocentric knee)
6. Condylar replacement supplemented by intramedullary stems (total hip stem, hinged knees, hinged elbows)

Besides the dimensional restrictions and the different possible forms, there are additional design criteria that determine and optimize the design. One criterion is that the postoperative stresses on the bone be as natural as possible, with abnormally high or low stresses avoided. This is required to avoid bone resorption as well as undesirable remodeling, both of which have occurred in many instances. The strength of the cancellous and cortical bone, including the directional effects, are key to this criterion.

Strength and structure of bone The articular cartilage, together with the close congruity of the joints (aided by the menisci in the case of the knee), spread the load over a wide surface area. Membrane stresses are set up in the surface and peripheral cortical shells, from which the loads perpendicular to the surface are carried by the trabeculae. These compressive loads are carried by the trabecular network to the cortices of the bone at some distance from the joint surfaces. From the other direction, the cortices can be considered to fan out into trabeculae to form the condyles of the joint.

The mechanical properties of compact bone depend on specimen orientation, the condition and location of the specimen, and the frequency of the test, the latter implying that bone is a viscoelastic material. A median value for the modulus of elasticity of bone is 10,000 N/mm^2 (1.4 × 10^6 lb/in^2), increasing from about 8000 to 13,000 N/mm^2 for 35 to 350 Hz, respectively [39]. Hence, the modulus is about one-twentieth that of stainless steel or cobalt-chrome alloy. The tensile strength of bone is 150 to 170 N/mm^2 at frequencies of 1 to 10 Hz, relevant to functional conditions. The compressive strength is about twice this value, and the shear strength 10 percent less than the tensile strength. In a rapid tensile test to failure, considerable plastic flow is exhibited, amounting to three to four times the elastic deformation at failure [40].

If a surface replacement prosthesis is used, the stresses in the cancellous bone and in the cortical shaft should be close to normal. However, in the case of a cemented intramedullary stem, the stresses in the bone will in general be less than normal. For example, for a bone of internal and external diameters of 27 and 16 mm, respectively, and a cobalt-chrome stem of 12 mm diameter, the bending stresses in the cortex will be 50 percent of normal. Failure of the bone by overstressing is therefore unlikely (with the possible exception of the tip area), but in regions where the stresses are considerably less than normal, bone resorption may be expected.

Cancellous bone is an intriguing material (Fig. 14). It consists of rods and sheets of bone, aligned according to the principal stresses. When uniaxial motion predominates, such as in the knee and the ankle joints, the trabeculae are arranged preferentially in the anterior-posterior direction, simulating a set of parallel disks. The cancellous bone has several unique functions: It helps in spreading the area of contact in joints by deflecting; it acts as an elastic shock absorber; and it acts as an inelastic shock absorber by trabecular microfractures [41]. It is not possible to quote single representative values for the mechanical properties of cancellous bone, as these depend on the location and orientation. Generally, the closer to the joint surface and the more oriented to the principal direction of force, the higher the modulus of elasticity and compressive strength. For the cancellous bone of the femoral and tibial condyles, perpendicular to and 5 mm below the surface, the average foundation compressive strength was 19.1 N/mm^2 [42]. In varus or valgus deformities, where sclerotic and porotic bone occurred, the strength was two times or one-tenth of normal. This factor is very important to the fixation of implant components. Ducheyne et al. [43] tested bone samples removed from the femoral condyles. The strength was again found to decrease with distance below the surface, with the elastic modulus in the range 0 to 1000 N/mm^2, and the strength up to 12 N/mm^2. In a study of the cancellous bone of the femoral head, contour maps were drawn of elastic modulus, showing a decrease from about 538 N/mm^2 around the periphery to a minimum of 103 N/mm^2 near the center [44]. The implication of all these results is that if a surface replacement prosthesis is used, the minimum amount of bone possible should be removed.

3 ANALYSIS OF DESIGNS

Many of the commonly used designs have been developed empirically, with gradual improvements based on morphological observations and clinical results, and to a

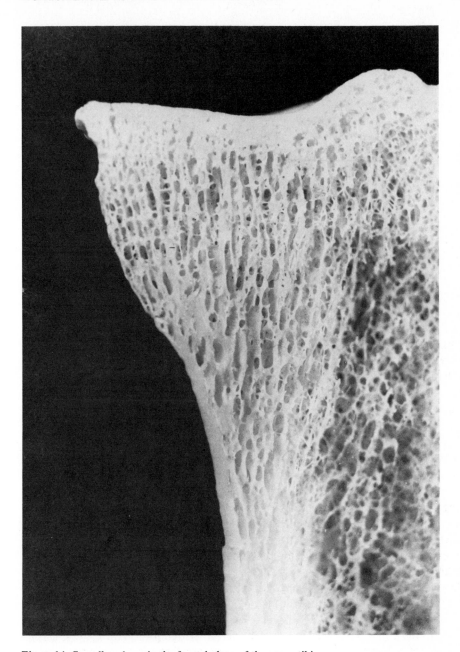

Figure 14 Cancellous bone in the frontal plane of the upper tibia.

lesser extent on laboratory tests and analysis. This picture is changing somewhat today in that the latter aspects are being given more attention. Until recently most prosthesis systems defied all but simple analysis because of the lack of detailed knowledge of joint forces, of interface conditions, and of analytic techniques to cope with the three-dimensional geometry and the varying mechanical properties of the biological materials. Finite-element techniques have now been applied to hip and knee prostheses, providing comparative and absolute data on the various stresses. Long-term testing of devices is hampered by the necessity to use dead bone, but some useful data concerning fatigue strength, wear, and fixation can be obtained nonetheless. Perhaps just as useful as dynamic simulator tests are experiments carried out on rigs, where strains, deformations, and the like are measured for various design parameters. Some of these analyses and tests will be discussed in the following pages.

3.1 Intramedullary Stems

Intramedullary stems can be used as the primary means of fixation, such as in total hips, or in combination with condylar attachment, such as in certain types of elbow prostheses (e.g., Ewald humeral component) and knee prostheses (Variable Axis, Guépar). Even with the hip, the provision of an effective collar can remove some of the load from the stem itself. The loads and moments carried by the stem will depend on the geometry, the elastic properties of the materials, and the interface conditions. Possible interfaces, together with the stresses they can transmit, are:

1. Smooth metal against bone (compressive, but not shear or tensile).
2. Smooth metal against cement (compressive, but not shear or tensile). If roughnesses or keyways are added, shear stresses can be transmitted.
3. Cement against rough cortical bone (compressive and shear but not tensile).
4. Cement against cancellous bone (compressive, shear, and tensile). Tensile depends on interdigitation.
5. Porous surfaces against bone (compressive, shear, and tensile).

Analyses and tests of all of these interfaces cannot be discussed here, and the following is directed most particularly to metal-cement-bone systems.

   In Fig. 15, the stresses resulting from three types of loading are shown. Axial loading results in shearing stresses at the stem-cement and cement-bone interfaces; axial torque results in circumferential shear stresses at each interface, whereas bending (produced, for example, by a horizontal force at the stem above the bone entry level) produces compressive and tensile stresses at opposite interfaces. Whether tension will actually be transmitted will depend on the interface conditions. On a macroscopic scale, with low friction between cement and bone, shear stresses must be transmitted on the faces of roughnesses on the endosteal surface, implying that the more roughnesses there are, the lower are the stresses on each roughness. Also, since the faces of the roughnesses will in general be inclined, hoop stresses will be developed in the bone. These comments apply to cases a and b in Fig. 15; in general, the internal surfaces of bones are not parallel, the upper femur, upper tibia, and metacarpal being examples. This implies load support because of the taper effect, again with hoop stresses (Fig. 15d). The opposite situation, a diverging bone canal, seems to apply at the distal humerus (Fig. 15e).

   The following remarks relate to the significance of different stresses in the

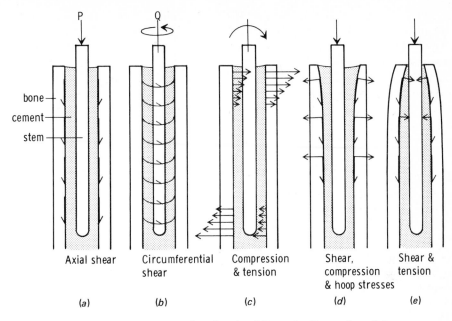

Figure 15 Stresses at the cement-bone interface for different loadings and canal shapes.

bone-cement-stem system. For the bone, the stresses after insertion of the prosthesis, compared with the normal state, will determine the extent of remodeling. For example, the longitudinal compressive stress in the calcar region resulting from direct load and from bending may reduce sufficiently to lead to bone resorption, reducing stem fixation. For the stem itself, the tensile stresses on the lateral surface must be lower than the fatigue limit of the material. The longitudinal and circumferential shear stresses at the cement-bone interface will affect the fixation. Direct normal stresses at the prosthesis-cement and cement-bone interfaces will relate to the compressive strength of the cement. The effect of normal stresses on the endosteal surface is not known with any certainty.

A composite of the above-mentioned stresses is shown for a hip stem in Fig. 16. It is emphasized that the stresses vary with the line of action of the femoral head, the position of the stem in the canal, and whether or not the abductor force is accounted for. Andriacchi et al. [45] determined the stresses on the lateral surface of the stem by using finite-element analysis, with particular reference to the stem breakage problem. When the femoral head force was parallel to the femoral axis, the stresses were tensile, being maximal in the middle third. As the force vector rotated toward the femoral axis, the stresses reduced, and could even become compressive below a certain point. A varus position of the stem gave increased stresses, but this would be at least partially compensated for by reduced force on the femoral head. The importance of support at the calcar by cortical bone was shown. If cement and trabecular bone were present, the stem stresses increased by 50 percent. Calculations based on the fatigue strength of cast cobalt-chrome showed

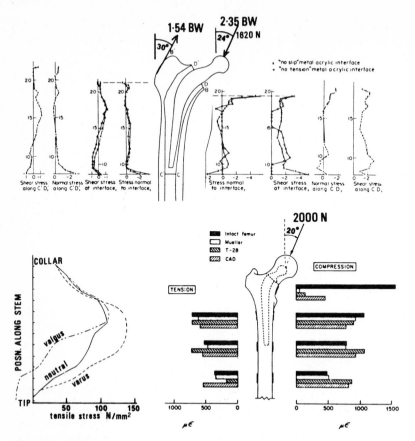

Figure 16 Stresses for a stem type of total hip cemented in the upper femur. (*Top, after Svensson et al. [46]; bottom left, after Andriacchi et al. [45]; bottom right, after Oh, [48].*)

that the life expectancy of a prosthesis was sensitive to the weight and activity level of the patient. For an adverse combination, the predicted life was less than a year. However, the expected life has been greatly increased with the recent introduction of strong metals such as forged nickel-cobalt-chrome, forged cobalt-chrome, and hot isostatically pressed cobalt-chrome powder, with fatigue lives 50 to 100 percent greater than that of cast cobalt-chrome.

Stresses at various interfaces of a Charnley prosthesis were calculated by Svensson et al. [46], using a two-dimensional finite-element analysis. They pointed out that for the bone and the stem, the bending stresses were most important; for the cement, the normal and shearing stresses. The shear stresses at the cement-bone interface were twice as high on the medial side as on the lateral, being a maximum of 2 N/mm². Even though the shear stresses varied considerably, depending on whether or not the stem-cement interface carried tension, the stresses in the stem itself and in the bone were not greatly affected. The normal stresses at the acrylic-bone interface showed a compressive peak of 2.5 N/mm² at the lateral tip, while on the medial side there was tension of about 1 N/mm^2. The tensile stresses down the lateral interface were small. The highest compressive stresses, however, were at the stem-cement interface, 2 and 6 N/mm^2 at the tip and medial edges, respectively. This emphasizes the importance of broad and contoured metallic surfaces in these areas. Different positionings of the stem in the bone canal were investigated. The "varus" position of the stem (neck against calcar, stem tip lateral) increased the stem tensile stress by 13 percent, whereas the more popularly recommended valgus position reduced the stresses in the stem but significantly increased the shear and tensile stresses at the cement-bone interface. A thickened stem decreased the maximum stresses without substantially decreasing the stresses in the bone. To simplify display of the six stresses at a given point in a material, Huiskes and Slooff [47] formulated an "equivalent stress." Several stresses were reduced by a low stem-to-bone modulus ratio, implying an advantage of titanium alloy, for example. The optimum modulus for the cement was midway between that of bone and stem.

The analytic methods described all have their limitations, including reliance on the input geometric, elastic, and interface data, and the variations among specimens. It is necessary, therefore, to compare experimental and analytic data, and to consider the results of each in the light of the assumptions and limitations. In a study carried out by Oh [48], strain gauges were attached to the outer surfaces of the femur to measure longitudinal tensile and compressive strain. Readings were taken both of intact femurs and after the insertion of different prosthetic stems. Different loads were applied in different directions, but the offsets of the femoral heads were compensated for by calculating the force that would be acting. The strains after prosthesis insertion were not greatly different from normal, except for a severe reduction in the longitudinal compressive strain in the calcar-lower neck area. They suggested that this was responsible for the bone resorption that occurs in this area. The strains were much higher with collar-calcar contact than without, but still lower than normal. However, this was contested on the grounds that the deflection of the prosthesis without a collar at the calcar region was so small that, even if a collar were present, any inaccuracy of fitting and any bone resorption would negate the effect [49]. This topic is thus still controversial. In comparing the strains in the bone with different prosthetic stems, the particular design of the stem and its bending stiffness made little difference to the strains, in agreement with the analysis of Svensson. A more recent study by Oh, Harris, and Bourne further investigated the effects of stem length, stem section, neck angle, and neck length.

For comparing the strength characteristics of different stems per se, there are a number of simple methods available. If material properties alone are required, a direct method is to machine-test specimens from the stem itself. One limitation is that if the properties of the lateral surface are required, it is not possible to machine a test specimen containing this surface for a rotating-beam test. One test method is to apply a load between the femoral head and the tip. The resulting bending moment on the stem will be a maximum at the point of maximum bowing, about one-quarter of the way down from the neck, reaching zero at the tip. This is a reasonable method, particularly in its simplicity. A variation of this method recognizes the clinical finding that fatigue breakage of the stem occurs mostly in the middle third, accompanied by loss of cement support in the proximal third. Hence, the stem is oriented vertically, with the lower third potted in acrylic cement, and a cyclic load is applied at the femoral head, giving a maximum stress just above the acrylic.

Another test method, used by Reuben et al. [50], was to hold the prosthesis in a fixture and apply a three-point bending load. For the stem, this was equivalent to a lateral force at the tip, the moment increasing linearly up the length of the stem. Since the sectional modulus increases up the stem, the failure point depended on the moment and the section modulus, but usually occurred somewhere in the middle third. Strain gauges were applied down the lateral face of the prosthesis, and strain versus load was plotted for increasing load, up to plastic deformation. Interesting discontinuities in yield were found along the stem in certain cast cobalt-chrome stems; they were attributed to large grain size or variations in the properties of different grains.

Four material classes were tested from contemporary off-the-shelf designs: cast cobalt-chrome, forged cobalt-chrome-nickel, wrought 316-L stainless steel, and Ti-6A1-4V. The microstrains at yield were, respectively, 2800, 6000, 3500, and 6600. The lower modulus of elasticity of the titanium alloy should be borne in mind here. The corresponding yield stresses were 350, 700, 340, and 390 N/mm². Further experiments on the new generation of materials, including forged cobalt-chrome alloy and cobalt-chrome formed by the hot isostatic pressing of powder, produced results up to two times the values quoted above.

In all these tests, the magnitude of a failure force is measured. This will clearly depend on the material itself, the geometry of the stem, the orientation of the force, and the offset distance of the neck. The stress at any point on a given stem can in fact be calculated if the stem geometry and the external forces are known. Hence the chief value of such experiments is to determine the material properties of production stems supplied by the manufacturers. The most important location at which to measure the properties is usually the lateral face. The next step, to specify some performance characteristics of different stems, with a given material, is not easy. The offset distance of the neck can be adequately accounted for by calculating the force vectors comparatively on the head, taking into account the lever arm of the body weight and the abductors. However, once the head-force vector has been determined, the proportion of the bending moment carried by the stem when cemented into a femur will depend on the parameters described earlier, leading to the importance of finite-element analysis and strain-gauge studies. In conclusion, the significance of bench tests on stems themselves, is first, to measure the material properties along the lateral face and elsewhere as appropriate, and secondarily, to measure the maximum bending stresses sustained by sections along the stem length. The significance of experimental and theoretical analysis is

1. To determine stresses in the materials under simulated *in vivo* loading conditions
2. To determine interface stresses under simulated *in vivo* loading conditions
3. To determine the effects of different variables, such as stem length, cross section, material modulus, and surface characteristics, on the strains and stresses

The overall aim of laboratory and clinical studies should be to optimize stem design and to clarify some of the still unknown factors.

3.2 Tibial Plateau Fixation

This section, although directed to knees, is relevant to the fixation of components onto condyles or surfaces of cancellous bone. Examples other than the upper tibia are the glenoid, the acetabulum, the phalanx at the MCP joint, the ulna at the elbow, and the talus. Loss of secure fixation of tibial components has occurred clinically in several ways. Excessive distortion of plastic components, especially of the thin modular type, has caused mechanical malfunction and fragmentation of the cement. Progressive sinkage has been attributed to weak bone, residual varus or valgus deformity, or components of inadequate surface area. Perhaps the most common is progressive radiolucency at the cement-bone interface, leading eventually to "symptomatic" loosening. The conditions that lead to these failure modes will include the following:

1. Excessive local or overall compressive stresses on the bone, causing failure of trabeculae
2. Tensile stresses at the implant-bone interface, producing relative micromovement
3. Excessive shear stresses on the bone, giving trabecular failure and micro-movement
4. Distortion of the tibial component sufficient to give excessive bending stresses in the cement

Implicit in the above is the assumption that there is a level of compressive stress and micromovement that will lead to bone resorption, replacement with fibrous tissue, and component loosening.

The different designs of tibial components can be reduced to a few reasonable possibilities (Fig. 17), if we recognize that each can have variations in shape, size, and location of the salient fixation features. In all these types, there is the choice of a solid plastic component, of enclosing the plastic in a metallic tray, or of using a different material such as a ceramic.

If the cruciate ligaments are preserved, modular components comprise one possibility. As little bone as possible should be removed. For the Charnley load angle inlay, which uses thin metal plates, the bone need barely be disturbed. The base of the plateaus can have a fin or posts to stiffen the support and to resist tilting. The major part of the load is transmitted as compression on the upper bone surface. A second possibility for cruciate preservation is to inset the component into a deep trough, such as in the polycentric design. In this case, the load is transmitted as shear, with some compression on the flanks of the tapered trough. An interesting possibility is to combine compressive and shear load support. A third possibility, which preserves the cruciates, is anteriorly joined modular components. This has been used on the Geomedic, the Anametric, and the Townley total knee. The crossbridge can have a spike or blade for fixation.

If only the posterior cruciate, or neither cruciate, is preserved, virtually the

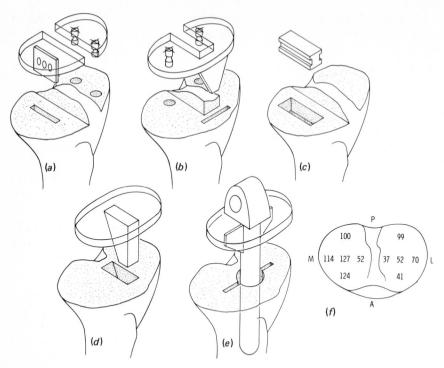

Figure 17 (*a* to *e*) Different basic designs of tibial component; (*f*) relative strength of the cancellous bone 5 mm below the surface.

whole of the upper tibia is available for fixation. The three-point fixation system can be used here also (Fig. 17*b*), or even two posts or blades, one on each side. Alternatively, since the bone is weaker at the center than at each side, the center can be used for a peg. Load support is in direct compression at each side, and as shear down the sides of the post. The post may additionally have some distal cortical support. An intramedullary stem uses a substantial length of the bone canal for fixation. The stem can be combined with a flat surface over the upper tibia, the amount of compressive load support from the latter depending on the elastic properties of the whole bone-component system. Other possibilities include incorporating a rim to fit over the tibia, inserting screws or staples anteriorly as in the Kodama-Yamamoto knee, or using the tibial spine as a saddle, as in the Deane knee prosthesis.

There have been only a few reported studies to date on tibial fixation per se. Compressive failure tests were carried out by Bargren et al. [51]. The failure forces for different types of components ranged from 3000 to 11,000 N, and they emphasized that it was important to cover the bone up to the periphery. This can be appreciated in part from Fig. 17, where the average values for bone strength 5 mm below the surface of a number of specimens are shown. However, the trabecular structure as a whole must be considered, such as the arch and plate arrangements well illustrated by Ikuhi [52].

The shear strength and stiffness of the cement-bone interface will depend on the cement interdigitation and the amount of fibrous tissue interposed. For an average-sized one-piece tibial component covering the whole of the upper tibia, and for a shear strength of 1.5 N/mm^2, the maximum torque that can be sustained is approximately 75 N m (660 lb/in^2), about 10 times that in level walking [33]. For comparison, a central peg 38 mm in length, similar to that of the Total Condylar, sustained an average torque of 33 N m before failure, the failure mode being trabecular compression. Returning now to compressive loading, the significance of the "strength" or "elastic" centrode was illustrated in some tests by Walker et al. [53]. By using a metal unicompartmental plateau, loads were applied at various positions along an anterior-posterior line, and the relative vertical movement between the plateau and bone was measured at the anterior and posterior. The load centrode when uniform compression occurred was not, in general, at the geometric center. Tensile tilting occurred for loads at positions even in the middle half. Short pegs or cement keyholes provide a resistance to tension, typical pull-out strengths of pegs shown in Fig. 17, *a* and *b*, being 1.4 to 1.7 times body weight, with a cement-bone shear strength of 1.2 to 2.9 N/mm^2. Walker et al. also tested plastic components for bowing for a force applied at the center. The bowing was greatest with soft bone, being 0.07 mm for the particular test, a value that could produce locally high compressive stresses.

An analytic approach to the problem was reported by Askew et al. [54]. They used a three-dimensional finite-element method to calculate the direct stresses at the cement-bone interface for different types of tibial component and loading (Fig. 18). Stiffness values for the cancellous bone at various locations were obtained by an area-fractions method. For a plateau consisting of an oval metal slab, tilting

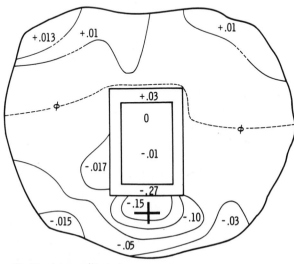

Plastic plateau with post

Bone-PMMA interface normal stresses (N/m^2) for 1N force

Figure 18 Stresses in a Total Condylar type of tibial component, for anterior loading at +. *(After Askew et al. [54].)*

occurred for either anterior or posterior loads. For a three-body-weight load, the compressive stresses were typically 4 N/mm², and the tensile stresses one-half and one-fourth this amount. The compression would be well tolerated by the bone with an average compressive strength of 19 N/mm² mentioned earlier. They compared metal and plastic components of the same configuration, concluding that the metal distributed localized loads more evenly, whereas the plastic concentrated the stress under the load 1.5 to 2 times under the loads. The tensile stresses caused by tilting were higher for metal by a factor of up to 2. The two conditions that reduced tilting, localized compressive stresses, and tensile stresses were a stiffened support such as a fixation post beneath the load and another fixation post at the opposite side to carry tension. An optimally designed component would have three or four posts evenly spaced around the periphery and as close to the periphery as possible.

Experiments were carried out by Walker and co-workers to measure the relative vertical movement between tibial components and the bone at points around the periphery, for different loading conditions. The tibia was mounted in a base, the upper tibia cut level, the trabecular spaces at the upper surface filled with modeling clay to simulate a nontensile bond, and the component cemented on. Different tibiae, representative of the types described earlier, were tested. Loads were applied sequentially to a simulated femoral component, in direct compression, and then compression combined with anterior and posterior forces, internal and external torques, and varus and valgus moments. Figure 19 shows a representative sample of the results. Tilting, in the form of distraction at one or more points around the periphery, was common. The amount of compression and distraction was consistently less with metal trays than with similar plastic

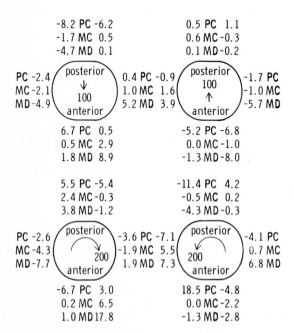

Figure 19 Relative vertical movements between a tibial component and the tibia at six points around the periphery. +ve = compression; −ve = distraction. PC = plastic component, central peg (Total Condylar type); MC = the same with a metal tray; MD = a metal tray with two short posts, on medial and lateral sides. Forces are pounds, and torques in pound inches.

components. In rotation, plastic components distorted significantly. A large central peg produced small compressions and distractions, even with varus-valgus loading. The finding that metal distracted less than plastic is not really contrary to the analytic results noted above, because the tensile stresses, as opposed to distractions, can be visualized as the force necessary to push that part of the component back onto the surface. It is likely, however, that if the cement-bone bond is weak in tension, the least distraction is an advantage.

An approach in some ways similar to the above was used by Chao [55] to evaluate the fixation of a Geomedic tibial component. The centrode of the component was determined geometrically, and moments about three axes defined in relation to this point. For example, if the resultant vertical force V in the frontal plane were displaced e to the medial side, the moment would be Ve. From available data for the force and moment cycles during the walking activity, the moments at specified small time intervals were summed for the whole walking cycle, giving a measure of the "loosening moment" on the component. One aim of the work was to examine the effects of component placement, such as tilting the component forward or backward, or placing it medially or laterally. This approach could be applied to assess the optimum locations of fixation posts, or to assess the loosening propensity of partially conforming types of tibial components.

In summary, some of the factors affecting tibial component fixation are:

1. Material used (if plastic, the thickness, or whether supported on a metallic tray)
2. Locations and sizes of fixation posts, blades, etc.
3. Amount of tibial bone removed, and the elastic and strength properties of the bone
4. Quality of cement fixation (or other fixation means)
5. Placement of the component
6. Alignment of the knee
7. Conformity of the component, or the forces and moments transmitted
8. Activity of the patient

3.3 Laxity, Stability, and Contact Stresses

It was illustrated in Fig. 6 that there are many possible forms for an artificial joint, ranging from nonconstrained to fully constrained. The degree of constrainment is, of course, load-dependent, in that the stability increases with the compressive load applied. However, the stability or constrainment of a given prosthesis can be expressed in geometric terms:

Stability = rate of distraction per unit displacement

In Fig. 20, for linear movements, the units of stability are millimeter per millimeter, and for rotations the units are millimeter per radian or millimeter per degree. It will be noted that in general the values for stability are not constant but must be expressed as a curve plotted as a function of linear or rotational displacement.

An example of stability for the ankle prosthesis was given by Pappas et al. [56]

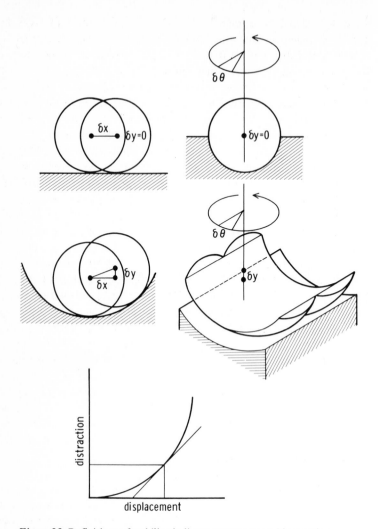

Figure 20 Definitions of stability in linear movement and in rotation.

(Fig. 21). Assume that in a certain activity a compressive force V and a moment M are acting. In the normal ankle, the talus is bound on one side by the fibula and on the other by the medial malleolus. If M is initially small and is increased gradually, the stress distribution shifts more and more to the medial side until, when $M = Va$, the ankle is on the point of tilting. The medial malleolus forms an effective pivot point, and the ligaments on the lateral side come into tension. The lever arm for the ligaments is a maximum at $2a$. For a moment in the other direction, a similar situation occurs. For a prosthesis that is domed in the frontal plane (Fig. 21), any moment will induce a tilting (ignoring friction), and the lateral or medial ligaments will be necessary. In this case the lever arm for the ligaments is only a. A prosthesis with cylindrical bearing surfaces has the advantage of the anatomic, that a moment of *Va* is needed before tilting occurs. However, on tilting there is a rather unstable pivot point, owing to the lack of restriction of medial-lateral sliding.

A design that provided pivoting on each side would have both advantages: a moment of about *Va* before tilting and a lever arm of nearly 2*a* for the resisting ligaments. These comments apply to varus-valgus tilting in the knee joint. A further example is in the MCP joint. Although in the anatomic joint, the joint surfaces are spherical, replacement by such is probably not optimal. The collateral ligaments are in no position to assist, because they only tighten after considerable rotation in the radial or ulnar direction. Hence, for motion in the sagittal plane only, the muscle balance about the pivot point *P* needs to be very accurate indeed. An alternative scheme is shown in Fig. 21, where there are effectively two pivot points so that as long as the resultant force passes between these two points, tilting will not occur.

Another way of defining stability is in terms of applied forces:

$$\text{Stability} = \frac{\text{displacement}}{\text{displacing force} \times \text{compressive force}}$$

Applied to condylar replacement knee prostheses, in the anterior-posterior directions, for a unit compressive force across the joint, this means the stability is the rate of change of a-p movement with the a-p force. An analogous definition applies in rotation. A modular knee with a flat tibial plateau provides the least stability, the only constraint being the friction forces. For other condylar replacement prostheses,

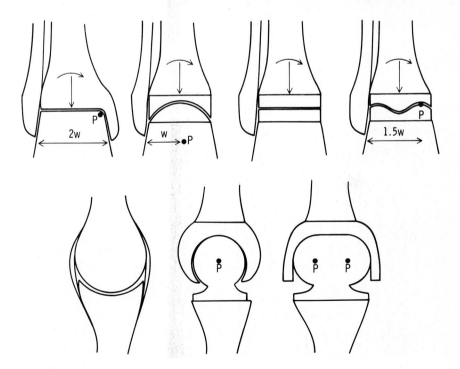

Figure 21 Stability in the ankle (top) and in the MCP (bottom) joints.

the inherent stability increases with increasing conformity of the femoral and tibial condylar surfaces.

The most important parameter in stability was shown [57, 58] to be $R - r$, the difference in the radii of curvature of the tibial and femoral condyles in the sagittal plane. A loading rig was constructed to apply any required combination of compressive, a-p, and rotatory forces (Fig. 22a). Part-cylindrical plastic tibial troughs and femoral rollers with two biconvex condylar surfaces simulated the prosthetic components. Different combinations of radii gave a range from full conformity $(R = r)$ to low conformity $(R \gg r)$. For a given pair of components, a compressive

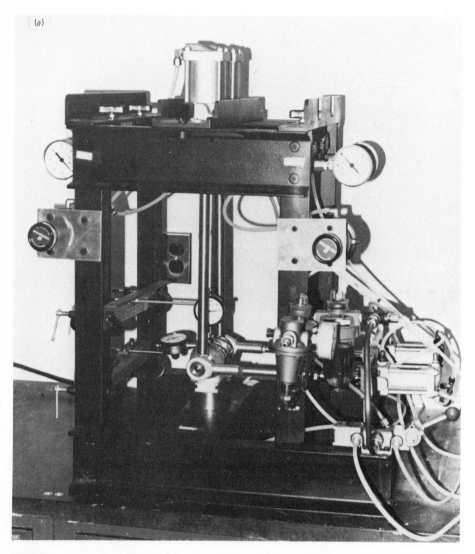

Figure 22 (*a*) Loading rig for studying the stability of knee prostheses.

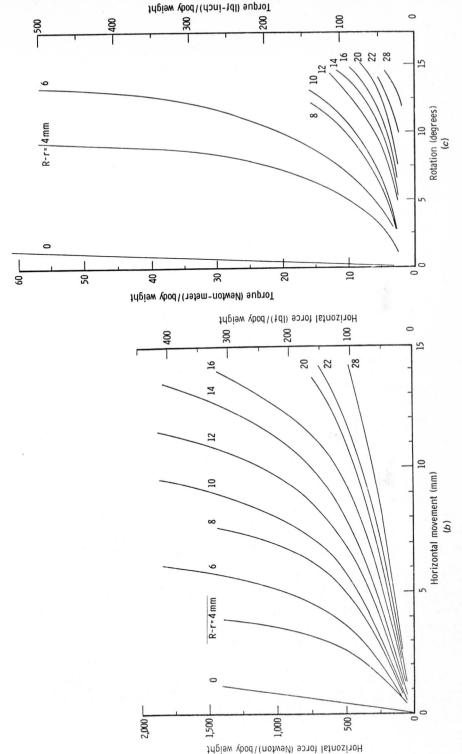

Figure 22 (*Continued*) (*b*) Laxity curves for an anterior force; (*c*) laxity curves for a torque.

load was applied (e.g., one body weight), and then a progressive anterior force or torque was applied, with displacement or rotation measured at each increment. Families of curves were thus obtained (Fig. 22b and c).

As examples, for a one-body-weight compressive force, with $R - r = 4$ mm, the ratio was about 1 mm per 200 N of force; with $R - r = 24$ mm, the ratio was about 8 mm per 200 N of force. For forces greater than one body weight, the ratios were reduced in proportion. It is evident that in walking, where the compressive force is about three body weights and the a-p shear force about 300 N, for $R - r = 4$ mm, the movement between the components is only 1 mm, whereas for $R - r = 24$ mm, the movement is only 3 mm.

This has implications regarding the function of the cruciate ligaments when a knee prosthesis is in place. If there is no compressive load across the joint, except where the condylar surfaces are closely conforming, the cruciates will provide most of the a-p restraint. However, in walking, if the condylar surfaces only allow 1 or 2 mm of movement, the cruciates will be almost inoperative, and most of the a-p force will be carried by the components. Calculations indicate that in the range of $R - r$ from 28 mm down to 8 mm, the posterior cruciate carries 45 percent down to 30 percent of the anterior force. For $R - r$ less than 8 mm, the percentage falls off rapidly toward zero. The latter case will apply to many prostheses, particularly with the knee toward extension, as Table 1 shows.

A further point about cruciate preservation relates to the backward movement of the contact point of the femur on the tibia with flexion. If the conformity is too great, there will be a conflict causing tenson in one or both cruciates, leading to restriction of motion and a tendency to loosening of the tibial component.

Rotation can be treated in essentially the same way as a-p force. The amount of rotation allowed by the condylar surfaces is proportional to the applied torque, inversely proportional to load, and increases with increasing $R - r$. As an example (Fig. 22c), for medium conformity with $R - r = 14$ mm, a load of three body weights, and a torque of 50 kg·cm, typical of normal level walking, the rotation is just over $2°$. This small amount of rotation indicates the inherent stiffness of condylar replacement prostheses to rotation. Almost all the torque will be transmitted through the components to the fixation. One method of eliminating rotational stiffness is to extend the tibial tracks on circular arcs, centered at the

Table 1 Percentage of a-p force carried by posterior cruciate

Prosthesis	Extension	Flexion
Geomedic 1	0.7%	0.7%
Freeman-Swanson	0.0	0.0
Total condylar	0.0	0.0
Anametric	16	29
Townley	25	46
Modular (approximate)	50	75

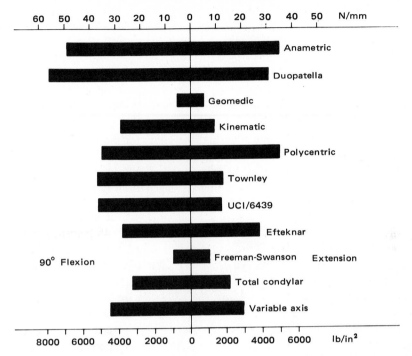

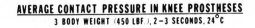

Figure 23 Contact stresses in knee prostheses in extension and flexion. The plastic was RCH-1000.

geometric center of the tibial component, as used at the U.C.I. and Eftekhar designs.

The subject of contact stress is included here because of its connection with laxity and stability: In general, the more laxity, the less the conformity, the less the contact area, and the greater the contact stress. For metal on high-molecular-weight polyethylene, excessive local stresses lead to cold flow and deformation, and to increased wear by surface cracking. An upper limit for design purposes has not yet been specified, partly owing to variations in what is nominally the same polyethylene [59], although 20 N/mm^2 has been suggested [60].

Using the same rollers and troughs as mentioned above, the contact areas were measured for short-term loadings of 10 s and long-term loadings of 10 min. The areas in the former case were less than the latter by 20 percent. For a Poisson's ratio of 0.4, the Hertzian elasticity equations show the effective moduli of elasticity to be 2148 and 1006 N/mm^2, respectively. At a load of three body weights the average contact stresses ranged from 10 to 38 N/mm^2.

Although the results could be transposed to knee prostheses by considering radii of curvature, tests were also done on samples of prostheses themselves, at three body weights and 2 to 3 s loading time (Fig. 23). In extension the stresses ranged from 5 to 35 N/mm^2, whereas in flexion the stresses were even higher, at 5 to 56

N/mm^2. It is evident, therefore, that the stresses are considerably higher than in the hip joint, for example, and in excess of what is considered to be the upper limit. Examination of removed low-conformity prostheses has shown stress cracking on the surfaces [60], although there are no reports as yet of catastrophic wear resulting from these high stresses.

3.4 Clinical Results

A group of contemporary artificial joints is shown in Fig. 24. The present types of total hip replacement using cemented metal on plastic components have been used for almost 15 yr, total knees for about 8 yr, and the joints for the upper extremity about 6 yr but in much smaller numbers than the hip and the knee.

   Most designs of total hip are similar in form, varying only in stem length and section, and in femoral head size. Dislocation has ranged from 0 to 4 percent in

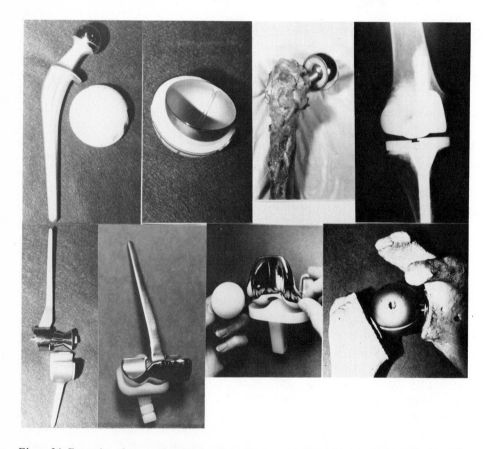

Figure 24 Examples of current prostheses. Top, left to right: HD-2 hip; surface replacement hip; Bateman proximal femur; Variable Axis knee. Bottom, left to right: Mayo elbow; Ewald elbow; Total Condylar knee; Gristina Trispherical shoulder.

different series [61]. Wear of the plastic socket has not shown itself to be a significant clinical problem, whether by penetrating the component, by reducing the range of motion to an unacceptable level, or via adverse affects of the wear particles. However, the latter may produce certain adverse affects, particularly in long-term follow-ups [62]. The most reliable long-term *in vivo* study available is that of Charnley and Halley [63]. In 9 to 10-yr follow-ups, 68 percent wore less than 1.5 mm, and the rest up to 4.5 mm. The average wear rate was 0.15 mm/yr. The rate in the second 5 yr was less than for the first 5 yr, which is surprising considering that surface fatigue is believed to be an important wear mechanism. In a series of 57 Müller 32-mm-diameter prostheses followed for 2 to 4 yr, the radiographically measured wear ranged from 0.05 to 4 mm/yr, seemingly a higher rate than for the Charnleys. This is contrary to the simple theory that indicates that the larger the head the lower the rate of depth penetration, but the greater the volumetric wear. Although the radiographic method for measuring wear has its drawbacks, Charnley's results were backed up by direct measurements of 26 removed sockets. The use of aluminum oxide ceramic on polyethylene and ceramic on ceramic has been shown [64] to reduce wear considerably. The wear rate of polyethylene was 20 times less against ceramic than against cobalt-chrome, attributed to the better wettability of ceramic and the fact that surface roughnessess were pits rather than asperities.

Radiolucency at the cement-bone interface in sockets is common, even up to a 100 percent incidence if partial lines are included. Most radiolucencies are non-progressive, however. Loosening with gradual migration of the socket has occurred in from 0.8 to 9.2 percent, the latter being in a 10-yr follow-up, the failures being mostly in cases of initial bony deficiency [61]. The bone preparation and cement technique must have an important effect also. Resorption of the lower neck and calcar has been a problem observed with long-term follow-ups. Based on the study of Oh [48], this is almost certainly caused by the abnormally low compressive stresses after stem insertion. It is still not known whether load transfer by a collar is maintained clinically. The surface replacement hips in current widespread use use thin-walled plastic shells. Theoretical and experimental analyses, as well as careful follow-ups, are needed to assess the viability of fixation, and whether metal shells for support would be an advantage.

Stem loosening is a more frequent complication than socket loosening. Stem breakage can be a secondary complication, and removal is not easy. The incidence up to 5 yr has been reported at 0 to 7 percent, with an average of 3.5 percent [61]. The failure modes were characterized by distal and/or medial migration of the stem, and cracking of the cement originating from the lateral bone interface and moving laterally. Medial migration and cement cracking in the proximal part was the most threatening condition for stem breakage [65]. New operative techniques and stem configurations should significantly reduce loosening and breakage: canal cleaning by abrasion or lavage, plugging of the canal and cement introduction by cement gun to increase pressure, stems with roughened surfaces or with "teardrops" for keying to the cement, and metals with 50 to 100 percent increase in fatigue strength. Time will tell whether there will be fewer problems with these new femoral components inserted in the optimal manner, than in the femoral components of surface replacements. It is well known that potential problems with the latter include necrosis of the head, loosening, and fracture of the femoral neck if the technique has been imperfect.

Bone ingrowth surfaces have been used for femoral stems, with apparent success after a few years [66]. However, such devices should be used cautiously at present, because of the potential problems of bone resorption resulting from stress protection if the fixation is too secure or, at the other extreme, loosening and abrasion of the endosteal surface.

Compared with total hips, there are a greater variety of total knees. In similar time periods, the knees have generally suffered from more problems than the hips. The modular types, with little or no dishing in the tibial component, have allowed medial or lateral subluxation [67]. Both tibial and femoral loosening have been a problem associated with components that are too thin, a residual varus or valgus deformity, or instability. With the polycentric design, tibial sinkage was a problem in a few percent of cases, whereas no femoral loosenings have occurred in hundreds of cases. The close conformity of the femoral and tibial tracks in the frontal plane has led to cold flow of the plastic (Fig. 25).

The effect of metal-plastic conformity on potential loosening was documented

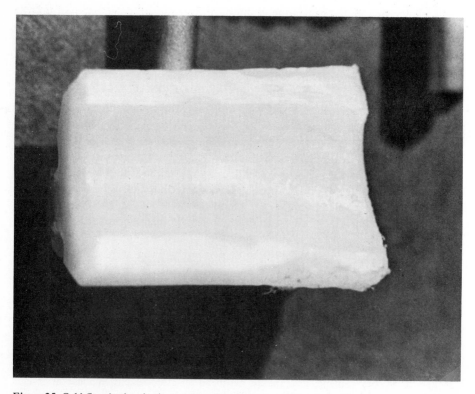

Figure 25 Cold flow in the plastic component of a polycentric knee prosthesis.

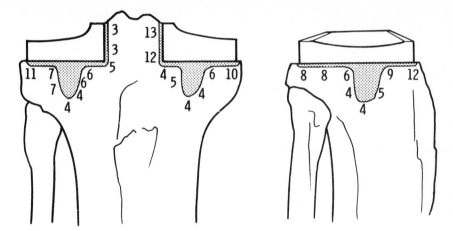

Figure 26 The locations of progressive radiolucency (numerals indicate frequency) at the cement-bone interface from radiographs of a series of condylar replacement knee prostheses.

in a comparable series of Duocondylars and Duopatellas. The only difference was that the tibial components were flat in the a-p direction in the former, and curved in the latter. The incidence of cement-bone radiolucency was as follows: complete and partial with the Duocondylars, 4.5 and 6.7 percent respectively; with the Duopatellas, the figures were 4.4 and 2.5 percent [68]. In the U.C.I. type, loosening and cold flow of the plastic have been significant problems in up to 14 percent [69]. In the conforming Geomedic prostheses, radiolucency has been reported at 80 percent [70], and reoperation for loosening after a 2-yr series at 10 percent [71]. By comparison, in a 1 to 3-yr series of 223 Total Condylars, only 22 percent of the tibial components showed any radiolucency [72]. P. S. Walker and H-H Hsieh (unpublished date, 1976) studied over 100 radiographs from patients with condylar replacement prostheses, mostly Duocondylars, in an attempt to correlate radiolucency with placement of the components. Although the correlations were not impressive, the locations of the radiolucency suggested a tilting mechanism for the development of radiolucency (Fig. 26). The pattern is consistent with tilting in both planes, with a resultant force on the knee in the frontal plane disposed medially. Conclusions from the above in terms of loosening are that plastic components seated on the bone with little or no fixation into the cancellous bone are inadequate; even moderate conformity will induce a greater tendency to loosening; and stronger fixation means that those currently existing are needed.

Metallic hinges are mostly used for severe cases or for reoperation, where a higher complication range would be expected. The infection rate has been quoted at 6 to 12 percent, and the loosening rate from 5 to 14 percent [70, 73]. In comparison, the infection rate for condylar replacement knees is usually 3 percent at most. Even though the aseptic loosening rate of hinges is no higher than that for many condylar replacements, the salvage procedure after a hinge is more difficult.

Because of the problems with all-metal fixed hinges, a new class of partially constrained "hinges" has emerged, such as the Stabilocondylar, the Spherocentric, and the Attenborough. These prostheses have not been without their problems, however, which have included loosening, recurvatum, and even bone fracture, caused in part by the short stems. Infection has been comparable to that with condylar replacements, however, suggesting a preference for metal on plastic and a less bulky prosthesis. New types of hinges that use metal on plastic to restrict varus-valgus but allow rotation about the tibial axis represent an interesting new approach.

Gait analysis and force-plate studies provide useful objective data on post-operative performance. A two-dimensional quasi-static force analysis was used in a study of the ankle. Five normal subjects and nine patients, before and 1 yr after total ankle replacement, were studied [35]. Total sagittal plane motion was 24.4°, 20°, and 23° in normal subjects, preoperative patients and postoperative patients, respectively. The fore-aft forces peaked to almost body weight in normal subjects, was close to zero for preoperative patients, but returned toward normal for postoperative patients. In contrast, the peak vertical force on the ankle, calculated to average 4.7 body weights in normals, did not change from the 3 body weights preoperatively. Simon and Mazur [74] studied patients with ankle fusions in follow-ups up to 10 yr. Ground-to-foot forces and gait patterns were compared between the operated and nonoperated sides, and with the patterns of normal subjects. There were minimal differences after fusion, attributed to the compensating factors of the subtalar and tarsal joints. There was some clinically observed limitation in walking up and down slopes, or on uneven ground. The work has been extended to a study of 21 patients with different types of prostheses, most of which were of the Mayo design. The results were inferior to fusion, with gait pattern, velocity, and step length as criteria; the difference was believed to result from joint instability. Ominous signs of progressive radiolucency were noted, a finding confirmed by Greenwald and Matejczyk [75].

For the upper extremity, there have been no long-term studies of a large number of prostheses for a particular joint, with the exception of the Silastic spacers for the MCP joint. There are literature reports of more than 4000 of these spacers, and many more thousands have been used in the field throughout the world. In late 1976, Swanson [76] reported on his own results, combined with those of several clinical collaborators. The passive ranges of motion were from about zero to 70°. From 1965 to 1973, of 868 implants, 66 were known to have fractured. Of those using the new improved Silastic rubber, from 1973 to 1976, 10 of 638 were known to have fractured. In another series of 530 consecutive arthroplasties [77], the average active motion was 38°, the fracture rate was 26 percent, and the recurrence of deformity 11 percent.

To date, the cemented metal-plastic types of prostheses, although promising greater strength, have so far not been without their problems. Dobyns [78] reported on a series of 411 Steffee joints performed at the Mayo Clinic, with up to $2\frac{1}{2}$ yr follow-up. The grip strength showed no improvement postoperatively. Forty-three percent had mild to moderate recurrence of ulnar drift. The range of motion was from about 25° to 70°. Of the first 250 cases, there was 11.2 percent reoperation, including 7 loose implants, 5 bent or broken implants, and 18 infections. Another cemented metal-plastic design was used in 104 joints in 28 patients and evaluated using a mechanical evaluation system [28]. The active range of motion was only 22°, but there were only a few instances of ulnar deviation. Pinch strength and radial and ulnar strengths were about the same preoperatively and postoperatively. Grip strength increased, however, to one-third of normal. Radiolucency was noted in one or more joints of 18 hands, and there were several cases of actual loosening. Overall, although the Silastic spacers have their shortcomings, the cemented metal-plastic type have not been shown to be significantly better, and the revision problems are more severe. It may be that a noncemented mechanical design could be an effective improvement.

A variety of elbow prostheses have been used, from a humeral condylar replacement to rigid metallic hinges [79]. The Street-Stevens humeral condyle replacement is a simple anatomically shaped metallic device that is hammered onto the condyles from the medial side, no cement being used. The developers have performed only 18 cases in 10 yr, mostly on ankylosed patients. Fixation has been reported as excellent, the main problems being poor range of motion in several cases and some pain in others.

The Ewald elbow is a condylar replacement of the nonlinked type, with anatomic metal-plastic bearing surfaces and intramedullary fixation stems. The humeral condyles overlap preserved bone for additional fixation. It should be pointed out that even nonlinked but conforming designs can transmit considerable torques when they are under the compressive loads of activity. In a report on 50 patients, mostly rheumatoids, followed for up to nearly 3 yr, alignment of the components was found to be critical for range of motion and stability. Although no frank loosening has yet occurred, radiolucencies around the plastic ulnar component have indicated redesign to include a metal shell with a longer stem.

The Pritchard elbow is based on spherical bearing surfaces, loosely linked to allow radial and ulnar motion. In 25 cases followed for 2 to 3 yr, no radiolucencies have been observed. If this situation is maintained, it suggests that laxity might transfer a useful amount of the moments from the components to muscles and soft tissues.

As for rigid all-metal hinges, it is generally accepted that the combination of the metal bearing and the rigidity leads to an unacceptable level of loosening. For the unstable elbow, therefore, attention has shifted to the use of plastic bushings and improvements in design and technique. The Stanmore hinged elbow has undergone several revisions in its 10-yr history. Presently it uses cobalt-chrome stemmed humeral and ulnar components, and an RCH-1000 bushing into which an axle is snapped at surgery. The prosthesis is narrow enough to fit within the distal humerus. Of 18 cases followed during these 10 yr, several have suffered infection and/or loosening, despite careful cleaning of the intramedullary canals for optimal cement filling. The Mayo elbow has been in use for several years and has undergone several design revisions. Many patients continue to have successful results, but several loosenings have been encountered of both humeral and ulnar components. A particular mode of failure of the humeral component has been gradual anterior migration of the end of the stem. This mode has also been observed on other hinged designs and suggests that the anterior-to-posterior component of the joint force may be a prime cause. To overcome loosening and instability problems, present design trends are to surface replacement types and linked types with lax metal-plastic bearings fitting between the humeral condyles and including "wings" or other means of attachment to the bone at each side.

Shoulder prostheses, particularly the linked type, are not used with great frequency, so that it is difficult to assess particular designs statistically. The Neer humeral head replacement is still the most commonly used device because of its simplicity, satisfactory results, and low complication rate. The addition of a plastic glenoid component has apparently enhanced the clinical result and is applicable when the glenoid is eroded. Fixation is not an easy problem, however, as mentioned earlier in this chapter. An example of such a design is the St. Georg used in 28 cases from 1974 to 1977. Two types of plastic glenoid were used, one with greater superior coverage than the other for the more stable shoulders. Particularly in rheumatoid arthritis, the results have been good and no loosening has been reported. The few complications included poor range of motion and infection. The linked types of shoulder prosthesis have had many serious problems. The locked-in ball-in-socket designs have suffered dislocation of the ball from the socket, wrenching out of the socket part from the glenoid, and breakage of the neck of the ball. Not only must the prosthesis sustain high forces and bending moments, but the inherent limitation of motion of a locked ball in socket means that impingement will inevitably be reached in some instances with high impact forces. Two ball-in-socket designs, the Stanmore and the Jefferson, are not securely locked in, but there are insufficient long-term data on these designs at this time. Two linked designs that allow a larger than anatomic range of motion are currently in clinical trials, the Trispherical [80] and the floating socket [81]. These are applicable to cases with no rotator cuff, and early clinical results are encouraging.

BIBLIOGRAPHY

Dowson, D., and V. Wright (eds.): "An Introduction to the Biomechanics of Joints and Joint Replacements," Publ. MEP, Bury St. Edmunds, England, 1978.

Dumbleton, J. H., and J. Black: "An Introduction to Orthopaedic Materials," Thomas, Springfield, Ill., 1975.

Swanson, S. A. V., and M. A. R. Freeman: "The Scientific Basis of Joint Replacement," Pitman, Tunbridge Wells, England, 1977.

Walker, P. S.: "Human Joints and Their Artificial Replacements," Thomas, Springfield, Ill., 1977.

REFERENCES

1. E. F. Haboush, A New Operation for Arthroplasty of the Hip Based on Biomechanics, Photoelasticity, Fast Settling Dental Acrylic, and Other Considerations, *Bull. Hosp. J. Dis.,* vol. 14, p. 2, 1953.

2. J. Charnley, Anchorage of the Femoral Head Prosthesis to the Shaft of the Femur, *J. Bone Jt. Surg.,* vol. 42B, p. 28, 1960.

3. B. Walldius, Arthroplasty of the Knee Using an Endoprosthesis, *Acta Orthop. Scand. Suppl.,* vol. 24, p. 5, 1957.

4. D. L. MacIntosh, Hemiarthroplasty of the Knee Using a Space Occupying Prosthesis for Painful Varus and Valgus Deformities, *J. Bone Jt. Surg.,* vol. 40A, p. 1431, 1958.

5. W. N. Jones, Mold Replacement in the Rheumatoid Knee, in R. L. Cruess and N. S. Mitchell (eds.), "Surgery of Rheumatoid Arthritis," chap. 6, Lippincott, Philadelphia, 1971.

6. F. H. Gunston, Polycentric Knee Arthroplasty, *J. Bone Jt. Surg.,* vol. 53B, p. 272, 1971.

7. P. Maquet, Valgus Osteotomy for Osteoarthritis of the Knee, *Clin. Orthop.,* vol. 120, p. 143, 1976.

8. E. J. Marey, "Animal Mechanism: A Treatise on Terrestrial and Aerial Locomotion," Appleton, New York, 1874.

9. M. P. Murray, Gait as a Total Pattern of Movement—Including a Bibliography on Gait, *J. Phys. Med.,* vol. 48, p. 290, 1967.

10. A. L. Nicol, "Elbow Prosthesis Design: Biomechanical Aspects," Ph.D. thesis, University of Strathclyde, Glasgow, U.K., 1977.

11. E. Schulz, S. P. Chan, and E. B. Marsolais, The Feasibility of the Selspot System for 3-D Gait Analysis, *Proc. Orthop. Res. Soc., Dallas, Tex.,* p. 115, February, 1978.

12. T. Andriacchi, G. Andersson, R. Fermier, D. Stern, and J. Galante, A Study of the Patterns of Lower Limb Mechanics during Stair Climbing, *Proc. Orthop. Res. Soc., Dallas, Tex.,* p. 116, February, 1978.

13. M. D. Lesh, J. M. Mansour, and S. R. Simon, Mechanical Energy Analysis of Pathological Gait, *Proc. Orthop. Res. Soc., Dallas, Tex.,* p. 118, February, 1978.

14. D. B. Kettelkamp, R. J. Johnson, G. L. Smidt, E. Y. S. Chao, and M. Walker, An Electrogoniometric Study of Knee Motion in Normal Gait, *J. Bone Jt. Surg.,* vol. 52A, p. 775, 1970.

15. W. C. Hayes, J. M. Feldman, C. Oatis, and J. E. Nixon, Gait Analysis by Multiaxial Accelerometry, *Proc. Orthop. Res. Soc., Dallas, Tex.,* p. 104, February, 1978.

16. J. E. Bateman, "Preliminary Report on Universal Proximal Femur," 3M Company, Surgical Products Division, Fair Lawn, N.J., 1977.

17. I. C. Clarke, H. C. Amstutuz, J. Christie, and A. Graff-Radford, THARIES Surface-Replacement Arthroplasty for the Arthritic Hip. *Proc. 5th Open Sci. Meet. Hip Soc.,* Mosby, St. Louis, 1977.

18. J. J. O'Connor and J. W. Goodfellow, Kinematics and Load-bearing in the Tibio-femoral Joint with Application to Prosthesis Design, *Proc. Orthop. Res. Soc., Las Vegas, Nev.,* p. 54, February, 1977.

19. B. F. Morrey and E. Y. S. Chao, Passive Motion at the Elbow Joint, *J. Bone Jt. Surg.,* vol. 58A, p. 501, 1976.

20. R. Contini, Body Segment Parameters, *Artif. Limbs,* vol. 16, p. 1, 1972.

21. P. S. Walker and W. Davidson, An Apparatus to Assess Function of the Hand, *J. Hand Surg.,* vol. 3, p. 189, 1978.

22. F. C. Hui, K. N. An, and E. Y. S. Chao, Three-dimensional Force Analysis of the Elbow under Isometric Functions, in "1977 Biomechanics Symposium," ASME, New York, 1977.

23. A. Seireg and R. J. Arvikar, The Prediction of Muscular Load Sharing and Joint Forces in the Lower Extremities during Walking, *J. Biomech.,* vol. 8, p. 89, 1975.

24. E. Y. S. Chao and K. N. An, Graphical Interpretation of the Solution to the Redundant Problem in Biomechanics, in "1977 Biomechanics Symposium," ASME, New York, 1977.

25. N. K. Poppen and P. S. Walker, Forces at the Glenohumeral Joint in Abduction, *Clin. Orthop.,* no. 135, p. 165, September, 1978.

26. E. Y. S. Chao, J. D. Opgrange, and F. E. Axmear, Three-dimensional Force Analysis of Finger Joints in Selected Isometric Hand Functions, *J. Biomech.,* vol. 9, p. 387, 1976.

27. N. Berme, J. P. Paul, and W. K. Purves, A Biomechanical Analysis of the Metacarpophalangeal Joint, *J. Biomech.,* vol. 10, p. 409, 1977.

28. P. S. Walker, L. R. Straub, W. Davidson, and M. S. Moneim, Development and Evaluation of a Mechanical Finger Prosthesis, in "Joint Replacement in the Upper Limb, p. 127, (I. Mech. E. Conf. Pub.) Institution of Mechanical Engineers, London, 1977.

29. N. Rydell, Forces in the Hip Joint II. "Intravital Studies in Biomechanics and Related Bio-Engineering Topics," R. M. Kenedi (ed.), Pergamon, London, 1965.

30. J. P. Paul, Forces Transmitted by Joints in the Human Body, *Proc. Inst. Mech. Eng., London,* vol. 181, part 3J, 1967.

31. A. Seireg and R. J. Arvikar, A Mathematical Model for Evaluation of Forces in Lower Extremities of the Musculoskeletal System, *J. Biomech.,* vol. 6, p. 313, 1973.

32. R. D. McLeish and J. Charnley, Abduction Forces in the One-legged Stance, *J. Biomech.,* vol. 3, p. 181, 1970.

33. J. B. Morrison, Function of the Knee Joint in Various Activities, *Med. Biol. Eng.,* vol. 4, p. 573, 1969.

34. J. B. Morrison, The Mechanics of the Knee Joint in Relation to Normal Walking, *J. Biomech.,* vol. 3, p. 51, 1970.

35. R. N. Stauffer, E. Y. S. Chao, and R. C. Brewster, Force and Motion Analysis of the Normal, Diseased and Prosthetic Ankle Joint, *Proc. Orthop. Res. Soc., Las Vegas, Nev.,* p. 44, February, 1977.

36. I. Oh and W. H. Harris, Anatomic Basis of Femoral Component Design for Total Hip Replacement, *Proc. Orthop. Res. Soc., Dallas, Tex.,* p. 275, February, 1978.

37. J. S. Mensch and H. C. Amstutz, Knee Morphology as a Guide to Knee Replacement, *Clin. Orthop.,* vol. 112, p. 231, 1975.

38. A. A. Amis, D. Dowson, A. Unsworth, J. H. Miller, and V. Wright, An Examination of the Elbow Articulation, with Particular Reference to Variation of the Carrying Angle, *Eng. Med.,* vol. 6, p. 76, 1977.

39. J. Black and E. Korostoff, Dynamic Mechanical Properties of Viable Human Cortical Bone, *J. Biomech.,* vol. 6, p. 435, 1973.

40. A. J. Burstein, J. D. Currey, V. H. Frankel, and D. T. Reily, The Ultimate Properties of Bone Tissue: The Effects of Yielding, *J. Biomech.,* vol. 5, p. 35, 1972.

41. J. Pugh, "Cancellous Bone," chap. 3, Thomas, Springfield, Ill., 1977.

42. J. C. Behrens, P. S. Walker, and H. Shoji, Variations in Strength and Structure of Cancellous Bone at the Knee, *J. Biomech.,* vol. 7, p. 201, 1974.

43. P. Ducheyne, L. Heymans, M. Martens, E. Aernoudt, P. deMeester, and J. C. Mulier, The Mechanical Behavior of Intracondylar Cancellous Bone of the Femur at Different Loading Rates, *J. Biomech.,* vol. 10, p. 747, 1977.

44. T. D. Brown and G. E. Graf, Material Property Distributions in the Human Femoral Head, *Proc. Orthop. Res. Soc., Dallas, Tex.,* p. 15, February, 1978.

45. T. P. Andriacchi, J. O. Galante, Belytschko, and S. Hampton, A Stress Analysis of the Femoral Stem in Total Hip Prostheses, *J. Bone Jt. Surg.,* vol. 58A, p. 618, 1976.

46. N. L. Svensson, S. Valliappan, and R. D. Wood, Stress Analysis of Human Femur with Implanted Charnley Prosthesis, *J. Biomech.,* vol. 10, p. 581, 1977.

47. R. Huiskes and T. J. J. H. Slooff, Mechanical Properties and Stress in Intramedullary Prostheses, *Proc. Orthop. Res. Soc., Dallas, Tex.,* p. 148, February, 1978.

48. I. Oh, Effect of Total Hip Replacement on the Distribution of Stress in the Proximal Femur, *Proc. 5th Open Meet. Hip Soc., 1977,* Mosby, St. Louis, 1977.

49. K. L. Markolf, D. Hirschowitz, and H. C. Amstutz, Mechanical Studies of Support Provided by the Collar of a Femoral Total Hip Component, *Proc. Orthop. Res. Soc., Dallas, Tex.,* February, 1978.

50. J. D. Reuben, F. J. Eismont, A. H. Burstein, and T. M. Wright. Comparative Mechanical Properties of Forty-Five Total Hip Stems, *Clin. Orthop.,* no. 41, pp. 55–65, June 1979.

51. J. H. Bargren, W. H. Day, M. A. R. Freeman, and S. A. V. Swanson, Mechanical Properties of Four Non-hinged Knee Prostheses, *Proc. Orthop. Res. Soc., Dallas, Tex.,* p. 155, February, 1978.

52. D. Ikuhi, Study on Trabecular Architecture of Distal End of the Femur, *J. Jpn. Orthop. Assoc.,* vol. 51, p. 1, 1977.

53. P. S. Walker, C. S. Ranawat, and J. N. Insall, Fixation of the Tibial Components of Condylar Replacement Knee Prostheses, *J. Biomech.,* vol. 9, p. 269, 1976.

54. M. J. Askew, J. L. Lewis, D. Jaycox, J. L. Williams, and Y. Hovik, Interface Stresses in a

Prosthesis-Tibia Structure with Varying Bone Properties, *Proc. Orthop. Res. Soc., Dallas, Tex.,* p. 17, February, 1978.

55. E. Y. S. Chao, private communication, 1977.

56. M. Pappas, F. F. Buechel, and A. F. DePalma, Cylindrical Total Ankle Joint Replacement, *Clin. Orthop.,* vol. 118, 1976.

57. P. S. Walker and D. Seitelman, The Interdependence of Rotational Stiffness and Contact Stress in Condylar Replacement Knee Prostheses, *Proc. Orthop. Res. Soc., Dallas, Tex.,* p. 152, February, 1978.

58. P. S. Walker and B. Wolf, The Control of A-P Movement in Condylar Replacement Knee Prostheses, *Proc. Orthop. Res. Soc., Dallas, Tex.,* p. 153, February, 1978.

59. R. M. Rose, A. N. Cviegnola, H. J. Nusbaum, I. L. Paul, S. R. Simon, and E. L. Radin, Comparative Evaluation of Müller-Type Acetabular Components for Total Hip Prosthesis, *Proc. 3rd Ann. Meet. Soc. Biomater. and 9th Ann. Int. Biomater. Symp., New Orleans, La.,* p. 116, April, 1977.

60. P. S. Walker and H-H Hsieh, Conformity in Concylar Replacement Knee Prostheses, *J. Bone Jt. Surg.,* vol. 59B, p. 222, 1977.

61. P. D. Wilson, Jr., E. A. Salvati, P. W. Hughes, H. J. Robinson, and D. M. Dines, Total Prosthetic Replacement of the Hip, *Proc. Workshop Internal Jt. Replacement,* sponsored by Rehabilitation Engineering Services Administration, U.S. Department of Health, Education, and Welfare, March, 1977.

62. H.-G. Willert and M. Semlitsch, Reactions of the Articular Capsule to Wear Products of Artificial Joint Prostheses, *J. Biomed. Mater. Res.,* vol. 11, p. 157, 1977.

63. J. Charnley and D. K. Halley, The Rate of Wear in Total Hip Replacement, *Clin. Orthop.,* vol. 112, p. 170, 1975.

64. M. Semlitsch, M. Lehmann, H. Weber, E. Doerne, and H. G. Willert, New Prospects for a Prolonged Functional Life-Span of Artificial Hip Joints, *J. Biomed. Mater. Res.,* vol. 11, p. 537, 1977.

65. G. M. McNeice and T. A. Gruen, Mechanical Failure Modes of Femoral Components, *Proc. Orthop. Res. Soc., New Orleans, La.,* January, 1976.

66. G. A. Lord and F. J. Kummer, Biological Uncemented Anchorage in Total Hip Replacement, *Proc. Am. Acad. Orthop. Surg., Dallas, Tex.,* paper 67, February, 1978.

67. J. D. Bloom and R. S. Bryan, Wide Track Polycentric Total Knee Arthroplasty, *Clin. Orthop.,* vol. 128, p. 210, 1977.

68. F. C. Ewald, W. H. Thomas, R. Poss, R. D. Scott, and C. B. Sledge, Duo-Patella Total Knee Arthroplasty, in "Rheumatoid Arthritis," *Proc. Am. Acad. Orthop. Surg., Dallas, Tex.,* paper 31, February, 1978.

69. J. A. Lacey, A Statistical Review of 10 Consecutive U.C.I. Knee Arthroplasties, *Proc. Am. Acad. Orthop. Surg., Las Vegas, Nev.,* paper 87, February, 1977.

70. J. N. Insall, C. S. Ranawat, P. Aglietti, and J. Shine, A Comparison of Four Models of Total Knee Replacement Prostheses, *J. Bone Jt. Surg.,* vol. 58A, p. 754, 1976.

71. M. D. Skolnick, M. B. Coventry, and D. M. Ilstrup, Geometric Total Knee Arthroplasty: A Two-Year Follow-up Study, *J. Bone Jt. Surg.,* vol. 58A, p. 740, 1976.

72. W. N. Scott, J. N. Insall, and C. S. Ranawat, Total Condylar Prostehsis, *Proc. Am. Acad. Orthop. Surg., Las Vegas, Nev.,* paper 86, February, 1977.

73. G. P. Arden and B. A. Kamdar, Complications of Arthroplasty of the Knee in "Total Knee Replacement," Inst. Mech. Eng. Conf. 1974, p. 118, *Inst. Mech. Eng. London,* Sept., 1974.

74. S. Simon and J. Mazur, private communication, 1978.

75. A. S. Greenwald and M.-B. Matejczyk, The Mechanics of Ankle Joint Function, *Am. Acad. Orthop. Surg., Sci. Exhibition, Dallas, Tex.,* February, 1978. Sci. Exhibit.

76. A. B. Swanson, Silastic Spacers for the MCP Joint, AAOS course, Surgery in the Upper Extremity, Hyannis, Mass., September, 1976.

77. R. D. Beckenbaugh, J. H. Dobyns, R. L. Linscheid, and R. S. Bryan, Review and Analysis of Silicone-Rubber MCP Implants. *J. Bone Jt. Surg.,* vol. 58A, p. 483, 1976.

78. J. H. Dobyns, Cemented Metal-Plastic MCP Prostheses, AAOS course, Surgery in the Upper Extremity, Hyannis, Mass., September, 1976.

79. Elbow Prostheses, in "Joint Replacement in the Upper Limb," Institution of Mechanical Engineers, London, 1977.

80. A. G. Gristina and M. R. Forte, The Trispherical Total Shoulder Prosthesis, *Proc. 3d Ann. Meet. Soc. Biomater. and 9th Ann. Int. Biomater. Symp., New Orleans, La.,* p. 128, April, 1977.

81. F. F. Buechel, M. J. Pappas, and A. F. DePalma, "Floating-Socket" Total Shoulder Replacement, *J. Biomed. Mater. Res.,* vol. 12, p. 89, 1978.

82. J. P. Paul, Approaches to Design—Force Actions Transmitted by Joints in the Human Body, *Proc. Roy. Soc., London, Ser. B,* vol. 192, p. 163, 1976.

MECHANICS OF THE SPINE: ANALYSIS OF ITS FLEXIBILITY AND RIGIDITY, POSTURAL CONTROL, AND CORRECTION OF THE PATHOLOGICAL SPINE

A. W. M. Schijvens
C. J. Snijders
J. M. Seroo
J. G. N. Snijder

The form of the human spine is expressed in a formula. As a consequence, curvature and rigidity can be calculated mathematically. Through scale factors and nondimensional parameters, an insight is gained into such phenomena as strength, elasticity, bone growth, and changes in curvature. Standing, sitting, and other postural mechanical problems are analyzed systematically. Finally, mechanical analyses of two new operational techniques, spondylolisthesis and scoliosis, are provided with the help of models.

1 INTRODUCTION

A mechanical structure can be analyzed for its strength or for its deformation. In the first case a comparison is made between active and admissible stresses in the material. In the second case, which is relative to what follows, three mutually related aspects of the problem (Fig. 1) are of interest: *load, rigidity* (to be derived from material properties and form, composition, and areas of cross sections), and *form* (or deformation). Given two of these three states, the third state can be determined. Let us demonstrate this concept with the aid of examples associated with the spinal structure.

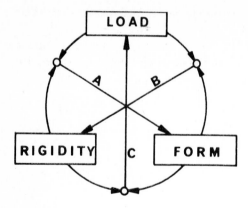

Figure 1 The mutual relationship among form, load, and rigidity. The arrows A, B, and C show the possible ways in which, by connecting two phenomena, the third can be found.

Example A. In the case of known material properties and a known load, the deformation that takes place can be calculated. In a child with a flexible spine and a low body weight, as well as in an adult with a stiffer spine and a higher body weight, the form of the spine will fit in as a third state. The adaptation of form could be elastic or even irreversible under certain circumstances, as in the case of scoliosis (wherein the normal material of the vertebral bodies deforms under too high and asymmetric a load, as shown in Fig. 2).

Example B. From form and load, an estimate can be made of unknown material magnitudes. Thus, the load might be normal, and yet an extreme form

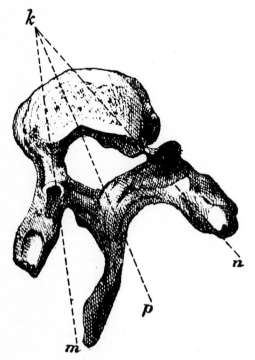

Figure 2 Deformation of a vertebra as a consequence of scoliosis.

might exist due to a degradation in material properties, as in the cases of vertebrae affected by tumors or tuberculosis (Fig. 3).

Example C. If form and material properties are known, the load can be calculated. Every deviation of form that is not caused by deviations of material is a consequence of the load.

2 DESCRIPTION OF FORM FOR THE SPINE

The form of the spine can be determined either from x-ray pictures or from the external dorsal contour. In both cases the form of the spine should be determined separately. Both methods imply specific advantages and disadvantages.

2.1 Form on X-Ray Pictures

The form of the spine is to be understood here as the smooth line passing through the geometric centers of the vertebral bodies and of the intervertebral disks. To determine the geometric centers, tangents are drawn at the ventralmost and dorsalmost limitations of the vertebral bodies; moreover, lines are drawn through the caudal and cranial limitations (Fig. 4). In this way quadrangles are obtained whose geometric centers are determined by connecting the midpoints of the opposite sides; the geometric centers are expressed in terms of the chosen

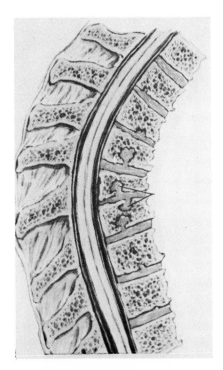

Figure 3 Deformation of a vertebra as a result of deviations of material in the case of Sheuermann's disease.

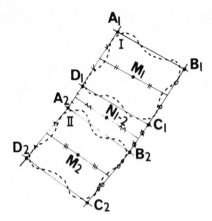

Figure 4 Determination of the geometric centers of vertebrae and intervertebral disks.

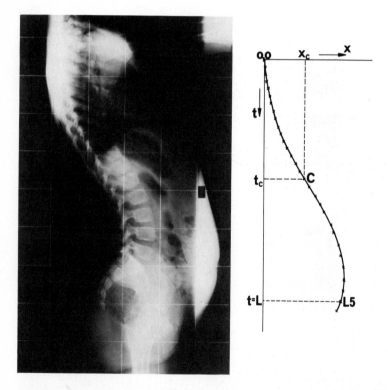

Figure 5 Description of the form of a lateral x-ray picture taken in the standing posture. The geometric centers of vertebrae and intervertebral disks are marked x. The origin of the system of axes is in the dorsalmost point of the kyphosis.

coordinate system. The form of the spine is obtained by connecting these geometric centers.

Figure 5 shows the form outline, in which the t axis is oriented in the direction of gravity and the x axis is oriented perpendicular to the t axis in the dorsalmost point of the kyphosis, taken to be the origin (0,0). A general point C has the coordinates (x_c, t_c). A measuring apparatus was developed by means of which the coordinates can be recorded directly onto a punched tape through electronics (Fig. 6).

The tape punched with the coordinates is the input tape for a computer program for the least-squares method, to fit the measured points to a curve $x = F(t)$ of the type

$$x = At^3 + Bt^2 + Ct + D \sin \frac{\pi t}{L} \tag{1}$$

The mathematical characterization of the form enables us to calculate the length of the curved line and the curvature at every point of the curve according to the formula

$$K = \frac{x''}{(1 + x'^2)^{3/2}} \tag{2}$$

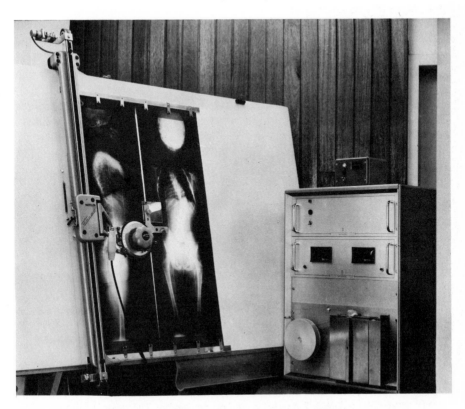

Figure 6 Apparatus developed for direct recording of geometric data on punched tape.

in which

$$x' = 3At^2 + 2Bt + C + \frac{\pi}{L} D \cos \frac{\pi t}{L} \qquad (3)$$

$$x'' = 6At + 2B - \left(\frac{\pi}{L}\right)^2 D \sin \frac{\pi t}{L} \qquad (4)$$

In cases of scoliosis the description of the form of the spine in anterior-posterior projection is also of interest. In this projection, a y axis is placed perpendicular to the xz plane (at the origin through the geometric centers of the first thoracic vertebra), Eq. (1) is again employed by replacing x with y, and a spatial system of coordinates is thereby obtained (see Fig. 7).

In Fig. 8, the descriptions of form in both planes of projection are shown for a scoliotic spine. By combining them mathematically, a space curve of the spine is obtained; Fig. 9 shows its top view, which is the projection on the xy plane.

2.2 Form of the Dorsal Contour

The smooth line connecting the points on the skin situated on the level of the dorsalmost points of the processus spinosi is taken as the form of the dorsal contour of the spine. This form cannot be recorded exactly on a lateral picture or projection, because it is hidden behind, i.a., the scapulae. Therefore, the back has to be approached from behind.

To avoid any mechanical contact with the back, which might disturb the unconstrained posture, an optical system (reflectometer) was used by Snijders [1]. By means of the apparatus shown in Fig. 10, the points on the skin are recorded successively on a recording roll. By placing the subject with the heels against a wooden block, a good reference line for the posture of the spine is obtained as the vertical through the hindmost limitation of the heels; this line represents the middle

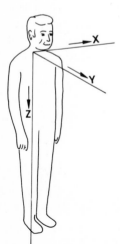

Figure 7 Spatial system of coordinates. The origin is situated in the geometric center of the first thoracic vertebra.

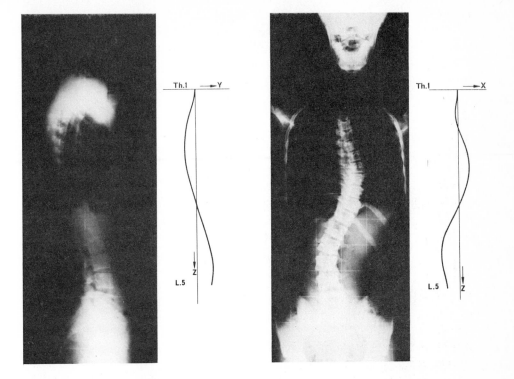

Figure 8 Descriptions of form of a lateral and an a-p projection of the spine in a case of scoliosis. Prior to the description of form, a correction is made as to the proportion of the x-ray projection.

of the recording roll. To be certain the subject stands still during the time of recording, approximately 45 s, a light support is applied at the shoulders and at the pelvis by means of the fixator mounted in front of the subject. It was ascertained that the form and the posture of the spine can be reproduced well in the unconstrained standing posture by reproducing the positions of the subject's feet and hands and the subject's viewing direction. It was also observed that in normal circumstances the form of the spine remained remarkably constant during several years.

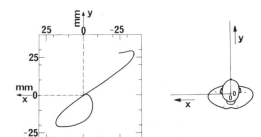

Figure 9 Top view of the spatially curved form of the spine in Fig. 8.

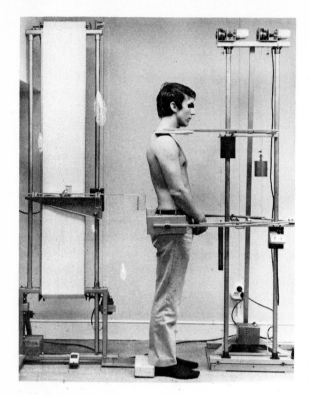

Figure 10 Recording the dorsal contour of the spine.

With this method, statistical research as well as research into alterations in form in special circumstances is very realizable. Particularly since x-ray pictures are not needed, this method is appropriate for examining healthy people and for examination in cases in which x-rays are undesirable. In Fig. 11 the spinal contours of two different subjects are shown. In both cases, the lines calculated by the computer are at most 1.7 mm from the measured points.

3 RIGIDITY, STRENGTH, AND MATERIAL PROPERTIES OF THE SPINE

Broadly speaking, the mechanical behavior of the spine can be compared with the behavior of an elastic rod, since its width and thickness are small in comparison with its length; its deformations due to moments of bending and of torsion are considered separately. As the deformation due to a load applied longitudinally (causing compression of the intervertebral disks) is proportionally small, this deformation is not taken into consideration.

3.1 Flexural Rigidity

The spine consists of a large number of vertebra-disk-vertebra segments (Fig. 12). We introduce a model to schematize the way in which elementary force phenomena are transferred. In this model, the spine is assumed to be a continuous, elastic thin-walled tube, reinforced internally by means of disks that are separated from each other by a medium (with hydrostatic behavior and a capacity for imbibition) surrounded by a stiff layer (as shown in Fig. 13). This model allows the transfer of tensile forces, compression, bending, and torsion. It is, however, not appropriate for the transfer of transverse forces, since the vertebral bodies will not remain "in line" (olisthesis). For a satisfactory description of the transfer of great transverse forces, the effects of the intervertebral joints must therefore be added. As 17 vertebra-disk-vertebra segments exist in the thoracolumbar area, the flexural rigidity (representing the average of the rigidities of the vertebral bodies and of the intervertebral disks and the ligaments) will be expressed in units of spine length.

To characterize rigidity, we employ the formula

$$K - K_0 = \frac{M}{EI} \qquad (5)$$

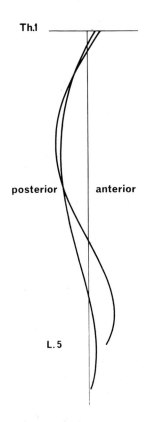

Th.1

posterior   anterior

L.5

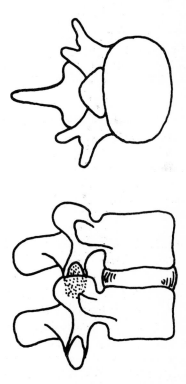

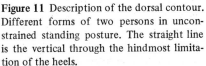

Figure 11 Description of the dorsal contour. Different forms of two persons in unconstrained standing posture. The straight line is the vertical through the hindmost limitation of the heels.

Figure 12 The spine consists of rigid vertebral elements and slack intervertebral elements.

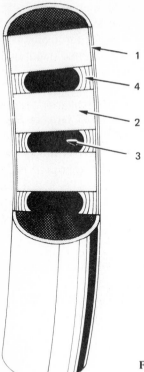

Figure 13 Model of vertebral motion segments. (1) Thin-walled tube; (2) disk; (3) hydrostatic medium; (4) stiff layer.

where K_0 = curvature in unloaded position (mm^{-1})

K = curvature after introducing the bending moment (mm^{-1})

M = bending moment (N mm)

I = second moment of area (mm^4), derived from form and area of the cross section at the section under consideration

and E is the modulus of elasticity in Newtons per square millimeter defined by

$$\epsilon = \frac{\sigma}{E} \qquad (6)$$

wherein ϵ is the strain of the material. For biological materials, E is not in proportion to σ (the stress). For small changes in σ, this relation may be considered linear.

To characterize the strength of the structure, we apply the formula

$$\sigma = \frac{Me}{I} < \sigma_b \qquad (7)$$

where σ = stress (N mm^{-2})

σ_b = stress beyond which fracture occurs (N mm^{-2})

e = ultimate distance of material (mm)

I = second moment of area (mm^4)

The physiological requirements of the spine are

1. Sufficient *strength*: Fracture is prevented.
2. Sufficient *rigidity*: Physiologically the spine must be sufficiently flexural and sufficiently elastic.

To gain an insight into the factors governing the construction of the human spine as well as spinal rigidity and strength, the spine may be compared with rods of solid bone and steel.

To compare the rigidities, we take the spinal rigidity in ventroflexion as $EI = 4 \times 10^6$ N mm^2 on the level of the third lumbar vertebra, at a vertebral body thickness of 39 mm [1], measured in the sagittal plane. Further, noting that the modulus of elasticity of compact bone is $E = 183 \times 10^6$ N/mm^2 [2], we can calculate how thick a bone rod (i.e., made of bone material) with a round cross section must be, to possess the same rigidity as the spine. We have

$$I_{\text{bone rod}} = \frac{\pi}{64} d^4 = \frac{EI_{\text{spine}}}{E_{\text{bone}}} = \frac{4 \times 10^6}{1.83 \times 10^4} = 218 \text{ mm}^4$$

Consequently the diameter of the bone rod must be

$$d_{\text{bone}} = 8.2 \text{ mm}$$

A similar calculation for a steel rod with a round cross section and $E = 2.1 \times 10^5$ N/mm^2 gives a diameter $d_{\text{steel}} = 4.4$ mm (Fig. 14).

For a comparison of strengths, we note that our equivalent rod of compact bone, with a diameter of 8.2 mm and having a tensile strength of 140 N/mm^2 [2], can only withstand a bending moment of 7578 N mm; for a length of 43 mm (the distance from center vertebra to center vertebra) fracture will occur for this rod of bone with a flexion of approximately 5.5°. However, the same length of human spine will transfer a bending moment at least twice as large (about 16,000 N mm), for which bending moment a bone rod would need a diameter of at least 10.3 mm. Thus, to be as strong as the spine the bone rod must be at least 2.5 times as rigid

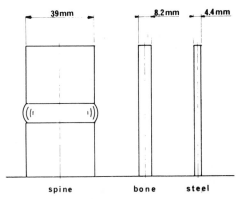

Figure 14 Comparison of spine, rod of bone, and rod of steel, all having the same flexural rigidity.

as the human spine. However, at the same time, to allow as much bending as the spine, the bone rod would have to be half as thick (3.25 mm).

Further, considering that spongy bone has a tensile strength of less than one-tenth that of compact bone, it can be postulated that a bone rod cannot produce the combined requirements of rigidity and bending strength (sufficient bending strength also guarantees sufficient compression strength). Figure 15 demonstrates that the degree of flexion afforded by the spine is far greater than that permitted by equivalent bone and steel rods having the same rigidity as the spine.

3.2 Material Properties

To relate the load to the form, it is necessary to know the material properties. As the flexibility of the spine is of importance in this chapter, we shall deal only with the modulus of elasticity and the second moment of area; the breaking strength, creep in structures, and elasticity of the individual parts of the spine, such as bone, ligaments, and disk tissue, are omitted. We are interested in the elasticity of the spine as a unit. The method for calculating the elasticity of spines presented in the following paragraphs is approximate. We are only interested in gaining insight into the characterization of the elastic behavior of the spine unit: stiff vertebral body and flexible disk.

To obtain quantitative information about the moduli of elasticity and shear of the spine, bending and torsion experiments have been made with autopsy specimens, using the measuring instrument shown in Fig. 16. In this instrument the topmost point of fixation of the spine can translate freely when the spine is loaded in torsion. The clamp D, within which the topmost vertebra is fixed, is connected to a large perspex disk that is placed on roller bearings. To load the spine with a torsional moment, equal weights are placed on the pans G. To load the spine with a bending moment, the spine is clasped at H and the glass disk is taken away; one of the wires is now directly attached to the topmost spine clamp. By placing weights on the corresponding pan G, a bending moment is imposed that is graphically represented in Fig. 17.

To determine the bending rigidity of the spine, nails are driven into the vertebral bodies (as shown in Fig. 18) to serve as reference lines. From the mutual

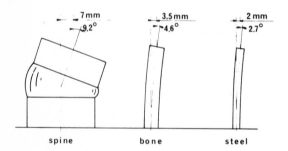

Figure 15 Rods of bone and steel with the same flexural rigidity as the spine, are, as compared with the spine, limited in their ventroflexural movement by their breaking strength (or elasticity).

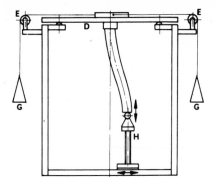

Figure 16 Schematic representation of a spine-loading instrument.

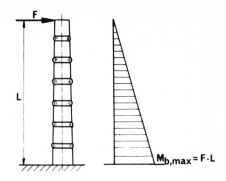

Figure 17 Bending moment during the loading experiments.

angular rotation ψ of these lines (at various loads), the rigidity of the spine can be obtained:

$$(EI)_d = \frac{M_b}{\psi/d} \tag{8}$$

Since it is the flexible disk (rather than the stiff vertebral body) that facilitates rotation, the stiffness $(EI)_d$, assessed with respect to the disk thickness d, is more amenable to measurement than $(EI)_l$; the latter can, however, be obtained from $(EI)_d$ with the help of the relation

$$(EI)_l = (EI)_d \frac{1}{d} \tag{9}$$

$(EI)_d$ can be calculated experimentally, but we should like to know the modulus E. As a first approach we assume that the second moment of area of the

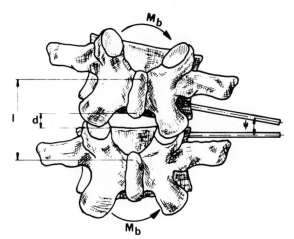

Figure 18 Relation between applied bending moment and mutual angular rotation.

cross section of the elliptical disk is proportionately represented as

$$I \propto a^3 b \qquad (10)$$

in which a is the diameter of the vertebral body concerned, lying in the plane in which the spine is bent, and b is the diameter perpendicular to this plane. When $(EI)_d$ is divided by $a^3 b$, a material constant E' is obtained, which is proportional to E, the modulus of elasticity of the disk and ligaments.

In Fig. 19 the spine is shown in the loaded and unloaded positions, bent forward and bent laterally. In Fig. 20 the calculated E' (along the spine) has been plotted for both forward and lateral bending. The stiffness $(EI)_l$ can be obtained from the E' as follows:

$$(EI)_l = E'a^3 b \frac{1}{d} \qquad (11)$$

where E' = constant of elasticity from Fig. 20
$\quad a$ = vertebral diameter in plane of bending
$\quad b$ = vertebral diameter perpendicular to plane of bending
$\quad l$ = distance between centers of two adjacent intervertebral disks
$\quad d$ = height of disk

Thus, by employing E' from Fig. 20 and by determining the dimensions a, b, l, and d from x-ray pictures (after applying appropriate correction factors for x-ray projection distortion), we can obtain the *in vivo* rigidity of the spine.

The E' given in Fig. 20 was obtained from measurements on the (nonpathological) cadaveric spine of an 18-yr-old subject. Thus, when we use formula (11) to get *an impression* of the rigidity of a particular patient with the help of x-rays, we

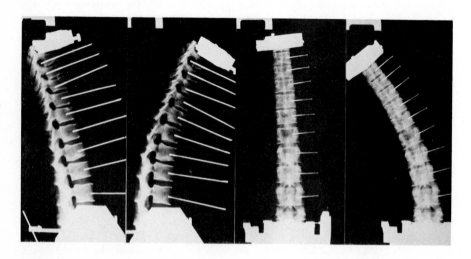

Figure 19 X-ray pictures of the load experiments before and after load (female, aged 18). Left, bent-forward position; right, bent-laterally position.

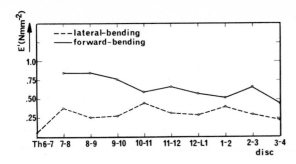

Figure 20 E' values for the spine of Fig. 21. Approximately linear for zero load up to the maximum ψ (female, aged 18).

get a nonpathological or a "nondegenerated" rigidity. For patients with specific pathological spine changes or when the disk may have degenerated, it is essential to develop curves such as that given in Fig. 20 for spines of varied etiologies.

To determine the torsional rigidity of the spine, we apply the method employed to calculate $(EI)_l$ and use the formula

$$GI_p = G' \frac{a^3 b^3}{a^2 + b^2} \frac{1}{d} \tag{12}$$

where G = modulus of shear (N mm^2)

I_p = second polar moment of area (mm^4)

The experimental setup for the torsion experiment, with clamped spine, is shown in Fig. 21. The orientations of the vertebral bodies relative to one another are designated by nails driven into them. By taking photographs from above, the angular rotations of these nails at various loads can be measured (Fig. 22). The values of G' calculated with the help of these photographs are graphed in Fig. 23. We note, from formulas (11) and (12), that spinal rigidity increases with (1) increasing vertebral diameter and (2) increasing l/d, the ratio of the distance between centers of successive vertebrae to the height of the disk.

4 DETERMINATION OF THE FORM AND LOAD–BEARING CAPACITY OF THE SPINE

To determine the form from the load and material properties, we employ the formula

$$K = \frac{M}{EI} \tag{13}$$

where K = curvature of material in a certain plane

M = bending moment exerted in that plane

EI = flexural rigidity of cross section considered

In employing Eq. (13), we imply that the influence of the transverse forces on the deformation is negligible. Alternatively, it is more pertinent to measure the form parameters and, with the help of known material properties, calculate the

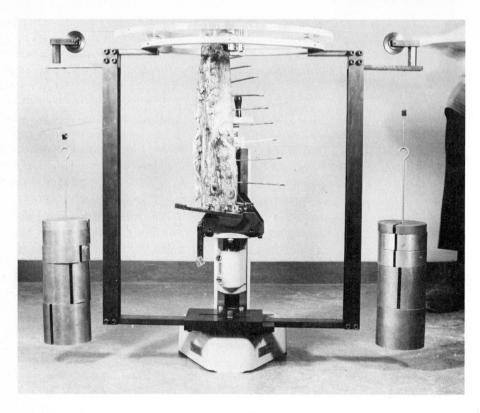

Figure 21 Torsion test.

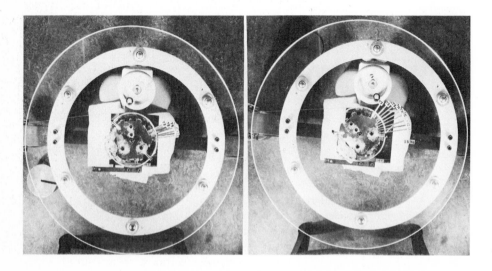

Figure 22 Photographs, taken from above, of the spine in an unloaded and loaded position.

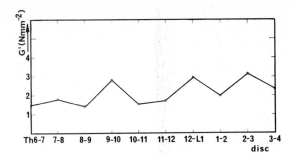

Figure 23 G' values for the spine of Fig. 21.

mechanical load on the spine responsible for producing the *in vivo* form. For this purpose, we employ the above equation to determine the bending moment

$$M = KEI \tag{14}$$

wherein K is the curvature of the deformed spine if it is straight in the unloaded state, and is the change in curvature if the spine is curved even in the unloaded state, as in the case of scoliosis. Of course, we need a mathematical description of the form of the spine (Fig. 24).

The determination of the form function $x = x(t)$ and the calculation of the curvature K therefrom have been discussed in Sec. 2. From Eqs. (14), (11), and (2), the bending moments are obtainable (*in vivo*) from the expression

$$M(t) = \frac{x''(t)}{[1 + x'(t)^2]^{3/2}} E'a^3 b \, \frac{1}{d} \tag{15}$$

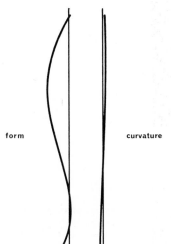

form   curvature

Figure 24 From the description of form, the curvature at any level can be calculated immediately.

5 PHENOMENOLOGICAL LAWS OF SKELETAL RESPONSE TO LOAD AND GROWTH

We noted earlier that a mechanical structure can be analyzed for its load-carrying capacity or for its form or deformed shape; of course, each property is related to the other by means of the rigidity of the structure. To compare the effectiveness or efficiency of skeletal structures, we need to obtain nondimensional parameters that incorporate both the load-bearing and form-characterizing properties of the structure. Alternatively, we can compare either the strengths or stresses of structures in terms of geometric dimensions. Thus, the internal stresses due to the weights of two structures of the same density are proportional to their characteristic lengths L, since the weight is proportional to the cube of the characteristic length, and the cross-sectional area is proportional to the square of the characteristic length.

In examining adult animals of the same form, we see that for smaller animals the skeleton constitutes a smaller percentage of the weight. The explanation is as follows: The muscular forces are proportional to L^2, and the forces due to weight are proportional to L^3. This means that the forces on the skeleton (due to the animal's weight) increase more than proportionally to the height or length, at a faster rate than the muscle forces. As a consequence (if the material properties remain the same), the loaded cross sections must increase more than proportionally; in other words, a bigger animal must have a thicker skeleton than a smaller animal would have if the latter were "blown up" to the same length as the former. Figure 25 illustrates this point.

Let us now determine the governing criterion for skeletal growth in the human body. One has to keep in mind that the construction material of the child is different from that of the adult; the child's skeleton, for the greater part, consists

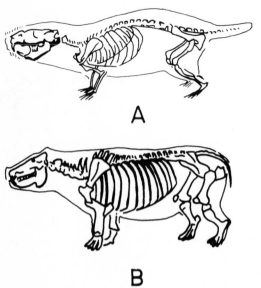

A

B

Figure 25 Skeletons of (A) a lemming and (B) a hippopotamus, both reduced to a same body length, to show the much greater robustness of the hippopotamus skeleton. Hence the troubles of bigger animals due to their own weight are ever increasing. *(After Hesse-Doflein [7]).*

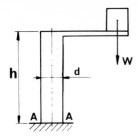

Figure 26 A part of the skeleton is loaded with the weight of the upper part. Every dimension in the horizontal direction depends on the growth in the direction of the width and hence is proportional to the dimension d.

of cartilage, whereas the adult's skeleton consists of hard bone. We shall first test the hypothesis that the process of growth takes place in such a way that the stresses in the bearing elements remain constant for increasing weight. To test this hypothesis, we take a bone cylinder (such as a spinal segment or even a femur) of dimensions h and d (Fig. 26), subject to a bending stress as a consequence of the upper torso weight W.

The bending moment M (cross section A-A) equals the weight W multiplied by the eccentricity or the lever arm; this arm is proportional to the width d (that is, $M \propto Wd$), according to Fig. 26. The weight W of the upper part of the skeleton equals the volume of this part multiplied by the specific mass ρ. The volume is proportional to $d^2 h$. Thus, $W \propto \rho d^2 h$, and

$$M \propto \rho d^2 h\, d \propto \rho d^3 h$$

The bending stress in cross section A-A is

$$\sigma \propto \frac{M}{Z}$$

where Z is the moment of resistance of the cross section and is proportional to d^3. Thus,

$$\sigma \propto \frac{\rho d^3 h}{d^3} \propto \rho h \qquad (16)$$

The bending stress σ consequently depends on the height h in the direction of gravity and does not depend on the diameter d. The assumption that the stresses in the bearing elements during growth remain constant implies that the height h of the bone structure (say, the femur) may not increase (provided, of course, that the material density remains constant), whereas width and thickness may increase. However, the height of the human does increase, which inevitably means that the stresses also increase, thereby violating our hypothesis of constant stress.

Another criterion that can be tested is that of the strains remaining constant. If the strain ϵ is to remain constant, the quantity σ/E also has to remain constant, for $\epsilon = \sigma/E$. However, since we have seen that stress σ increases, E must also increase. This implies that the bone must grow more rigid and stronger. The admissible stress and the modulus of elasticity of the bone, taken as a composite of hydroxyapatite and collagen, are given by

$$\sigma_c = \sigma_H V_H + \sigma_M(1 - V_H)$$

$$E_c = E_H V_H + E_M(1 - V_H) \tag{17}$$

where σ_c, E_c = admissible stress, modulus of elasticity of composite

σ_H, E_H = admissible stress, modulus of elasticity of hydroxyapatite

σ_M, E_M = admissible stress, modulus of elasticity of matrix collagen

V_H = degree of filling, or ratio of area of hydroxyapatite to entire area of composite in cross section perpendicular to axis of bone

The total strain,

$$\epsilon_c = \frac{\sigma_H V_H + \sigma_M(1 - V_H)}{E_H V_H + E_M(1 - V_H)} = \frac{\sigma_c}{E_c} \tag{18}$$

thus depends on the degree of filling, which will have to be adjusted in such a way (to maintain constancy) that the right combination of stress and E is maintained. If such a mechanism is to be effective in the human body, there must exist an element (in the bone) recording the strain and emitting a signal that increases the degree of filling, so as to return the strain to its original value. It is plausible that this process occurs because piezoelectric phenomena in the bone have been detected by several researchers, with an electric signal emitted when the bone is loaded (or strained). Thus the hypothesis that growth occurs according to consistent strains is probable.

Let us finally test the hypothesis that in the case of similar loads the bone elements bend into identical forms. In Fig. 27 we have

$$\phi = \frac{Mh}{EI} \tag{19a}$$

According to Eq. (16), M is proportional to $\rho\, d^3 h$. Also, EI is proportional to $\sigma\, d^4$ and hence to $\rho h\, d^4$. On substituting for M and EI in the above equation, we obtain

$$\phi \propto \frac{\rho\, d^3 h^2}{\rho h\, d^4} \propto \frac{h}{d} \tag{19b}$$

Furthermore, according to the hypothesis of identical form, the angular rotations are the same for both small and large skeletal constructions. Hence, ϕ = constant implies that h/d is constant; that is, h is proportional to d. This means that the

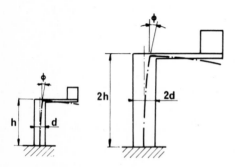

Figure 27 Deformed spine with the upper torso weight acting eccentrically at height h.

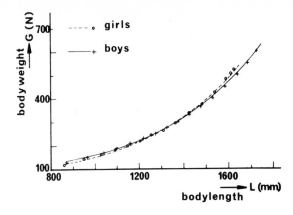

Figure 28 Weights of children between 2 and 17 yr of age versus these children's lengths. Equations (21) fit the data quite well.

thickness of the parts of the skeleton increases (grows) proportionately to the growth in length. Hence the volume of the skeleton, which is proportional to d^2h, is now proportional to h^3; that is,

$$V \propto d^2h \propto h^3 \tag{20}$$

The weight of the skeleton G is hence proportional to ρh^3. We have seen that during growth the bone changes structurally under the influence of the degree of filling. For this reason we cannot assume that ρ is constant.

In Fig. 28, the measured weights of boys and girls are plotted as functions of their lengths. On fitting a weight function (polynomial in h) to this data, we obtain, with h in meters,

For boys:

$$G = 56.0h^4 + 102.0 \text{ N}$$

For girls: $\hspace{8cm}$ (21)

$$G = 59.8h^4 + 93.1 \text{ N}$$

It is seen that the weight G is proportional to h^4. Consequently the specific mass of the skeleton ρ must be proportional to h. Thus, for adults the bone must not only be stronger and more rigid, but, moreover, it must also have a larger specific mass than the bones of children.

To verify that $G \propto h^4$ in a different way, we measured, with the help of x-ray pictures, the vertebral diameters (at the same level) of a number of persons. On plotting their weights versus the fourth power of their vertebral diameters (Fig. 29), a good linear relation was noted. Now, the curvature K of the parts of the skeleton is proportional to ϕ/L. Since our identical-form hypothesis requires that ϕ is constant, we have $K \propto 1/L$. In other words, the spine of the child (having a small L) will be curved more than the spine of the adult (Fig. 30).

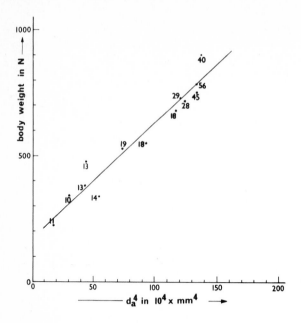

Figure 29 Weights of a number of persons plotted as the fourth power of the corresponding vertebral diameters.

6 STANDING AND SITTING AS MECHANICAL PROBLEMS

6.1 Load on the Spine

The loads affecting the spine can be divided into three types:

1. The load as a consequence of one's own weight
2. The load due to the affecting muscles and ligaments
3. The external load, such as the extra weight during lifting, or accelerating forces

The proportionate weights of the various parts of the skeleton are shown schematically in Fig. 31 [3].

The load due to the affecting muscles is unknown; a correlation between

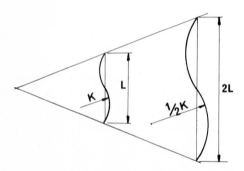

Figure 30 Identical form development results in less curvature.

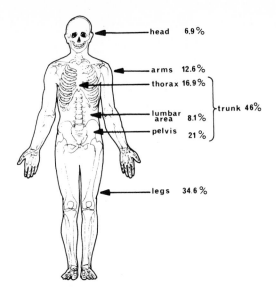

head   6.9 %

arms   12.6 %

thorax 16.9 %

lumbar
area   8.1 %   } trunk 46 %

pelvis   21 %

legs   34.6 %

Figure 31 Weights of body parts as percentages of body weight.

electromyogram-measured and occurring muscular force good enough to yield this information has not proved to be possible thus far. On the other hand, we can often readily calculate the magnitude of the unknown muscular force with the help of a simple vector diagram, provided the direction of this force is known (Fig. 32). When dealing with the influence of the load on the posture, we omit the inertia forces and consider only the posture in the unconstrained standing position. In this position only a few groups of muscles are active, and they regulate the equilibrium with minimal exertion around the joints, such as ankle, knee, and hip joint. The collective term for those muscles that regulate standing is *postural* muscles, as opposed to the *phasic* musculature that causes movements and reflex movements. The phasic musculature has a different function, and consequently different behavior and structure, from the postural muscles.

To gain an insight into the load on the spine and the forces acting on it due to the postural muscles, consider Fig. 33. There, A is a point at which the bending moment in the spine is zero. F is the weight of the part that lies above A. Point B

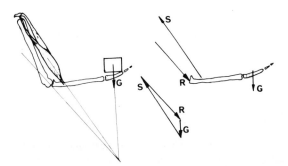

Figure 32 From a simple vector diagram the unknown muscular force can be calculated, provided its direction is known. (For simplicity the weight of the arm is omitted here with respect to the weight carried by the hand.)

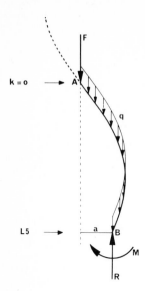

Figure 33 Forces and moments affecting a part of the spine.

is the transition from the lumbar vertebrae to the sacrum and thus is the clasp in the pelvis. The load q represents the equally divided weight of the part of the spine between A and B. The clasp reactions have been drawn at point B. The reaction force R provides vertical equilibrium; the clasping moment M can be calculated from the equilibrium of moments and is caused at B by muscles; the most important muscle causing the moment at B is M. psoas (Fig. 34). Basmajian [4] monitored its activity during standing. Whereas in quadrupeds its function is phasic, in the erect-going human it is postural and procures the equilibrating moment around the pelvis. As a result, it is also the cause of lumbar lordosis; it can immediately be seen that when M. psoas is activated more, lumbar lordosis increases. Consequently, the cause of increased lordosis must generally be sought in connection with the existence of a shortened or slightly hypertonic M. psoas.

6.2 Mechanics of Standing

To systematically build up a mechanical model of the skeleton, with the influences of its forces, we start from a model that contains only the principal joints. These are (1) the ankle joint, (2) the hip joint, and (3) the lumbar spine, which is a complex of joints. Displacements of the lumbar spine will be characterized by its curvature, whereas displacements at the ankle and knee joints will be characterized by rotations. The curvature of the lumbar spine is the consequence of rotations in every lumbar joint (Fig. 35). The knee joint is considered to be "locked" in the frontal plane.

   The method to be applied aims at gaining an insight into the posture as a whole and into the relations contributing to the equilibrium around voluntary joints. Our analysis starts at the ankle joint. To analyze the equilibrium at this joint, we separate it and build a free-body diagram of the foot (Fig. 36).

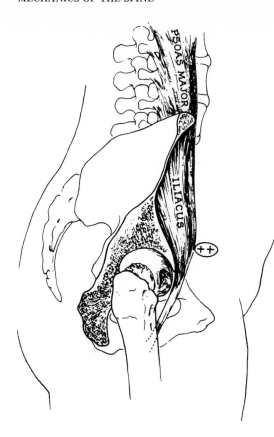

Figure 34 In the erect posture the M. psoas is activated positively. *(After Basmajian [4].)*

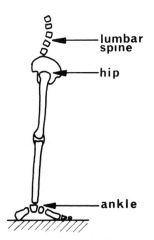

Figure 35 Principal joints related to standing.

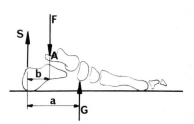

Figure 36 Equilibrium around the ankle joint. For simplicity S is assumed to be parallel to G.

The ankle joint can be considered as a hinge that is able to sustain forces in the horizontal and vertical directions only, but no moments. The position and magnitude of the ground reaction G (equal to one-half the weight) can be determined by a stabilograph [5]. For the equilibrium of moments around A, we find that

$$bS = (a - b)G \qquad (22)$$

from which the force S in the triceps surae group is given by

$$S = \frac{a - b}{b} G \qquad (23)$$

For the representative data $G = 380$ N, $a = 115$ mm, and $b = 60$ mm, we obtain $S = 347$ N. Thus, in symmetric standing, the triceps surae will have to tighten to 347 N in each leg to guarantee equilibrium around the ankle joint.

The reaction force at the ankle joint is obtained from vertical equilibrium considerations as

$$F = S + G = 347 + 380 = 727 \text{ N} \qquad (24)$$

In this example, the load on one ankle joint has, for standing in unconstrained posture, the same order of magnitude as the body weight. When the body is inclining forward (in which case the magnitude of a increases), this load becomes still larger.

To analyze the equilibrium around the head of the hip, we consider the complete leg as a free body and analyze the forces acting on it. The force system in Fig. 37 can be defined by means of an x-ray picture of the leg in combination with a stabilogram. There, G is half the body weight, B is the weight of one leg acting through its center of mass, H is the reaction force on the head of the femur, M is the reaction moment around the head of the femur, and p and q are the distances between the vertical A-A through the center of mass of the body and the lines of action of forces B and H.

From anatomical considerations, we have

$$B = 0.17G$$

Equilibrium of the forces in Fig. 37 results in

$$H = G - 0.17G = 0.83G \qquad (25)$$

The equilibrium of moments around the head of the femur provides

$$M = qG - (q - p)B \qquad (26)$$

Combining Eqs. (25) and (26), we obtain

$$M = qH + \frac{0.17}{0.83} pH$$

This can be written as

$$M = eH \qquad (27)$$

where
$$e = q + \frac{0.17}{0.83} p \qquad (28)$$

As the reaction force on the acetabulum (and its direction) are the same as these on the head of the femur, we can analyze the equilibrium of the pelvis readily in Fig. 38, whence we obtain $M = eH$. Another consequence is that, should the reaction force H lie behind the acetabulum, the moment around this acetabulum is clockwise. The muscles contributing to the moment around the acetabulum are as follows:

1. Those causing (in Fig. 38) a clockwise moment: M. rectus femoris, M. psoas major, M. iliacus, M. pectineus, M. gracilis, M. adductor longus
2. Those causing (in Fig. 38) a counterclockwise moment: M. gluteus maximus, M. adductor magnus, M. adductor brevis, M. ischiocrural

Both these types of muscle groups link the pelvis and femur and effect the posture of the pelvis with respect to the femur. In unconstrained standing a certain adjustment of these muscle groups occurs around the hip joint. Collectively, these muscles produce a moment M given by $M = eH$.

When the body is inclining backward, e increases. To provide equilibrium, M

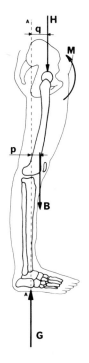

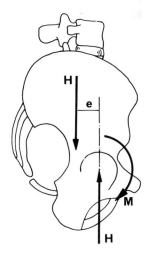

Figure 37 Forces and moments on the free-body leg.

Figure 38 Equilibrium of forces and of moments in the pelvis.

(acting clockwise and counterclockwise on the acetabulum and femur head, respectively) should increase proportionally; to effect this, the muscle group 1 above should be activated to a larger extent, so that the increased associated muscular strength F (see Fig. 39) provides an increased moment.

In unconstrained standing, the distance e (Fig. 38) is manipulated so that M lies in an appropriate range of control. Imagine that, in an unconstrained standing posture, H runs exactly through the hip joint. Then $e = 0$ and $M = 0$. A slight deviation from equilibrium results in a small value for e, say a positive value. When e reaches a certain threshold value, the muscles around the hip joint react and provide an opposite moment M(threshold). After having attained this threshold value, the muscular group F pulls back again on the head of the femur; e now becomes negative as M becomes counterclockwise. At this point the muscular groups acting to the left are tightened to again decrease e.

We thus see that postural control is in this case effected by H shifting and causing e to oscillate from positive to negative values; the positive value is defined in Fig. 38. In conjunction with this oscillation, an oscillatory rotation in the hip joint occurs that can result in early wear of the hip joint (e.g., coxarthrosis). The condition for this early wear consequently is average $e = 0$, or, according to Eq. (28) for two legs,

$$q + \frac{0.35}{0.65} p = 0 \tag{29}$$

Postural control around the hip joint entails continuous switching over from a clockwise moment to a counterclockwise moment and, in turn, switching over from muscular group 1 to muscular group 2, which contributes to fatigue. For this reason, in unconstrained standing the postural muscles are more effective than the phasic muscles since the postural muscles do not get tired as quickly and are irritated less easily; moreover, these muscles are stronger and have a better supply of blood. This means that group 1 of which M. psoas and M. rectus femoris are

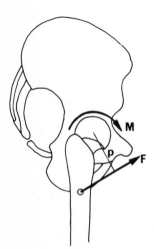

Figure 39 Equilibrium of moments around the head of the femur. This is not a free-body diagram.

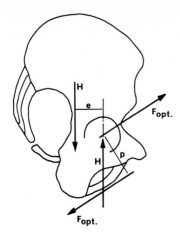

Figure 40 Equilibrium of moments around the acetabulum.

explicitly postural, is continuously active and that, according to Fig. 38, H lies constantly behind the head of the femur.

For good posture, e is continuously positive (positive to the left), and the adjustment then takes place between $e - \Delta e$ and $e + \Delta e$. The characteristics of the postural muscles are such that a small change in activation can effect a big change in force immediately. An increase in the value of e can immediately be compensated for by a small change in the activation, without a rotation in the hip joint. The muscles constantly yield a tensile force around the hip joint and arrange e in an equilibrium. This tensile force is the consequence of an activation of these muscles.

In unconstrained standing in a certain posture, the length of the muscle is almost constant; the degree of activation will be optimal for that specific muscle, so that it will not get tired soon. Moreover, it can adjust well around this optimal activation. If the corresponding optimal tensile force is called F_{opt}, the moment around the hip joint will be (Fig. 40)

$$M = pF_{opt}$$

In fact, the above formula must read

$$M = p_1 F_{1,opt} + p_2 F_{2,opt} + p_3 F_{3,opt} + \cdots$$

in which $F_{1,opt}$, $F_{2,opt}$, ... are the various contributing optimal muscular forces. All these forces can be combined into a resulting F_{opt} that acts at a distance p from the head of the femur.

In Fig. 40, the pelvis has been drawn in equilibrium; we can observe therefrom that

$$eH = pF_{opt} \tag{30}$$

When the activation of one of the muscles that compensates for the moment around the head of the femur (e.g., the M. psoas) increases above normal, the force F_{opt} also increases. From formula (30), if p and H remain constant, it follows that e must also increase. This means that the weight of the upper part of the body must be displaced further backward. This can be done by turning the pelvis backward, so that the sacrum will stand steeper. This is not possible, unless the M. psoas is made longer. A second possibility is to increase the lordosis. People with a contraction or shortening of the muscles that provides a clockwise moment will continuously lordosize their lumbar spines to a greater extent. When the shortening of the muscles increases, the moment of the hip also increases, and the lumbar spine lordosizes more, until it is no longer possible to produce equilibrium with one's own weight alone; the muscular groups that provide a counterclockwise moment of the hip also need to be tightened. If the muscle that has been shortened runs from femur to lumbar spine (like the M. psoas), the pelvis will turn forward in the first instance and a substantial tensile force will be exerted on the lumbar spine.

Good posture implies that the line of gravity lies behind the head of the femur. In this case the principal postural muscles, such as the M. psoas and the M. rectus femoris, are slightly tightened and ensure equilibrium around the hip joint. Should these muscles be shortened or hypertonic, then the equilibrium is disturbed. Mostly an increased lordosis is the consequence of this, along with a tightening of the phasic gluteal muslces, which lie on the other side of the head of the femur. In its turn, this results in low back complaints and tiredness that occurs sooner during standing.

6.3 Postural Mechanics for Pregnant Women

To study the postural control system (as described above) with application to some real-life problems, research was conducted into the posture of women who were in the last month of pregnancy, and into the alteration of this posture two weeks after partus. For this purpose the contours, stabilograms, weights, and lengths of 16 women were measured before and after childbirth. To observe high percentage changes in body weight, women having a normal weight before pregnancy were studied. The first remarkable result of this research was that, after partus, all women were about 1 to 2 cm shorter in height than before partus. The cause was the larger curvature of the spine after partus. Continually, after partus, a thoracic and a lumbar increase in the curvature of the spine (indicated by points A and C in Fig. 41) were observed. This is contrary to the generally accepted opinion. From this contour picture, this curvature was calculated mathematically. Thoracic and lumbar curvature mean here the curvature of the most dorsal and most ventral parts of the kyphosis and lordosis, respectively. The increases in curvature (measured after childbirth) for the 16 women are shown in Table 1.

This increase in curvature can easily be explained in terms of the equilibrium conditions around the head of the femur. In Fig. 42 this equilibrium condition is schematized once again. There, H represents the head of the femur, and B the pelvis. The pelvis balances on the head of the hip, and the two principal forces affecting the pelvis are F and P, respectively the weight of the body above the head of the femur and the muscular force. The force F lies behind the head of the femur (see Fig. 40); to obtain equilibrium around this head, the muscular groups on the ventral side must tighten. In this respect the most important muscular group is the M. psoas.

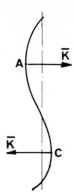

Figure 41 Increase in curvature after childbirth was measured at the points *A* and *C*.

The above described situation exists in most cases. When, however, an extra weight *G* is added on the right side of the head of the femur, e.g., in the case of pregnancy, Fig. 43 shows that there are two possible ways to effect a new equilibrium. The first possibility is to displace the weight *F* of the trunk, head, and arms further backward. This results in an increase in the counterclockwise moment about *H* in proportion to the clockwise moment due to the added force *G*. Consequently, extra muscles must be employed to take the line of action *F* further backward.

The second possibility, to effect equilibrium by a relaxation of the M. psoas, is more plausible, because the M. psoas has already been tightened. As a consequence, less energy is employed and the total reaction force *R* on the head of the femur does not increase. On relaxation of the M. psoas, such that the decrease in the clockwise moment due to a decrease in *P* is as large as the increase in the

Table 1 Increases in curvature ΔK after childbirth

Subject	Thoracic ΔK (mm^{-1} × 10^4)	Lumbar ΔK (mm^{-1} × 10^4)
1	6.4	20.0
2	5.3	15.9
3	5.5	16.5
4	5.3	8.8
5	7.3	20.2
6	7.2	14.0
7	11.3	22.6
8	9.2	21.1
9	6.3	22.9
10	7.2	22.5
11	8.0	20.0
12	3.9	15.4
13	5.2	10.5
14	4.8	25.8
15	4.3	17.0
16	8.1	24.2

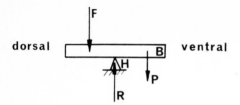

Figure 42 Equilibrium of the pelvis B on the head H of the femur.

counterclockwise moment due to the added force G, equilibrium will exist again.

Thus, in unconstrained standing during pregnancy, the tightening of the M. psoas will be less than normal. This relaxation has an immediate consequence for the lumbar spine, the M. psoas having its origin here. Refer Fig. 44, where A is the clasp point of the spine in the pelvis, R is the resulting force due to body weight, the muscles lying behind A, and the muscles lying between the spine and the pelvis (such as the dorsal extensors and the M. quadratus lumborum), and P is the force due to the M. psoas (causing a clockwise moment). For equilibrium with P, the force R adapts so that its counterclockwise moment about A will balance the clockwise moment of P about A. Consequently, the sacrum-iliacum joint (clasp point A) will have as small a bending load as possible. Thus, when the M. psoas, as a result of pregnancy, tightens less, the whole lumbar spine will be loaded less in bending. This change in bending moment will increase linearly with the change of weight G in the abdomen, because the muscle sites do not vary. Consequently, every change in moment will depend only on the changes in force, so that we can write

$$\text{Change in moment} \propto \text{change in force}$$

or
$$\Delta M \propto \Delta P$$

However, according to Fig. 43, $\Delta P \propto \Delta G$, due to the increased abdominal weight. Hence,

$$\Delta M \propto \Delta G \tag{31}$$

The corresponding change in curvature ΔK due to ΔM is determined with the formula

$$\Delta K = \frac{\Delta M}{EI} \tag{32}$$

in which EI represents the rigidity of the lumbar spine. For adults, $E = \text{constant}$

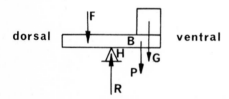

Figure 43 In pregnancy, P must decrease to effect equilibrium, owing to the extra weight in the abdomen.

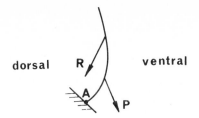

dorsal   **R**   **ventral**

Figure 44 Clasping of the lumbar spine in the pelvis A with the help of the effecting forces P and R.

and $I \propto d^4$. Hence, $EI \propto d^4$. Figure 29 implies that the weight $G \propto d^4$, so that

$$EI \propto G \qquad (33)$$

[Equation (33) can only be used for adults.]

Equation (32) can now be written as

$$\Delta K \propto \frac{\Delta M}{G} \qquad (34)$$

With Eq. (31), this becomes

$$\Delta K \propto \frac{\Delta G}{G}$$

or $\qquad\qquad\qquad\qquad \Delta KG \propto \Delta G \qquad (35)$

From this formula and from the above it appears that the product of lumbar change in curvature and weight is proportional to the increase in weight in the abdomen, when the equilibrium around the head of the femur is determined by the M. psoas.

For the 16 women examined, ΔKG and ΔG are listed in Table 2. In Fig. 45

Table 2 Change in curvature, weight, and their product $G\,\Delta K$ for 16 women

Subject	G (N)	ΔK (mm$^{-1} \times 10^4$)	$G\,\Delta K$ (N mm$^{-1} \times 10^3$)	ΔG (N)
1	704	20.0	1408	87
2	587	15.9	933	72
3	629	16.5	1036	64
4	622	8.8	547	56
5	714	20.0	1440	91
6	704	14.0	984	49
7	603	22.6	1360	146
8	618	21.1	1298	136
9	697	22.9	1596	145
10	625	22.5	1406	78
11	653	20.0	1306	103
12	603	15.4	922	87
13	619	10.5	647	58
14	539	25.8	1394	95
15	682	17.0	1159	99
16	530	24.2	1281	85

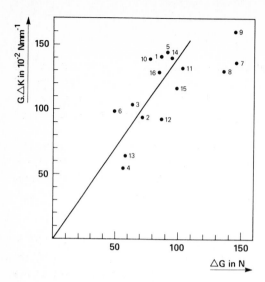

Figure 45 Product $G \Delta K$ plotted against the change in body weight. It is mandatory for the line to begin at the origin, since at zero weight there can be no curvature change.

these data are presented graphically. A linear regression has been fitted to the data. Thirteen of the 16 points are well represented by the equation of the regression line; points 7, 8, and 9 are exceptions and do not conform to the rectilinear relation of formula (35); for these subjects another mechanism must contribute to the equilibrium around the head of the femur.

With respect to subject 7, the first thing that strikes us is the large ΔG (twins!). Contour pictures of this woman, taken before and after childbirth (Fig. 46), show that in the lumbar area the curvature after childbirth has flattened appreciably. Also in the lumbar region, it seems that during pregnancy the woman could not decrease her lumbar lordosis any further, and consequently, reached an upper limit of ΔK (the order of magnitude is the same as in cases 1 and 5). The explanation for this is that, according to Fig. 44, the M. psoas is entirely relaxed. Yet, to have equilibrium with the very large weight in the abdomen, this muscle cannot relax further; consequently those muscles that provide a counterclockwise moment around the hip would have to be tightened. The most important muscle of this group is the M. gluteus maximus. This muscle runs from the upper side of the hip to the dorsal side of the pelvis and is not attached to the lumbar spine. As a result, the tightening of the gluteus has no direct bearing on the curvature K of the lumbar spine. Hence this case does not fall on the linear regression line of Fig. 45.

In summary it can be noted that as a consequence of pregnancy, as the weight in the abdominal cavity increases, the lumbar spine will be proportionately less curved. This results in an increase in length of 1 to 2 cm and in a flat back. The above discussion may imply that, should a woman's lumbar lordosis not decrease, it would be due to shortened muscles, particularly those of the M. psoas. In such a case, the woman will have difficulty in arranging a favorable equilibrium around the pelvis, resulting in an excessive load on the sacrum-iliacum joint.

6.4 Mechanics of Sitting Posture;
Implication for Comfortable Chair Design

The form taken by the spine during sitting with only one support at the level of the shoulders can be compared with a spring column that is hinged at the base and clamped at the top to a support that can move freely in the vertical directions (Fig. 47, left). This column has two stable positions, viz., one on the left side and one on the right, that can be retained without external forces.

To move the column from one of these stable positions to the other, an auxiliary moment needs to be applied momentarily at the bottom hinge. To confirm this, two contour pictures were taken of a very flexible girl (aged 22) in sitting posture (Fig. 47, right). These pictures show clearly the bistable behavior, or so-called "click-clack" phenomenon.

Transition from sitting posture to lying posture and vice versa For an enduring sitting posture, stable position 1 in Fig. 47 must be preferred (for good circulation and to avoid strained ligaments) to position 2. During a transition from sitting posture to lying posture, as in the case of a reclining chair, this stable position must

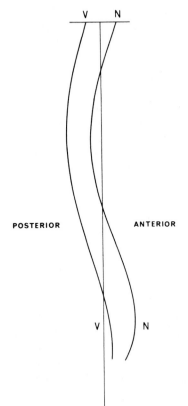

Figure 46 Contour pictures of a twins-carrying woman in standing posture. V, during pregnancy; N, after partus.

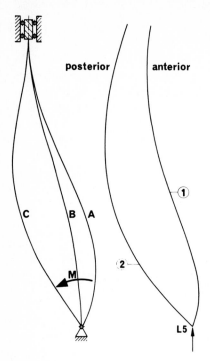

Figure 47 Click-clack phenomenon. The spine (right) has two stable positions, just like the spring column (left). By momentarily exerting a moment at the bottommost point, the form can "click" from one stable position to the other.

be maintained as long as possible. In Fig. 48, G is the total weight of the trunk, the head, and the arms. This force G can be divided into two forces, G_1 and G_2, which act respectively, perpendicular to and parallel to the back of the chair. When the back support of the chair is tilted backward, the component G_1 increases. This component G_1 produces the moment M of Fig 47, which is the cause of the transition from stable position 1 to stable position 2 (click-clack). To maintain stable position 1, it is necessary to introduce an extra force F on the back, which

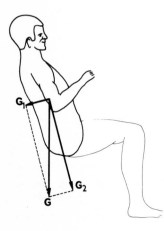

Figure 48 Components G_1 and G_2 of the upper torso weight G. G is the total weight of trunk, arms, and head. G_1 and G_2 are, respectively, perpendicular and parallel to the back of the chair.

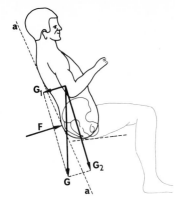

Figure 49 *F*, an extra force on the back, ensures the equilibrium of the moments, so that the stable position 1 of Fig. 47 is maintained.

must be in the direction opposite that of the force G_1 (Fig. 49). This force F must act on the upper edge of the pelvis. Now, there are two points of support at the back, one at the height of the shoulders and the other at the upper edge of the pelvis. These points of support exist if an even tangent plane is placed behind and against the back in stable position 1 (line a–a in Fig. 49). In practice, this plane is represented by the back of a chair. Now, both points of support must be maintained during the transition to the lying posture, and for this reason the back of the chair must follow and conduct the back and the pelvis. This means that the mechanical rotation axis of the back of the chair must coincide with the biomechanical rotation axis between the back and the upper legs.

In general, to maintain good support, the condition to be fulfilled is that the mechanical rotation axis between two planes of support should coincide with the biomechanical rotation axis between the corresponding rotating parts of the body. During the transition from sitting posture to lying posture and vice versa, this means that

The rotation axis between the back of the chair and the seat should coincide with the biomechanical rotation axis between the trunk and the upper legs.

The rotation axis between the leg rest and the seat should coincide with the biomechanical rotation axis between the lower legs and the upper legs.

These conditions have been determined experimentally [6]. Figure 50 is a sketch of the measuring equipment and the geometric parameters. The back of the chair and the seat consist of even planes upholstered with foam rubber (15 mm thick). The edge of the plane of the back of the chair lies 10 cm above the seat, so that the possibility of sagging of the soft parts (buttocks) exists. The back of the chair can rotate around the point A that lies at the same height as the seat and can produce an angle ϕ $(0° \leqslant \phi \leqslant 90°)$; it can also translate over a distance x_1 along a horizontal axis PQ. By adjusting ϕ and x_1 independently, the back of the chair can be placed in any desired position. When the back of the chair is tilted, the knee displaces. This displacement, which equals the displacement of the femur-tibia

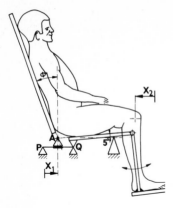

Figure 50 Sketch of the measuring setup and the geometric parameters.

rotation axis, is expressed by the coordinate x_2 in Fig. 50. The feet are supported by an even plane in such a way that the upper legs distinctly touch the seat.

To effect an unconstrained sitting posture for small values of ϕ, the seat was mounted at an angle of 5° to the horizontal. For large ϕ values, this angle does not exert any influence; hence the 5° seat angle was maintained during the whole measuring procedure.

Measurements were made as follows: Starting from the initial position $\phi = 0°$, the angle of the back of the chair was changed, in steps of 4° to 6° from $\phi = 0°$ to 90°. After each adjustment of ϕ, x_1 was also adjusted until the desired support of the pelvis was provided, and the patient said that he or she was sitting comfortably. After this, x_2 was measured. Starting from $\phi = 60°$, the pelvic orientation was effected by the biarticular muscles operating the pelvis, of which the M. psoas and M. rectus femoris are the most important. As the lying posture (with stretched legs) was reached, both lower legs were placed at an angle of 45° to the vertical, starting from $\phi = 50°$. Starting from $\phi = 90°$, the measurements were repeated in the opposite direction, again in steps of 4° to 6°. Figure 51 shows the measured results

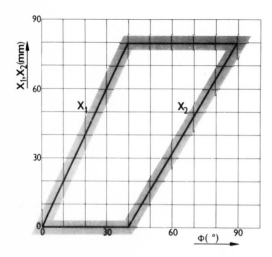

Figure 51 x_1 and x_2 as a function of ϕ, for 12 measurements. For $0° \leqslant \phi \leqslant 40°$, x_1 is a linear function of ϕ, and x_2 is a constant. For $40° < \phi \leqslant 90°$, x_2 is a linear function of ϕ, and x_1 is a constant.

graphically. We note that no distinct correlation exists between build or sex, and x_1, x_2. For $30° \leqslant \phi \leqslant 50°$ it appeared to be difficult to find an unconstrained, comfortable sitting posture (patient's subjective remark).

An explanation of the results must take into account a sliding down and slipping of the pelvis combined with a bending of the spine. In Fig. 52 the pelvis has been drawn for the case of $\phi = 0°$ (line 1). Point C is the hip joint (a fixed point in the pelvis). Points B and D, respectively, are the points of contact with the seat and the back of the chair in the case $\phi = 0°$. Measurements (Fig. 51) indicate that for $0° \leqslant \phi \leqslant 40°$, x_2 is constant. We can draw the back of the chair, moving along a distance x_1, and depending on ϕ, according to Fig. 51. On the other hand, Fig. 52 shows these situations in the case of $\phi = 20°$ (line 2) and in the case of $\phi = 35°$ (line 3). It appears that in the case of $0° \leqslant \phi \leqslant 25°$, the lines defining $x_1(\phi)$ in Fig. 51 will touch the pelvis at point D (Fig. 52). Consequently, there are two points of the pelvis, namely C and D, that do not move. This means that the pelvis remains in the same position and consequently does not rotate or translate in the area $0° \leqslant \phi \leqslant 25°$. The rotation of the back of the chair is followed by the rotation of the lowermost lumbar vertebrae. In Fig. 53 these vertebrae have been drawn for the case of ϕ being $20°$. After reaching the maximum rotation of the lowermost vertebrae (approximately $14°$ rotation with respect to each other), the back of the chair does not touch the pelvis (Fig. 52, line 3). Then the pelvis rotates around the hip axis C in the case of $25° \leqslant \phi \leqslant 40°$ until it touches the back of the chair again after each step of ϕ. This appears from the measured results: x_1 increases, x_2 remains constant. Herein, the seat-bones slide over the seat. The frictional forces and the less stable position of the pelvis are as was noted before ($30° \leqslant \phi \leqslant 50°$), the cause of the difficult sitting posture. This rotation of the pelvis continues until the sacrum-coccyx touches the seat (Fig. 54) at point E. This occurs at $\phi = 40°$.

From this position the pelvis rolls over the sacrum ($40° \leqslant \phi \leqslant 90°$) to a stable

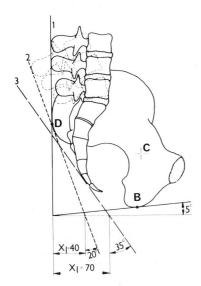

Figure 52 Pelvis with some lumbar vertebrae in the case $\phi = 0°$ (line 1). B is the point of contact of the pelvis and the seat; C is the hip joint (fixed point in the pelvis); D is the point of contact of the pelvis and the back of the chair in the case of $\phi = 0°$.

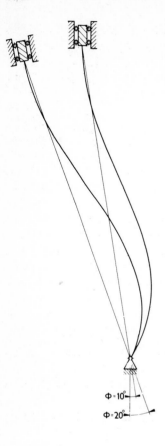

$\Phi = 10°$
$\Phi = 20°$

Figure 53 Spine (as per Fig. 47) for $\phi = 10°$ and $\phi = 20°$.

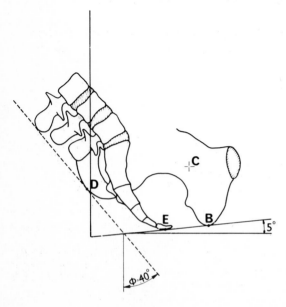

Figure 54 Starting from $\phi = 25°$, the pelvis topples over until the sacrum/coccyx touches the seat at point E ($\phi = 40°$).

position in which the edge of the pelvis and the lumbar vertebrae are supported by the back of the chair and the seat ($\phi = 90°$). During this last phase, the hip axis C moves backwards (Fig. 51: $x_2 = 0 \rightarrow 75$ mm). Initiating from pure rolling this shift in a horizontal direction is 80 mm. Notwithstanding negligence of the occurring slip, this corresponds well with the measurement (75 mm).

Summary The desired support for the back as well as the biomechanical rotation axis of the trunk with respect to the upper legs have now been determined. The site of this rotation axis depends on ϕ (Fig. 55):

$$0° \leqslant \phi \leqslant 25° \qquad D \text{ (upper edge of pelvis)}$$

$$25° \leqslant \phi \leqslant 40° \qquad C \text{ (hip joint)}$$

$$40° \leqslant \phi \leqslant 90° \qquad \text{according to shaded line from } E \text{ to } F$$

For $40° \leqslant \phi \leqslant 90°$, the biomechanical knee axis moves linearly with ϕ from G to H (75 mm).

Conclusions; rules for the design of a reclining chair

1. For good sitting posture, the support of the pelvis is a prime necessity.
2. For good support while tilting, the back of the chair should rotate about an axis like the one in Fig. 54.
3. A relatively short transition stretch may be observed between the two sites of the rotation axis.
4. It is necessary that the back of the chair's lowest edge lie approximately 10 cm above the seat (line 2 in Fig. 52).
5. The range of $30° \leqslant \phi \leqslant 50°$ should be avoided because the position of the pelvis is unstable in this range.
6. If an adjustable leg support is included, this support ought to rotate around an axis running through the knee joint. This axis should translate parallel to the knee joint ($G \rightarrow H$ in Fig. 55).

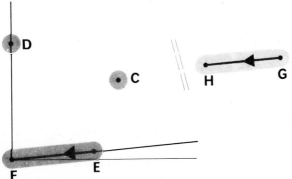

Figure 55 The site of the rotation axis depends on the position of the back of the chair (see text).

7 TWO SURGICAL APPLICATIONS

Our mechanical and mathematical analyses of the spine provide the foundations for the development of new methods of treatment of the pathological spine. Here we shall discuss two operative methods: (1) the correction of spondylolisthesis, and (2) the correction of scoliosis.

7.1 Spondylolisthesis

Spondylolisthesis occurs in approximately 2 to 4 percent of the population of developed countries. As a consequence of a defect (spondylolysis) in the inter-articular part of the neural arch (Fig. 56), the vertebral body, together with the above-lying spine, slips forward (olisthesis). Besides irritation of the cauda and the nerve roots, particularly bad posture can result, which in the long run can give rise to several complaints.

Every therapy applied so far has resulted only for the most part in temporary or partial removal of the pain, without normalizing the mechanical situation and improving the posture. For normalization of the mechanical situation (in cases of spondylolisthesis), the olisthetic vertebra must be replaced in its original position. The necessary force (calculated for this purpose) is introduced with the help of stainless steel wires that are attached to the processus spinosi of the two vertebrae lying above the olisthetic vertebra (Fig. 57). The wires are run through small holes made in the processus spinosi with the aid of a pair of punching tongs. The isotonic tensile force is applied to the wires by means of a spring motor that has been hung in a frame (Fig. 58). By changing the wire pulley on the shaft driven by the spring motor, the force can easily be changed.

The direction of the force exerted on the olisthetic vertebra by the wires is adjusted by means of conducting wheels that can be transposed with respect to the frame. A winding mechanism for the wires and a system of pulleys enables tension

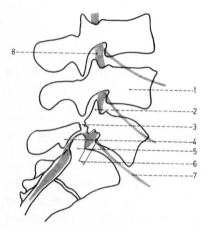

Figure 56 As a result of a fracture in the neural arch, the vertebral body slips to the ventral side. (1) Vertebral body; (2) superior articular process of L5; (3) lysis; (4) neural arch; (5) superior articular process of S1; (6) olisthesis; (7) neural root; (8) cauda (spinal marrow).

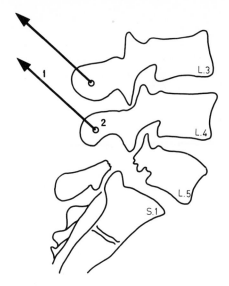

Figure 57 Traction is applied to the processus spinosi of L3 and L4.

to be applied to the steel wires simultaneously and gradually. The frame is positioned on the body by means of a Milwaukee brace.

The magnitude of the force needed for the repositioning is calculated with the help of a biomechanical analytical (shear) model, for which purpose the grade of olisthesis, disk diameter, and height are measured in a lateral x-ray picture. At the level of the olisthesis (which, in 80 percent of the cases, is the level of the fifth lumbar vertebra-first sacral vertebra) the disk diameter, the disk height, and the extent of shear are measured and corrected by the x-ray projection factor. The shear is measured with respect to the vertebra lying beneath, and expressed as a percentage of the diameter of this vertebra (Fig. 59). The procedure distinguishes between the following cases:

1. Olisthesis smaller than approximately 30 percent
2. Olisthesis larger than approximately 30 percent

If the olisthesis is smaller than approximately 30 percent, then relatively small forces (of magnitude approximately 40 N) on the processus spinosi of the two vertebrae lying above are adequate to stretch the tissue of the annulus fibrosis and of the surrounding ligaments to reposition the olisthetic vertebra completely. In the case of a spondylolisthesis on the level L5-S1, the disks L4-L5 and L3-L4 transmit the correction force through to the olisthetic levels. The correction process takes approximately 36 h and is performed with a fully conscious patient. For repositioning the olisthetic vertebra during the operation, when the wires are introduced, an intercorporal spondylodesis is applied from dorsal (Fig. 60). To this end, two bone grafts from the crista are put into the intervertebral space, along both sides of the dura. To provide compatible growing together with the vertebral bodies, grooves

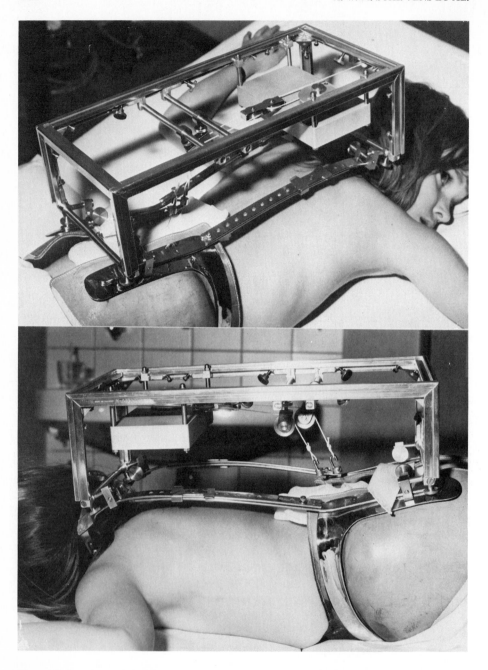

Figure 58 Traction apparatus for the repositioning of spondylolisthesis. Isotonic forces are exerted by a spring motor directly on the spine, by means of wires passing through the skin.

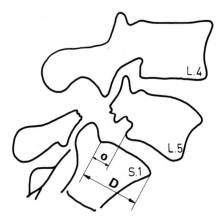

$$\text{Shear} = \frac{O}{D} \times 100 \ \%$$

Figure 59 Shear is measured with respect to the vertebra lying beneath, and expressed as a percentage of the diameter of this vertebra.

are milled in both boundary plates of the intervertebral space. During the time of growing together of the bone grafts, traction is maintained through the frame of Fig. 58.

If the olisthesis is larger than approximately 30 percent, the required repositioning force is too large to be sustained by the allowable fracture strength of the spinous processi. In such cases, the major part of the annulus fibrosis and the ligaments on the olisthetic level are cut; the traction required for a complete correction need not be larger than the lumbar spine's own weight. In this case, it is practical to prepare the vertebral bodies in such a way that these can grow together immediately (by milling off the cartilage layers of S1 and L5), so that no bone grafts need be introduced for fixation. During the postoperative phase, the patient is rehabilitated to obtain a nonpathological posture of the body. In this connection

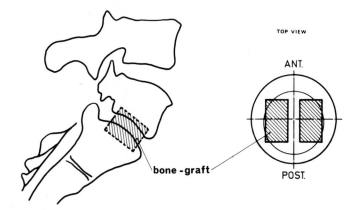

Figure 60 Lateral and top views of the position of the grafts in the intervertebral disk.

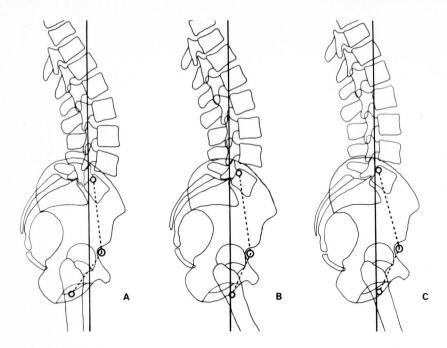

Figure 61 Lumbosacral region in the case of spondylolisthesis. The dashed line gives the position of the M. psoas. (*A*) Situation before operation; (*B*) state directly after operation; (*C*) state after some stretching of the M. psoas.

especially, the M. psoas plays an important part (Fig. 61). This muscle must be lengthened by exercises, in most cases. Figure 62 illustrates repositioning and fixation for the case of spondylolisthesis greater than 30 percent.

During all operations performed, in addition to the redressing of complaints, the excessive lordosis (if any), the steep sacrum base incline, and the psoas contracture were also corrected.

7.2 Scoliosis

Scoliosis is a lateral curvature of the spine accompanied by an axial rotation of the vertebrae (Fig. 63). The correction method corrects this deformation, provides an erect posture, and thereafter maintains the corrected form without hindrance to growth. The principle of the correction method involves correction of scoliosis with the help of transverse forces.

Figure 64 shows the bending-moment distribution (in the spine of a certain scoliosis patient) that is needed to correct the scoliosis completely, and the bending moment introduced by corrective transverse forces on the spine at three levels. The bending moments correspond well; therefore these three transverse forces are sufficient to correct the scoliosis The forces are exerted directly on the three vertebrae by means of bars (Fig. 65). In the thoracic region, these bars are attached to the processus transversi by means of a clamping device. In the lumbar region, attachment is made to the neural arch and the processus spinosus.

The forces are introduced from outside the skin (Fig. 66). Two forces are introduced into each bar, to apply the moment needed for the rotational correction. To generate these six forces (two for each vertebra), an external frame of two extra rods is designed to connect the uppermost and lowermost vertebral bar. Between these rods and the middle vertebral bar are two screw-thread connections (Fig. 67). By gradually turning the nuts on the screw threads, the centrally located vertebra can be placed fully in line with the other two. The turning of the correction nuts takes place with the help of a moment-producing device from which (by means of a calibrated scale) the transverse force introduced can be read directly. When the correction force reaches a value of about 50 N, the correction is stopped; the next phase of the correction does not take place until the transverse force has dropped to half the 50 N due to relaxation of the spine and the thorax. After that, the turning of the nuts is started again.

The correction process occurs very gradually. For the patient of Fig. 68, with a scoliosis of 46°, it took one week for complete correction. The process is performed with the full knowledge of the patient; the patient does not experience any inconvenience as a result.

When the spine has been overcorrected by approximately 5°, fixation is effected. This fixation is necessary to prevent the spine from again taking up the

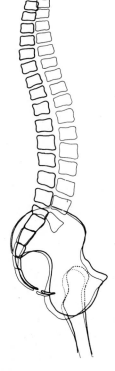

Figure 62 Case of spondylolisthesis greater than 30 percent, before and after repositioning and fixation.

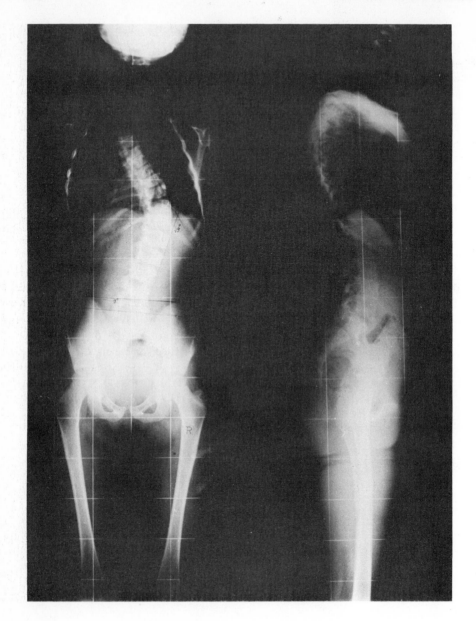

Figure 63 X-rays of a patient with scoliosis.

scoliotic form. The straightened spine is fixed with the help of the existing Harrington apparatus (Fig. 68).

This method for correcting scoliosis is not an optimal one. Severe cases have presented problems. The treatment consists of two operations, viz., (1) implantation of corrector and (2) implantation of fixator. A change in treatment, requiring only one operation to effect both correction and fixation, is an ambition yet to be realized.

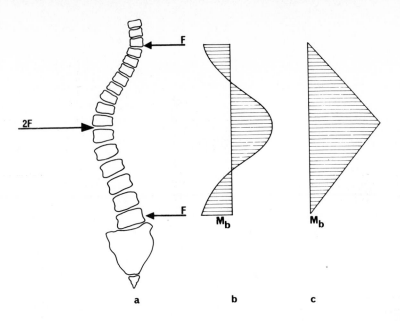

Figure 64 (*a*) Transverse forces needed to correct scoliosis; (*b*) graphic representation of the bending-moment variation needed to correct scoliosis; (*c*) bending moment caused by the transverse forces.

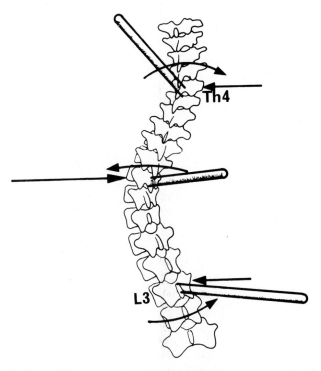

Figure 65 Spatial view of scoliosis with the three bars to correct the curve.

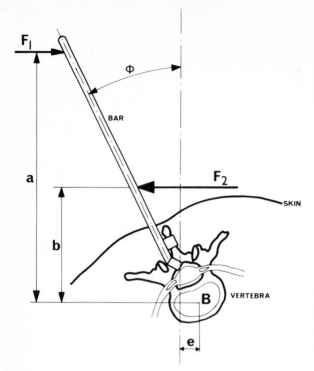

Figure 66 Two forces are needed to bring the vertebra back to its initial position. $F_2 - F_1$ causes the transverse force. M, the torsional moment around B, is $F_1 a - F_2 b$.

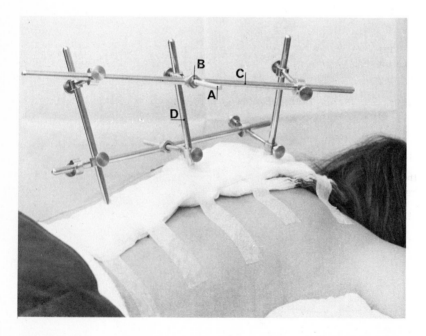

Figure 67 Patient with scoliosis corrector. The function of the external frame is to place the vertebrae "in line." A screw-thread; B, correction nut; C, connection rod; D, bar connected with the vertebra.

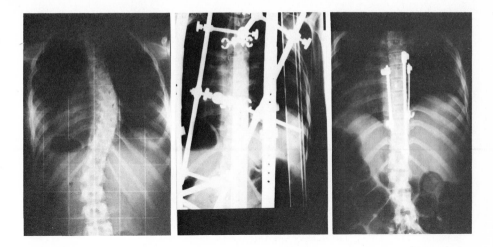

Figure 68 Patient of 16 yr with a scoliosis of 46°. Left, x-ray before operation; middle, during the correction period of one week; right, after implantation of the Harrington equipment to fixate the spine.

GLOSSARY

Annulus fibrosus: part of the intervertebral disk; fibrous ring enclosing the nucleus pulposus.

Curvature: a curve can be approximated by an arc of a circle at any arbitrary point; the curvature is the reciprocal of the radius of such a circle. A circle with a short radius has a relatively large curvature.

Dorsal contour: the dorsal contour of the spine is the fluent line passing through the points on the skin considered to represent the most dorsal points of the processus spinosi.

Flexural rigidity: resistance against bending; bending stiffness.

Form of the spine: the fluent line passing through the geometric centers of the vertebral bodies and the intervertebral disks.

Kyphosis: thoracic part of the spine which, seen from the ventral side, is concave.

Lordosis: part of the spine which, seen from the ventral side, is convex.

Nucleus pulposus: gelatinous central portion of an intervertebral disk.

Processus spinosus: process of the vertebra directed backward.

Sacrum(os): bone composed of connated caudal vertebrae.

Scoliosis: laterally crooked spine.

Spondylolisthesis: shifting of vertebrae in consequence of a fracture in the interarticular part of the vertebral arch.

Torsional rigidity: resistance against torque; torsional stiffness.

Vertebral body: rigid portion of a vertebra, being virtually rectangular in lateral aspect.

REFERENCES

1. C. J. Snijders, "On the Form of the Human Thoracolumbar Spine and Some Aspects of Its Mechanical Behaviour," Stichting, Voorschoten, Holland, 1971.
2. H. Yamada, "Strength of Biological Materials," Williams and Wilkins, Baltimore, 1970.
3. M. Williams and H. R. Lissner, "Biomechanics of Human Motion," Saunders, Philadelphia, 1962.
4. J. V. Basmajian, "Muscles Alive, Their Function Revealed by Electromyography," Williams and Wilkins, Baltimore, 1967.
5. C. J. Snijders and M. Verduin, Stabilograph, an Accurate Instrument for Sciences Interested in Postural Equilibrium, *Agressologie,* vol. 14C, pp. 15–20, 1973.
6. T. H. M. Bougie and L. M. K. Meeuwissen, De Rolstoel, report, University of Technology, Eindhoven, Holland, 1972.
7. R. Hesse and F. Doflein, "Tierbau und Tierleben in ihrem Zusammenhang betrachtet," 2nd ed., Fischer, Jena, 1943.

STRESS AND STRAIN
IN THE INTERVERTEBRAL DISK
IN RELATION TO SPINAL DISORDERS

Lars Sonnerup

The structure of the human intervertebral disk in relation to its mechanical functions is briefly described. Emphasis is placed on the relation between mechanical loads and disk injuries. The general mechanical behavior of the disk and its components is delineated, and on this basis the stress-strain situation in the disk is studied theoretically. Both a continuum approach and a discrete-element structural model are employed. The latter method enables fluid flow within and out of the disk to be taken into account, thus describing some of its rate-dependent response. With the mechanical models of the disk as a background, the mechanisms of failure of the annulus fibrosus are discussed, and an explanation is offered as to how observed concentric fissures between the annular layers are initiated.

1 INTRODUCTION: ANATOMY AND COMMON INJURIES
OF THE INTERVERTEBRAL JOINT COMPLEX

The intervertebral joint is a structural complex connecting adjacent vertebrae of the spine. It consists of the intervertebral disk with the anterior and posterior longitudinal ligaments, together forming the joint between the vertebral bodies, and the synovial joints between the vertebral arches. The anatomy of the lumbar intervertebral joint is shown in Figs. 1 and 2. The main features of a typical lumbar vertebra,

This work was done while the author, on a fellowship from The Royal Society, spent an academic year at the Biomechanics Unit of the Department of Mechanical Engineering, Imperial College, London.

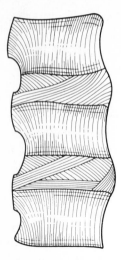

Figure 1 Lumbar intervertebral joints, lateral view. Lower disk dissected to show arrangements of fibers.

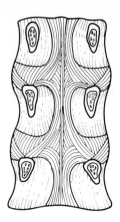

Figure 2 Lumbar intervertebral joints, posterior view.

the vertebral body and the vertebral arch, are illustrated in Fig. 3. A vertebra is composed of spongy bone covered with a thin layer of compact bone except at the top and bottom surfaces of the vertebral body, where the spongiosa forms a perforated area, peripherally bounded by the bony epiphyseal ring (Fig. 3). This perforated surface is covered by a cartilage plate, forming the boundary between the intervertebral disk and the vertebral body.

Gross injuries of the intervertebral joint are generally caused either by impact situations, as in car crashes and special courses like the ejection of an aircraft pilot, or by excess loading under the more static conditions of everyday life.

The spinal response to impact has received increasing attention in recent years, and the state of knowledge of the subject is reviewed by Orne and Liu [1], who also present a mathematical treatment of the problem with particular reference to

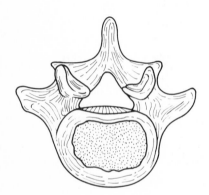

Figure 3 Lumbar vertebra.

the pilot ejection situation. The most common injuries caused by ejection are the more or less pure compression fracture of a vertebra and the so-called anterior lip fracture, where the anterior bony edge of a vertebra is sheared off in a fashion suggesting that extensive bending in the sagittal plane has played a major role.

Injuries produced by excess loading under normal conditions show a more variable pattern. It is, however, obvious from the extensive report on the normal and morbid anatomy of the intervertebral disks by Beadle [2] that, in general, the spongy vertebral bodies fail rather than the intervertebral disks. Failure of the spongiosa often results in fractures of the cartilage plates above and below the intervertebral disk. Commonly observed fractures of the epiphyseal ring, to which the peripheral parts of the disk are firmly attached, is probably also a result of failure of the underlying spongiosa. Figure 4 shows a typical compression fracture of a vertebral body.

In his early report on disks, Beadle correlated disk lesions with spinal deformities. The mechanics of the spine related to such problems has been extensively investigated since then, and recently mathematical models simulating the kinematics and kinetics of the spine have been developed to elucidate the causes of these

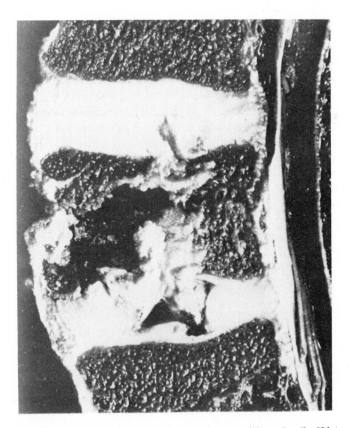

Figure 4 Compression fracture of vertebral body. *(From Beadle [2].)*

deformities (Schultz and Galante [3], Panjabi and White [4], White [5], and Schultz et al. [6]). The subject is treated by Snijders in this volume.

Although it is evident, from both Beadle's findings and later experimental investigations, that failure of the intervertebral joint under excess loading in compression and bending generally is due to incomplete fractures or collapse of the vertebral bodies, the intervertebral disk is still the key component of the joint. It is the mechanical properties of the fibrous disk structure that determine how the load on the spine is transmitted from one vertebra to the other, because the distribution of stress within the disk yields the load distribution on the vertebral bodies. In a recent investigation by Farfan et al. [7] it is further shown that torsional loads play a significant role in the production of injury to the joint. In this case the damage is observed primarily in the peripheral fibrous part of the disk itself, whereas the vertebrae remain virtually intact. Finally, the disk also gives the joint its specific deformation properties, needed for mathematical modeling. This forms the background for the interest in the mechanics of the intervertebral disk.

2 STRUCTURE OF THE DISK

The anatomy of the intervertebral disk has been described at length by Beadle [2], who divides it into three main parts: the cartilage plates bounding it above and below, the nucleus pulposus in the center, and the annulus fibrosus forming its peripheral boundary. Figure 5 shows these components schematically, and Fig. 6 displays the horizontal section of a typical lumbar intervertebral disk.

The cartilage plates are dense plates of hyaline cartilage. They cover the perforated areas of the vertebral surfaces and delimit the tissue of the nucleus pulposus from the spongiosa of the vertebral bodies (Fig. 3).

The nucleus pulposus is a fluidlike tissue mass composed of a three-dimensional network of fine collagen fibers in a gel matrix of ground substance. It occupies 30 to 50 percent of the disk.

The annulus fibrosus consists of a series of concentric, ring-shaped layers made up of rather coarse, parallel collagen fiber bundles with little matrix of ground substance between them. The fibers of each layer run in a well-defined direction, generally obliquely from one vertebral end surface to the other. The fiber directions

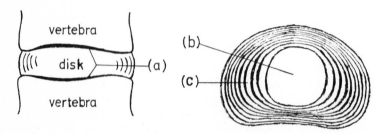

Figure 5 Components of the disk: (*a*) cartilage plates; (*b*) nucleus pulposus; (*c*) annulus fibrosus.

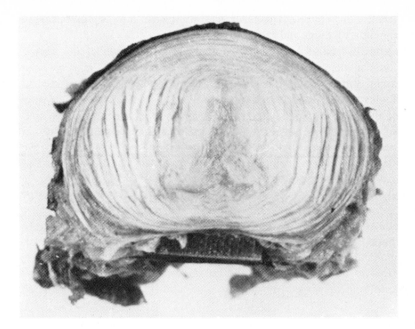

Figure 6 Horizontal section of lumbar disk. Note the lamellar appearance of the annulus fibrosus. *(From Beadle [2].)*

of adjacent layers cross each other, as indicated in Figs. 1 and 2. The concentric layers are interconnected, and the space between them is occupied by a looser, moister tissue of fibers and amorphous ground substance. The fibers of the annulus attach themselves peripherally to the epiphyseal ring and in the interior to the cartilage plates.

There is no absolutely distinct border between the nucleus and the annulus, the inner layers of which are fainter and more widely spaced than the peripheral ones (Figs. 5 and 6). Beadle estimates the number of layers in a lumbar disk to be between 10 and 12. Apparently, then, the structural arrangement of the disk could be thought of as interconnected, ringshaped, fibrous layers with a gel of ground substance and tissue fluid in the center and in the interspaces between the layers (Fig. 5). The fluid content of the normal disk is high (70 to 80 percent).

3 FEATURES OF DISK DEGENERATION AND INJURY

Degenerative change of the intervertebral disk is a common phenomenon, even at an early age. Beadle gives a comprehensive survey and points out the significance of mechanical stress and strain as initiating and accelerating factors in disk degeneration. Here only a short account of the most common structural changes in the disk associated with injurious mechanical loads, i.e., the various kinds of fissures and tears of the tissues, will be given. These damages are divided into two groups, concentric (circumferential) fissures and radiating tears.

The concentric fissures are most common and could be thought of as a separation between two annular fibrous layers through breakage of the links between them for a certain distance along the circumference. They are most often seen in the anterior annulus. Farfan et al. [7] have been able to produce similar separation of the layers of the annulus experimentally in torsion tests and hence suggest that torsion is a chief mechanical factor in the production of disk degeneration.

The radiating tears often start in the nucleus region and run out into the annulus, in some cases producing complete communication between the nucleus and the outside. They are tensile ruptures of the nucleus tissue and the layers of the annulus fibrosus. Farfan et al. [7] postulate that the radiating tear is the last stage in a degeneration chain starting with the concentric fissures. Farfan et al. [8] have studied the geometry of radial, annular ruptures in detail and found five basic patterns of rupture location: posterolateral, posterior bilateral, posterocentral, lateral, and anterior. The posterior ruptures were the most commonly observed.

In later stages of disk degeneration, the nucleus and annulus successively lose their fluid content, and the disk ultimately becomes a rather desiccated, disordered fibrous mass.

4 MECHANICAL BEHAVIOR OF THE DISK

The intervertebral disk shows the typical mechanical properties of soft connective tissue structures. It displays nonlinearity (increase in stiffness with deformation) as well as rate dependency (increase in stiffness with rate of deformation) in its load deformation characteristics. The rate dependency implies in turn the phenomena of stress relaxation, strain retardation, and hysteresis.

Experimental investigations of the past often fail to take into account the rate dependency when presenting load deformation data. Indeed, to the knowledge of the author, no thorough investigation of the disk response to different load or deformation histories has been published. The above-mentioned general features are, however, implicit from knowledge about the mechanical behavior of other soft connective tissues (cf. Viidik [9]) and have been partly confirmed experimentally in the past. Thus, Virgin [10] pointed out the influence on the mechanical response of fluid flow into and out of the disk and reported significant fluid exchange during a cycle of compression and recovery. He also noted the creep phenomenon for disks under constant compressive load. Brown et al. [11] made further investigations of the disk in compression and measured the fluid exchange in this context. Their results indicate a definite gradual decrease in volume of the disk with increasing compressive load. This volume reduction is explained as initially due to collapse of voids in the disk and then due to flow of fluid from the disk through the cartilage plates into the vertebral bodies. The experimental technique did not permit measurement of radial flow through the annulus fibrosus. They further observed load relaxation in their specimens. Both Virgin and Brown et al. demonstrated the

nonlinearity of the disk, manifested by the stiffness increasing gradually with deformation.

Recently Farfan et al. [7] have demonstrated the response, including sensitivity
to rate of deformation, of the disk in torsion. Figure 7 is redrawn after their results
and shows the nonlinearity and rate dependency. The dynamic response of the
intervertebral joint as a whole and of the isolated disk has been investigated by
Markolf and Steidel [12] and Fitzgerald and Freeland [13]. Markolf and Steidel
used free vibration tests to determine the stiffness and damping of the intervertebral
joint in bending and torsion. For the corresponding measurements of axial stiffness
and damping they conducted resonance tests on the isolated disk. Their main objective was to produce engineering data on the mechanical characteristics of the intervertebral joints, useful in mathematical treatments of the spinal response to dynamic
loads. Thus they give numerical values of stiffnesses and damping factors in the
mentioned modes of deformation for the joints of the lower portion of the spine.
In all tests small amplitudes were used, limiting the applicability of the data to
models of the initial (small deformation) dynamic response of the vertebral column.
Fitzgerald and Freeland conducted forced vibration tests (small amplitude) in pure
shear on isolated disks from dogs with the main aim of comparing the dynamic
response of the disk with that of some synthetic elastomers, believed to be suitable
for disk replacements in humans. Their results show significant damping in the disk
and indicate that a certain silicone rubber is a possible candidate as a disk replacement material. Markolf [14] has also studied the static characteristics of the joint in
bending, torsion, shear, and compression.

The conclusions concerning the static mechanical behavior of the disk itself, to
be drawn from these investigations, are that in compression and bending there are a
marked nonlinearity and rate dependency, in torsion the nonlinearity is less but the
rate dependency prevails, and finally in shear the response is much more linear.

In a current experimental investigation, Moont [15] has studied the rate

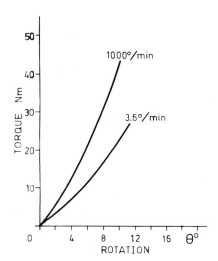

Figure 7 Mechanical response of the lumbar disk in torsion at two extreme rates of deformation. *(Data from Farfan et al. [7].)*

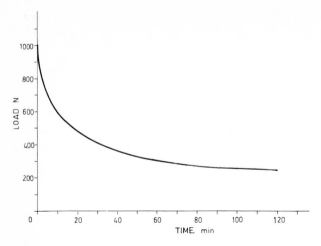

Figure 8 Relaxation curve for lumbar disk. Three consecutive tests with a time lapse of 8 h between the first and second and 16 h between second and third gave virtually the same curve. *(Data from Moont [15].)*

dependency of the load deformation characteristics of the disk in compression. As will be discussed further in the next section, a closer examination of load deformation curves for soft, parallel-fiber connective tissue reveals that the stiffness, with increasing rate of deformation, soon approaches an upper limit. Thus the load deformation relationship becomes rate independent for speeds of deformation above a certain value, and a maximum stiffness response is obtained for all such speeds. To determine, for instance, the total amount of load relaxation possible at a certain deformation level, it is then only necessary to bring the specimen to that deformation sufficiently fast. The necessary speed is usually quite low (cf. next section and Fig. 12). This turns out to be valid also for the intervertebral disk, and by first determining the rate of deformation necessary to produce the maximum stiffness response, Moont is able to show a considerable amount of load relaxation from the "instantaneously" developed value at a fast deformation to a fixed level. Figure 8 shows such a relaxation curve. The fact that the load diminishes so rapidly and drastically under constant deformation again suggests that fluid flow out of the disk can play a significant role, at least in the initial phase of the relaxation process.

5 TENSILE PROPERTIES OF THE DISK MATERIAL

In view of the fiber arrangement in the disk, tensile data obtained from excised specimens of the disk material must be used with caution. The material in such a specimen does not function exactly as it does *in situ* in the disk. Brown et al. [11] performed tests of this kind, cutting out test specimens vertically through the disk and leaving a piece of bone attached to the fibers in each end of the specimen. Specimens were taken from various parts of the disk. The results show, as could be expected, that the nucleus pulposus is very weak in tension, and that the strength increases gradually toward the periphery, being highest at the anterior and posterior boundaries of the disk.

5.1 Nucleus Pulposus

Nachemson [16] showed that the weak nucleus pulposus, in the intact disk, in fact behaves hydrostatically like a fluid when the disk is loaded in compression. No detailed information about the viscoelastic properties of the nucleus is known to the author at present, but it seems obvious that the shear modulus must be very low.

5.2 Parallel-Fiber Material

In turning to the detailed tensile properties of the annulus fibrosus, it is necessary to take into account the structural arrangement of the fiber bundles in the concentric annular layers. In each layer the bundles run in parallel (Fig. 1). It is therefore of interest to consider, generally, the tensile properties of soft, parallel-fiber connective tissues.

From investigations by Viidik and others on such material (cf. Viidik [9]), it is apparent that the characteristic shape of the load elongation curve (Fig. 9) is a result of a straightening of the wavy fiber bundles, during the initial stage of low but increasing stiffness, to a final parallel arrangement of higher stiffness and more linear response. Figure 9 shows typical curves for the anterior cruciate ligament of the rabbit. The linear part of the curves starts at a rather low load level, but when a considerable amount of deformation has taken place. The waviness of the fiber bundles disappears entirely well before this load has been reached. The failure of a

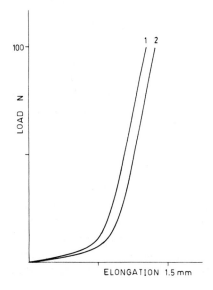

Figure 9 Load elongation curves for the anterior cruciate ligament of the rabbit. Numbers 1 and 2 denote first and second loading of the same specimen. *(Data from Viidik [9].)*

specimen is a gradual process, starting as part ruptures in the upper linear region and leading to decreasing stiffness and eventually complete rupture.

The rate dependency of the load elongation relationship was studied by Frisén et al. [17]. Load elongation tests on the anterior cruciate ligament at different rates of deformation were performed. For each rate a different curve was obtained. Figure 10 illustrates these curves schematically. It appears that there exists an upper limiting response that is rapidly approached with increasing speed of deformation (curve $v \approx \infty$ in Fig. 10). This behavior is more evident from the experimental results of Fig. 11, where the vertical distance between a curve at speed v and the curve at infinitely slow speed $v \approx 0$ is plotted as a function of elongation. This distance clearly corresponds to the amount of load that would relax if the deformation motion were suddenly stopped and the elongation kept constant. Each curve in Fig. 10 gives a corresponding curve in Fig. 11. The curves of Fig. 11 are seen to cluster together as the rate of deformation increases, indicating that the maximum stiffness response is approached. The details of these findings were considered by Sonnerup [18], who showed that the slope of the linear part of the load elongation curve rapidly tends to its upper limit as illustrated in Fig. 12.

As was pointed out in the previous section, this feature of rate dependency holds also for the intervertebral disk as a whole and is an important factor to control in creep and relaxation experiments on connective tissues and structures. The rate of deformation necessary to obtain the maximum stiffness must be determined, to ensure that load or deformation is imposed sufficiently fast in these tests.

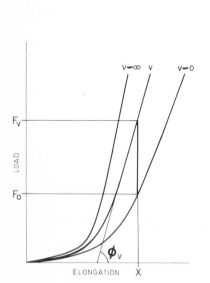

Figure 10 Schematic load elongation curves at different rates of deformation v.

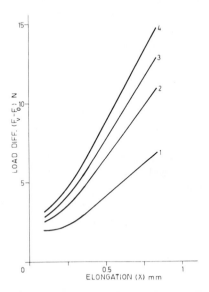

Figure 11 Influence of rate of deformation for anterior cruciate ligament specimens from rabbit. Speeds: 1, 0.5 mm/min; 2, 1.0 mm/min; 3, 5.0 mm/min; 4, 20.0 mm/min. *(Data from Frisén et al. [17].)*

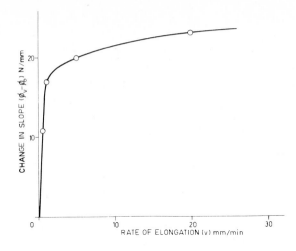

Figure 12 Influence of rate of deformation. Data from Fig. 11 replotted.

5.3 Annulus Fibrosus

It is reasonable to assume that the tensile properties of the layers of the annulus fibrosus, in the fiber direction, are similar to those of parallel-fiber tissue in general. It is, however, difficult to perform tests to confirm this, as the specimens have to be cut out from the structure, instead of being available in a natural, suitable shape as in the case of tendons and ligaments. Tests on the annulus layers have, however, been performed by Galante [19]. He tested specimens from various parts of the annulus, cut out in different directions according to Fig. 13. A typical cyclic load elongation diagram for a specimen cut out horizontally is shown in Fig. 14. Apparently, this specimen consists of a number of layers, the fibers of which cross each other in a symmetrical, oblique fashion, thus forming a trellis structure (Fig. 14). The properties of such a specimen must inevitably be quite different from those of the parallel-fiber material: lower stiffness and strength, larger nonlinearity, and more hysteresis. *In situ* in the annulus, however, this piece of material will perform differently, the cut fibers along the edges of the specimen then being intact and running between firm attachments at both ends

In light of these considerations, it is to be expected that the intact layers of the annulus will show a stiffer and more linear behavior than the excised specimens (cf. Sonnerup [18]). The difference in stiffness between the horizontal and vertical directions, i.e., the anisotropy of the layers, is nevertheless clearly demonstrated by Galante and shown in Fig. 15. This difference is due to the fact that the fibers run at an acute angle to the horizontal direction (Fig. 1). The variation of stiffness with position, i.e., the inhomogeneity of the annulus, is likewise demonstrated by

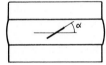
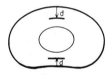

Figure 13 Sampling of specimens from annulus fibrosus.

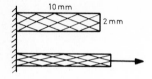

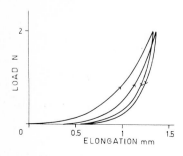

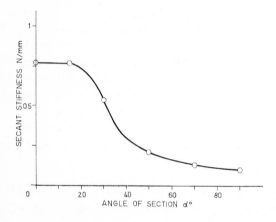

Figure 14 Cyclic load elongation curves for horizontally excised annulus specimen. Trellis structure of the specimen indicated. *(Data from Galante [19].)*

Galante and illustrated in Fig. 16. Here the variation is probably caused by the change in spacing of the annular layers from the inside toward the periphery (Fig. 5).

6 ANALYSIS OF STRESS AND STRAIN IN THE DISK

From the considerations of previous sections, it is obvious that a detailed analysis of the disk is necessary for an understanding of both its normal mechanical response and the mechanisms of disk failure. The distribution of stress and strain in the disk for various cases of loading is then of fundamental importance and will now be discussed with particular reference to pure compression and torsion of the disk.

In attacking the problem of stress and strain analysis, two main approaches could be employed: (1) The material of the disk is assumed to be a continuous medium (although not necessarily a homogeneous and isotropic one), and the

Figure 15 Anisotropy of the annulus material. *(Data from Galante [19].)*

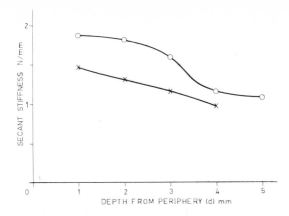

Figure 16 Inhomogeneity of the annulus material, anterior ○ and posterior ✕. *(Data from Galante [19].)*

methods of continuum mechanics are used to determine what is then to be understood as average stress and strain distributions. (2) The multiphase character of the disk structure, with tissue fluid, amorphous ground substance, and fiber bundles, is taken into account in an arrangement of interacting, discrete structural elements and fluid substance, and the methods of structural mechanics are applied. In both cases, the main structural features of the disk must be incorporated in the models subject to analysis, and even in the continuum treatment a certain division into idealized components is feasible.

6.1 Continuum Analysis

The most apparent structural characteristic of the disk is the variable mechanical response of the tissue in different parts. In the center there is the gel of the nucleus pulposus, reinforced by a fine, three-dimensional fibrous network. Toward the periphery, the tissue transforms into a more two-dimensional arrangement of coarse fibrous layers and less amorphous ground substance. As mentioned earlier, Nachemson [16] showed that under static load conditions the disk develops a uniform hydrostatic pressure in the central region. This pressure in the nucleus is generally in excess of the applied compressive load per unit cross-sectional area of the disk. In the peripheral fibrous annulus, however, a nonuniform distribution of stress will arise. If the annulus is considered as a continuous, solid ring, normal stresses according to Fig. 17 are implicit from the pressure in the nucleus region. These stresses are not equal and will vary from point to point through the annulus. Depending on loading conditions, shear stresses may also appear. The division of the disk into two continuous components, the nucleus considered as a fluid and the annulus considered as a solid ring, is thus a reasonable starting point in the continuum approach and has been used to estimate the stresses of the annulus fibrosus for pure compression and torsion of the disk.

Compression The case of pure compression was studied by Sonnerup [20, 21] with the aim of elucidating how the variation of stiffness through the annulus fibrosus

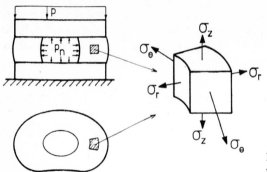

Figure 17 State of stress in the compressed disk.

influences the distribution of stress in it. Since the investigation was intended as a qualitative estimation of the stress situation, geometric simplifications to cylindrical symmetry were introduced, and only stresses in the central horizontal plane of symmetry of the disk were determined. The idealized problem is illustrated in Fig. 18. A ring-shaped thin slice of the annulus is considered, and the nucleus pressure p_n together with the varying lateral pressure p_z are taken as the outer loads creating the radial and tangential stresses in this ring. These pressures are estimated experimentally.

The nonlinearity of the annulus material is neglected in accordance with the considerations of the previous section and by taking into account the fact that, in the intact normal disk, there is a certain amount of internal stress, even when the disk is unloaded (cf. Beadle [2]). *In situ* in the spine, there is, further, a preload on the disk due to the action of muscles and ligaments. The prestress of the material results in a more linear response to additional loading (Fig. 9). The anisotropy of the material in the annulus is probably more important than the nonlinearity. However, compared to the inhomogeneity (variation of stiffness through the annulus),

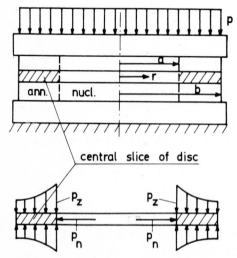

Figure 18 Continuum model of the disk in compression. Circular symmetry assumed. Stresses in the central slice are according to Fig. 17. *(From Sonnerup [21].)*

even the anisotropy is neglected in this first approximation. Thus the material is assumed to be isotropic and linearly elastic, with a stiffness increasing radially through the annulus fibrosus. Finally, the annulus material is also considered as incompressible, an assumption generally valid for soft tissues.

Governing Equations The fundamental equations of the problem for the tangential stress determination are given below. The detailed solution is presented in App. A (cf. also Sonnerup [21]). The notation employed in the equations is delineated in Figs. 17 and 18. Standard notation for stress and strain is used.

Equation of equilibrium:

$$\frac{d(r\sigma_r)}{dr} - \sigma_\theta = 0 \tag{1}$$

Equation of compatibility:

$$\frac{d(r\epsilon_\theta)}{dr} - \epsilon_r = 0 \tag{2}$$

Constitutive equations:

$$\epsilon_r = \frac{\sigma_r - \frac{1}{2}(\sigma_\theta + \sigma_z)}{\psi(r)}$$

$$\epsilon_\theta = \frac{\sigma_\theta - \frac{1}{2}(\sigma_r + \sigma_z)}{\psi(r)} \tag{3}$$

$$\epsilon_z = \frac{\sigma_z - \frac{1}{2}(\sigma_r + \sigma_\theta)}{\psi(r)}$$

According to experiments (Fig. 16), the quantity $1/\psi(r)$, where $\psi(r)$ is the variable stiffness, is assumed to be a linear function

$$\frac{1}{\psi(r)} = \lambda \left(1 - \frac{\mu r}{b}\right) \tag{4}$$

where the constants λ and μ are material parameters.

Boundary conditions:

$$\sigma_r(a) = -p_n \qquad \sigma_r(b) = 0 \qquad \sigma_z(r) = -p_z(r) \tag{5}$$

Solution and Results The solution for the tangential stress has the general form

$$\frac{\sigma_\theta}{p_n} = \frac{p_m}{p_n}[(x + k)y' + y - 1] \tag{6}$$

where

$$y = A \sum_{\nu=0}^{\infty} \alpha_\nu x^\nu + B \sum_{\nu=0}^{\infty} \beta_\nu x^\nu + \sum_{\nu=0}^{n} B_\nu(x + k)^\nu$$

$$x = \frac{r - a}{b - a}$$

$$k = \frac{a}{b - a}$$

$$p_m = \frac{2 \displaystyle\int_a^b p_z \, r \, dr}{b^2 - a^2} = \text{mean lateral pressure across annulus}$$

The coefficients A and B are determined from the boundary conditions (5), and the coefficients B_ν are given by the form of the function $p_z(r)$ (cf. App. A). As a simple estimation, this function is assumed to be linear according to the expression

$$\frac{p_z}{p_m} = C(x - x_m) + 1 \tag{7}$$

where

$$x = \frac{r - a}{b - a}$$

$$x_m = \frac{2 + a/b}{3(1 + a/b)}$$

This function is based on the experimental studies of Sonnerup [21], summarized in Fig. 22; we shall return to this relationship later.

Two special cases were evaluated numerically. First, the pressure p_z was put constant ($C = 0$; $p_z = p_m$), and a detailed investigation was made of the influence of the parameters μ and p_n/p_m on the stress distribution. The results for a disk of normal geometry (the nucleus 50 percent of the disk) are shown in Figs. 19 and 20. Figure 19 shows the influence of the variable stiffness. The value $\mu = 0$ corresponds to constant stiffness [Eq. (4)]. Experiments show that values of μ as high as 0.7 could well be expected (Fig. 16). From Fig. 20 it is seen that the ratio p_n/p_m does not influence the tangential stress to any significant degree in this model. It is the value of the nucleus pressure p_n, rather than the applied pressure p, that determines the magnitude of the tangential stress. The ratio p_n/p can vary considerably, which is the reason for expressing the tangential stress in terms of p_n here. Thus Fig. 19, in which p_n/p_m is given the value 3 according to experiments, quite generally illustrates the influence of variable stiffness.

In the second case, the influence of a lateral pressure gradient C was investigated by substituting expression (7) for p_z. The influence of C on the tangential stress distribution in a normal disk is shown in Fig. 21. The value of μ here is 0.7. It is seen that even for the rather heavy pressure gradient of $C = -2$, corresponding approximately to zero pressure at the outer boundary of the annulus ($r = b$), the deviation from the stress values for $C = 0$, that is, $p_z = $ constant, is less than 10 percent.

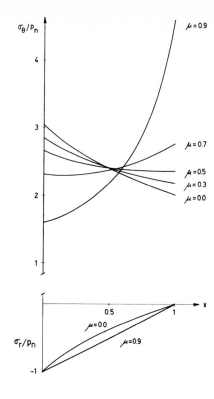

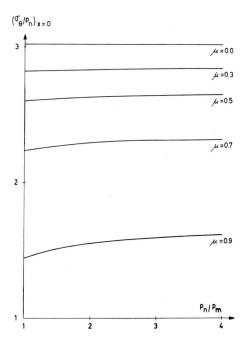

Figure 19 Distribution of stress through the annulus for various degrees of material inhomogeneity. *(From Sonnerup [21].)*

Figure 20 Influence of lateral pressure ratio p_n/p_m on tangential stress for various degrees of material inhomogeneity. *(From Sonnerup [21].)*

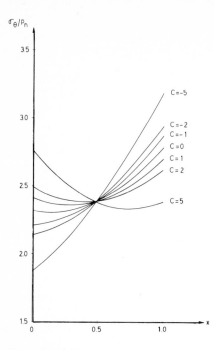

Figure 21 Distribution of tangential stress through the annulus for different lateral pressure gradients C; $\mu = 0.7$. *(From Sonnerup [21].)*

Lateral Pressure Distribution To obtain information about the lateral pressure distribution p_z, pressure measurements through the middle plane of the disk were performed. The details of these experiments are described by Sonnerup [21]. Figure 22 shows results for a normal lumbar disk under various external loads. The slope of the straight lines between the experimental points of Fig. 22 gives an estimation of the lateral pressure gradient. The steepest slope in Fig. 22 corresponds to the value $C = -2.5$ (slope of the line between points $x = 0.5$ and $x = 0.9$ for load value 200 N). However, the experimental procedure disturbed the normal functioning of the disk in such a way that the characteristic excess pressure in the nucleus could not develop, leading probably to lower lateral pressures in the inner parts of the annulus and hence to lower gradients through the annulus. It is thus quite possible that pressure gradients with a significant influence on the tangential stress distribution (cf. Fig. 21 with $-C > 2$) develop under real conditions.

Discussion The analytical solution presented here takes the boundary conditions at the vertebral end plates into account through the pressure distribution $p_z(r)$. If, in the simplified geometry of Fig. 18, the firm attachment of the annulus fibrosus to the plane end plates were neglected and perfectly frictionless contact assumed, then a state of plane strain ($\epsilon_z = $ constant) would arise. This would in turn lead to a radially increasing lateral pressure p_z, since the stiffness through the annulus is radially increasing [Eq. (4)], and for the case of constant stiffness the classical solution of this problem yields $p_z = $ constant for plane strain (see the solution for the problem of a thick-walled tube under internal pressure in any textbook on the theory of elasticity). Obviously, the real boundary conditions lead to a lateral

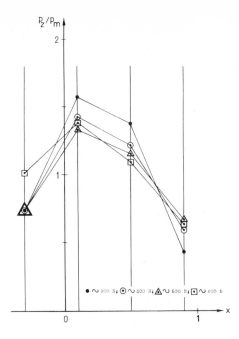

Figure 22 Pressure distribution through the annulus of a normal lumbar disk for various external loads. *(From Sonnerup [21].)*

bulging of the disk rather than a pure expansion, and the compressive strain in the axial (z) direction will decrease radially as is shown in Fig. 23, instead of being constant as in plane strain. Thus, the conditions with attachment at the end plates tend to produce a deviation from plane strain, yielding a lowering of the values of p_z toward the periphery of the disk. According to the experimental results of Fig. 22, the effect is strong enough to give a radially decreasing lateral pressure p_z.

In the central plane of the disk, where the stresses are determined, this is the main influence of the constraints at the end plates, since by symmetry the shear stresses vanish here. However, the radial shear stresses set up close to the end plates, according to Fig. 23, will produce a shear-stress gradient in the axial direction that is nonzero across the central plane of symmetry and hence influences the equilibrium equation (1). With this taken into account, the equilibrium equation becomes

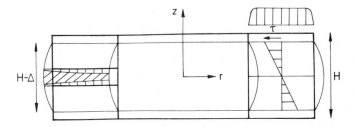

Figure 23 Influence of constraints at the vertebral end plates on strain and stress in the central plane of symmetry of the disk. Left side illustrates deviation from plane strain. Right side illustrates axial shear-stress gradient set up by radial shear stresses τ at the end plates.

$$\frac{\partial (r\sigma_r)}{\partial r} - \sigma_\theta + r\frac{\partial \tau_{zr}}{\partial z} = 0 \tag{8}$$

The shear-stress gradient $\partial \tau_{zr}/\partial z$ is difficult to determine experimentally and was thus neglected in the above simplified analysis. As is shown in App. A, it is, however, possible to estimate its qualitative influence by assuming it to be approximately constant across the central plane of symmetry. Figure 24 shows the result of such an analysis for the value $C = -3$ of the lateral pressure gradient. The parameter D is proportional to $(-\partial \tau_{zr}/\partial z)_{z=0}$ according to App. A. It is seen that the effect of D is to lower the values of the tangential stress throughout the annulus, as could be expected.

In a recent finite-element analysis of the intervertebral disk, Belytschko et al. [22] arrive at a more complete picture of the various stress distributions in the annulus fibrosus. They show that the excess pressure in the nucleus pulposus is a result of the anisotropy of the annulus (Fig. 15). Their stress distributions in the central plane of symmetry for a normal disk are similar to those obtained here, although their tangential stress values on the inner boundary of the annulus are considerably lower—a result probably of including more accurately the details of the disk geometry with a slightly barrel-shaped annulus (Fig. 17). Their lateral pressure distribution for a normal disk corresponds to the gradient value $C = -3$ approximately. In Fig. 24 their tangential stress distribution for this case is shown, and it is seen that for $D = 2$ the maximum values at the outer boundary are the same for the two analyses. The value $D = 2$ corresponds to a ratio between average shear stress at the vertebral end plates (Fig. 23) and average lateral pressure across the annulus of $\tau/p_m = 0.4$, which yields a reasonable order of magnitude for the average shear stress at the end plates.

Torsion As mentioned, Farfan et al. [7] studied the effects of torsion on the lumbar intervertebral joint in an extensive experimental investigation. They also

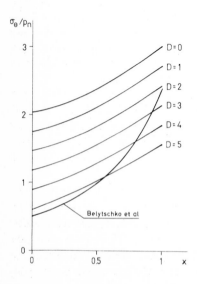

Figure 24 Influence of axial shear-stress gradients on the tangential stress distribution through the annulus; $\mu = 0.7, C = -3$.

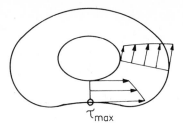

Figure 25 Distribution of shear stress in the annulus for torsional loads. Maximum stress appears in the most narrow part of the annulus.

performed experiments on the isolated disk, determined the failure torque, and calculated the shear stress at failure, assuming a linearly elastic response for the annulus fibrosus and a zero resistance for the nucleus pulposus. The strain of the annulus fibers at failure was estimated from the gross angle of rotation. In a recent article Kraus [23] reviews and analyses these results.

They used two methods to determine the shear-stress distribution in the annulus. In the first, the cross section of the disk, as well as the nucleus region, was assumed to be elliptical, and the stress distribution was obtained from the classic solution of the problem of torsion in a hollow, elastic shaft with this cross section. The maximum shear stress was thus calculated from the formula

$$\tau_{\max} = \frac{M_t}{W_t} \tag{9}$$

where M_t = torque
W_t = torsional section modulus for hollow elliptical cross section
The stress distribution across the narrowest part of the cross section is, in this case, linear according to the equation

$$\tau = \frac{r}{r_b} \tau_{\max}$$

where r_b is the minor outer radius of the elliptical cross section.

In the second method, the more detailed shape of the disk was taken into account using an electrical analog, the "conducting sheet" analog, to determine the stress distribution. The method is described generally by Dally and Riley [24] and summarized for torsion of the intervertebral disk by Kraus [23]. Briefly, the procedure is to cut an enlarged copy of the cross section of the disk out of electrically conducting *Teledeltos* paper and apply voltages to a gridwork of conducting lines on this model of the cross section, thus obtaining a voltage map, analogous to the real shear-stress distribution. The shear stress is, at each point of the cross section, proportional to the corresponding voltage of the map. The conversion factor involves the shear modulus of the annulus material.

Both methods are based on the theory of elastic torsion. This theory gives generally, for a hollow shaft, a stress pattern like that in Fig. 25. In the narrowest parts of the cross section the stresses will be highest, and they increase radially, always taking their maximum values on the outer boundary. Thus the narrow posterior part of the annulus will experience the highest torsional stresses, the maximum being in the most peripheral layers (Fig. 25). The strain distribution will, for purely geometric reasons, show a similar pattern, with maximum strain values on the outer boundary.

This pattern of stress and strain is valid for a long, hollow elastic shaft, and it seems at first that the picture must be different here due to the short vertical height of the disk as pointed out by Kraus [23]. Obviously, the restraints from the vertebral bodies tend to place the maximum strain (and hence stress) at the most remote point from the axis of rotation rather than in the narrowest portion of the cross section. However, the vertebral end plates are not plane so that the height of the disk varies from point to point usually with lowest values posteriorly (Figs. 1 and 2). As a result, it is still likely that the maximum strain and stress appear in the posterior region as shown in Fig. 25, and values determined by the methods described could be used for comparative purposes. This also conforms to the previously mentioned fact that posterior ruptures are the most common type of radiating tears through the annulus (cf. Farfan, Huberdeau and Dubow [8]).

6.2 Structural Analysis

In the structural approach to the problem of stress and strain analysis, the aim is to create a model with a closer resemblance to the actual disk structure. Such a model will then enable a more realistic study of the mechanical functioning of the disk. In particular, the rate dependency will be more easily incorporated. It is the macroscopic arrangement of interconnected fibrous layers in a matrix of ground substance and tissue fluid that should be modeled. By considering these layers as discrete structural elements, the anisotropy of the disk material is readily taken into account.

The model is analyzed for both compression and torsion, these loadings being compatible with the assumed circular symmetry. The basic formulation of the problem will be presented here. For details of the theoretical analysis, refer to App. B (cf. also Sonnerup [25]). The notation may be found in Figs. 26 to 28.

Model Properties The disk is simplified to a circular cylindrical structure of interconnected walls, representing the fiber layers of the annulus, according to Fig. 26. The space between the cylindrical walls is occupied by a fluid, representing the fluidlike matrix. The main properties of the model are:

Cylindrical symmetry. Circular cylindrical walls interconnected by evenly distributed radial links, symbolizing the loose, fibrous tissue between the layers of the annulus fibrosus and other links between these layers.

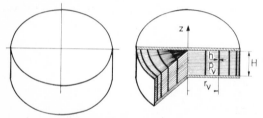

Figure 26 Structural model of the disk. Circular symmetry assumed.

Inhomogeneity. Increasing number of walls per unit length radially, symbolizing the actual radially increasing tangential stiffness of the annulus material; a variable stiffness of the radial links from one annular interspace to the other.

Anisotropy. Thin cylindrical walls with different stiffnesses axially and tangentially; radial links responding only to radial strain.

Fluid flow. Fluid-filled interspaces in the structure and permeable cylindrical walls, allowing fluid transport from one interspace to another due to pressure differences in the fluid across the walls.

Analysis for Compression *Constitutive Equations* The constitutive relations for the structural elements are as follows:

For the cylindrical walls, anisotropic, linearly elastic properties are assumed according to the matrix equation

$$E \begin{bmatrix} \epsilon_\theta \\ \epsilon_z \end{bmatrix} = \begin{bmatrix} c_{11} & -c \\ -c & c_{22} \end{bmatrix} \begin{bmatrix} S_\theta \\ S_z \end{bmatrix} \rightarrow E\epsilon = CS \tag{10}$$

wherein the constants E and c_{ij} are material parameters (Fig. 27). A cylindrical wall in this model is to be thought of as two adjacent layers of the annulus fibrosus, lumped together to render the axial and tangential directions the principal directions of anisotropy.

For the radial links, uniaxial, linearly elastic properties are assumed according to the equation

$$E \epsilon_r^\nu = k_\nu^{-1} S_r^\nu \tag{11}$$

wherein the constant k_ν is a material parameter for the links of the annular interspace ν (Fig. 27).

The cylindrical walls are assumed to be *permeable* according to the equation

$$v_\nu = \kappa_\nu(p_{\nu+1} - p_\nu) = \kappa_\nu \Delta p_\nu \tag{12}$$

wherein the constant κ_ν is a coefficient of permeability for the wall ν (Fig. 27).

Equations of Equilibrium and Compatibility Apart from the above constitutive equations, fundamental structural equations of equilibrium and compatibility must be established. This is done under the simplifying assumption of small deformations in the system and neglecting the fact that the radial expansion of the cylindrical walls is restrained by the attachment to the end plates (again simulating, in principle, the conditions across the central horizontal plane of symmetry of the disk).

Radial equations of equilibrium (Fig. 28):

$$S_\theta^\nu = (\Delta\sigma_r^\nu - \Delta p_\nu) r_\nu \qquad \nu = 1, 2, \ldots, n \tag{13}$$

where n is the number of layers, and

$$\Delta\sigma_r^\nu = \frac{S_r^{\nu+1} - S_r^\nu}{2\pi r_\nu} = \frac{\Delta S_r^\nu}{2\pi r_\nu} \qquad \Delta p_\nu = p_{\nu+1} - p_\nu$$

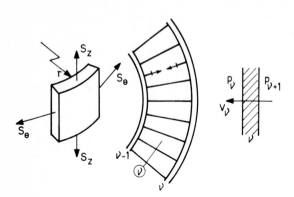

Figure 27 Stresses in the structural elements and fluid flow through the cylindrical walls at compression. The quantities S_θ and S_z are section forces per unit length in the cylindrical walls in the usual manner, whereas S_r is the total force per unit height of the disk between two walls, i.e., the sum of the forces in all the links between two adjacent walls. The fluid flow v expresses the volume of fluid per unit time through one unit of wall area. Fluid pressures are denoted p, and the index v refers to either a certain wall or a certain interspace according to the figure.

Axial equation of equilibrium (Fig. 28):

$$\bar{p} = \frac{1}{r_n^2} \sum_{v=1}^{n} [p_v(r_v + r_{v-1}) \Delta r_{v-1} \, \phi_v - 2S_z^v r_v] \tag{14}$$

where $\bar{p}$ is the average applied pressure on the model, and

$$\Delta r_v = r_{v+1} - r_v \qquad \phi_{v+1} = \frac{\Delta r_v - h}{\Delta r_v} \qquad r_0 = 0$$

In this equation, the wall thickness h is included to account for the fact that although the cylindrical walls are assumed thin and h is neglected in Eqs. (13), in summing across the structure, the fibrous skeleton occupies a nonnegligible part of the total cross-sectional area.

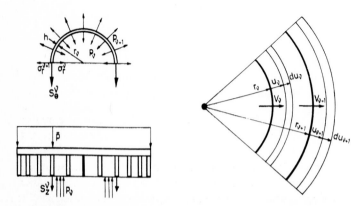

Figure 28 To illustrate the equilibrium and compatibility relations for the structural model at compression. The stress from the radial links is denoted σ_r, and u is the radial displacement. The quantity V denotes the volume of fluid passing through a wall in the radial direction, per unit height of the model and time.

Equations of compatibility (Fig. 28):

$$\epsilon_r^\nu = \frac{\Delta u_{\nu - 1}}{\Delta r_{\nu - 1}} \qquad \epsilon_\theta^\nu = \frac{u_\nu}{r_\nu} \qquad \nu = 1, 2, \ldots, n \tag{15}$$

where $\qquad \Delta u_\nu = u_{\nu + 1} - u_\nu \qquad u_0 = 0$

Boundary conditions (Fig. 26):

$$\epsilon_z = \text{constant (plane, rigid end plates)} \tag{16}$$
$$p_{n+1} = 0 \qquad k_{n+1} = 0$$

Solution Two special states in compression lend themselves to immediate discussion. If the model is given an instantaneous compression $\epsilon_z = -\delta$, an initial state of stress and strain, characterized by the fact that no flow through the walls has had time to take place, will develop. If overall volume constancy is assumed, and the walls can expand freely, it is evident that the tangential and radial strains will be equal and constant throughout the structure in this initial state: $\epsilon_\theta^\nu = \epsilon_r^\nu = \delta/2$. Depending on the elastic characteristics of the radial links in relation to those of the walls, various pressure distributions in the fluid of the disk will be created. Equations (10) to (16) yield, for the initial state, the pressure distribution

$$p_\nu = p_1 + \sum_{i=1}^{\nu - 1} \Delta p_i = p_1 + \frac{E\delta}{4\pi} \sum_{i=1}^{\nu - 1} \frac{1}{r_i} (\Delta k_i - 4\pi K_\theta)$$

$$= \frac{E\delta}{4\pi} \sum_{i=\nu}^{n} \frac{1}{r_i} (4\pi K_\theta - \Delta k_i) \tag{17}$$

where

$$\Delta k_\nu = k_{\nu+1} - k_\nu \qquad K_\theta = \frac{c_{22}/2 - c}{\det C}$$

and $p_{n+1} = 0$ gives

$$p_1 = \frac{E\delta}{4\pi} \sum_{i=1}^{n} \frac{1}{r_i} (4\pi K_\theta - \Delta k_i)$$

Two extreme cases of Eq. (17), for $\Delta k_\nu \gg 4\pi K_\theta$ and $k_\nu = \Delta k_\nu = 0$, are illustrated in Fig. 29. It is seen that the pressure can both increase and decrease toward the periphery.

From the initial state, a period of transient rearrangements within the structure takes the disk to a final stationary state of stress and strain. Here two possibilities arise: Either the disk could be assumed to be completely sealed at its boundaries, so that no fluid can escape out of it, or (in the case of a constant outer load) there is a steady flow of fluid through the outer boundary of the annulus, and perhaps also through the cartilage plates. It is the first of these situations that is easily surveyed.

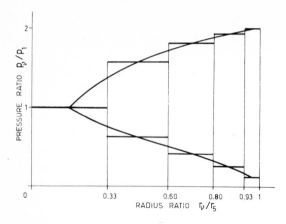

Figure 29 Extreme pressure distributions through the structural model in the initial state. Upper curve corresponds to strong radial linking, $\Delta k_\nu \gg 4\pi K_\theta$. Lower curve corresponds to no radial linking, $k_\nu = \Delta k_\nu = 0$.

The fluid pressure differences will then be evened out by flow so that $p_\nu = p$. At the same time the overall volume constancy will prevail so that $\epsilon_\theta^n = \delta/2$. These two conditions are sufficient to determine the stresses and strains in the fibrous structure as modeled here. Equations (10) to (15) yield for the final state the following set of difference equations:

$$\frac{u_\nu}{r_\nu} - \left(\frac{k_{\nu+1}}{\Delta r_\nu} \Delta u_\nu - \frac{k_\nu}{\Delta r_{\nu-1}} \Delta u_{\nu-1}\right) \frac{\det C}{2\pi c_{22}} = \frac{c}{c_{22}} \delta \qquad (18)$$

Equations (18) determine the radial displacements u_ν through the structure and hence, by Eqs. (15), (10), (11), and (16), the strains and stresses. The redistribution of tangential stress from the initial state with equal values in all the walls ($\epsilon_\theta^\nu = \delta/2$) to the final state is shown in Fig. 30 for the case of weak radial links. It is seen that the tangential stress has relaxed in the inner layers.

The transition from an initial to a final state apparently implies the phenomena of creep, relaxation, and rate dependency as observed for the real disk and is not

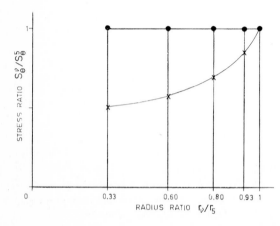

Figure 30 Tangential stress redistribution in the cylindrical walls from initial to final state for weak radial linking. Final values are marked ×.

dependent on the assumption of linear relations in Eqs. (10) to (12). On the contrary, it is possible to introduce nonlinearities reasonably simply in these equations, to mimic the real behavior more closely.

The situation in which the disk loses fluid can also be accounted for analytically. The transient state is governed by a set of differential equations, which are derived in App. B for the linear case.

Analysis for Torsion For the case of torsion, different assumptions about the properties of the cylindrical walls have to be made. In view of the arrangement of the obliquely running fiber bundles in the layers of the annulus, as previously described (Figs. 1 and 2), it could be expected that only every second layer bears a torsion load. Further, the inclined fibers of these layers will induce compression of the disk even when a pure torque is applied. A very simple estimation of the stationary state in torsion could be obtained by assuming the load-bearing layers to be stressed only in the fiber direction α according to Fig. 31. The radial links, and in transient states pressure differences, will maintain the curved shape of the fiber bundles of the layers (Fig. 31). An equilibrium consideration for this case yields the following formulas for fiber stress S_f and fluid pressure p in terms of the applied torque M_t:

$$S_f = \frac{M_t}{K_t} r_\nu \tag{19}$$

$$p = \frac{M_t}{V_t} \tag{20}$$

where

$$K_t = \pi(\sin 2\alpha) \sum_{\nu=1}^{n} r_\nu^3$$

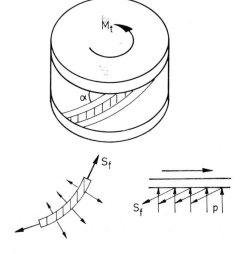

Figure 31 Fiber stress and fluid pressure in torsion of the structural model.

$$V_t = \pi(\cot \alpha) \left[\sum_{\nu=1}^{n} (r_\nu + r_{\nu-1}) \, \Delta r_{\nu-1} \, \phi_\nu \right] \frac{\sum\limits_{\nu=1}^{n} r_\nu^3}{\sum\limits_{\nu=1}^{n} r_\nu^2}$$

It is seen that for a given torque the fluid pressure p increases with the angle of inclination α of the fiber bundles. The fiber stress S_f assumes a minimum value for $\alpha = 45°$. The fluid pressure is created by compression of the disk, a secondary effect of the torsion (Fig. 31).

6.3 Comments

In his report on lumbar intradiskal pressure, Nachemson [16] also estimated the tangential stress in the annulus fibrosus by considering it as a statically determinate (thin) ring, loaded by the nucleus pressure on the inside. Depending on disk geometry, he found that this average tangential stress was in the range $2p_n < \sigma_\theta^{av} < 4p_n$. Taking into account his finding that there is a linear relationship between applied load per unit cross-sectional area of the disk and nucleus pressure $p_n = cp$, with a statistical mean value for c of 1.5 for normal disks, the range in terms of external load becomes $3p < \sigma_\theta^{av} < 6p$. In tests to failure in compression, he found the ultimate applied pressure to be about 3 N/mm^2, and hence a nucleus pressure of about 4.5 N/mm^2 at failure is to be expected. However, since failures occur through end plate fractures, and these fractures can arise gradually, the nucleus pressure at complete failure can be lower than this figure owing to leakage through the end plates. Finally, in a later investigation, he also showed that the nucleus pressure under certain maneuvers may well rise as high as 3 N/mm^2, corresponding to an external total load on a normal lumbar disk (cross-sectional area 1500 mm^2) of 3000 N (Nachemson and Elfström [26]). This gives an average tangential stress of 9 N/mm^2, a value close to those found by Galante [19] for the tensile strength in the fiber direction of the annulus layers, and well in excess of those found by Brown et al. [11] for the vertical direction and by Galante for the horizontal direction.

For reasons pointed out in the previous section (trellis action and low strength for specimens of the type shown in Fig. 14), only the values from specimens taken in the fiber direction are relevant for the intact annulus fibrosus. In these specimens, however, only about 50 percent of the fibers are load bearing, the fibers with a direction transverse to the long axis of the specimen being almost nonfunctioning. This means that the tensile strength calculated on the basis of "effective" load-bearing area of the specimens should be roughly twice Galante's values for the fiber direction, or on the order of 20 N/mm^2. The tangential stress σ_θ^{av} is then well below the actual tensile strength of the intact annulus tissue, even at failure of the disk, a result confirming the previously mentioned fact that gross rupture of the normal annulus is difficult to produce experimentally and does not generally occur as a result of occupational maneuvers.

The average tangential stress just discussed corresponds to the skeletal point of intersection between the curves in Figs. 19 and 21. From these curves, however, it is seen that considerably higher values can develop on the outer boundary, as a result of variable material stiffness and lateral pressure through the annulus fibrosus. According to the curve $\mu = 0.9$ of Fig. 19, $\sigma_\theta^{max} > 4.5p_n$ when $\sigma_\theta^{av} = 2.4p_n$. With the end conditions taken into account, these values are lowered as is shown in Fig. 24, but still the tangential stress on the outer boundary is at least 30 percent higher than the average value and as much as 100 percent higher according to Belytschko et al. [22] (Fig. 24). However, for the realistic case $D = 2$ in Fig. 24, the peak value is $\sigma_\theta^{max} = 2.4p_n$, which is still well below the tensile strength of the annulus at failure of the disk ($p_n \leqslant 4.5$ N/mm^2).

The above considerations apply mainly to the stationary situation in the loaded disk and are, as pointed out, concerned with the average tangential stresses and continuous stress distributions necessary to support the pressure of the nucleus, i.e., stresses calculated under the assumption that the material of the annulus fibrosus is a continuous medium. In the structural model of the disk, however, the distinction is not primarily made between the nucleus and the continuous annulus, but rather between the fibrous skeleton and the fluidlike matrix. This leads to discontinuous stress distributions through the disk, with pressure in the fluid and tension in the fibrous structure. With an instantaneous loading in compression, equal and constant radial and tangential strains will develop throughout the disk as a result of the overall incompressibility. To this strain situation corresponds a pattern of pressures in the fluid-filled interspaces [Eq. (17) and Fig. 29] and tensile stresses in the fibrous network, determined by the stiffnesses of the latter structure. In the model, all the cylindrical walls are given the same properties, which means that the instantaneously developed tangential stress will be equal in them, as mentioned (Fig. 30). Via the flow of fluid within the disk, this initial pattern of variable pressures and equal tangential stresses will be transformed into a final one, with equal pressures and variable tangential stresses, provided no fluid flows out of the disk (Fig. 30). This redistribution is, of course, accompanied by a corresponding change in radial stresses in the links between the walls. The question as to whether redistribution due to flow *within* the disk or gross flow of fluid *out through* the annulus and the cartilage plates is the prime mechanism of the transient behavior of the disk remains to be solved experimentally.

For compressive loads approaching the ultimate value at gross failure, leakage through the end plates has to be considered, as pointed out above. In such a case, the load in a stationary state must eventually be carried by the more firm components of the interfibrous matrix of, in particular, the annulus fibrosus. That this is the situation in stationary compressive loading is in fact suggested by Kraus [23]. Also, in degenerated disks with less fluid content, there is evidently a tendency for the annulus to carry a larger portion of the compressive load.

In torsion, the fiber stress assumes a minimum value for the fiber direction $\alpha = 45°$ [Eq. (19)]. In compression it is apparent from the previous analyses that the fiber direction $\alpha = 0$ would be most favorable, since the tangential stress is the dominating stress in the fibrous structure (Figs. 19 and 28). The actual main fiber direction in the annulus fibrosus, $\alpha \approx 25°$, is thus a reasonable optimum for combined torsion and compression.

In the context of the structural model, the excess pressure in the nucleus ($p_n = 1.5\bar{p}$), measured by Nachemson (cf. Nachemson [16]), is explained by the fact that the fibrous structure occupies part of the cross-sectional area. If, for example, only 70 percent of the cross section is subject to fluid pressure p_f (corresponding roughly to the water content of the disk), then approximately $0.7p_f = \bar{p}$ and $p_f = 1.4\bar{p}$. Since some axial tensile stress also may be present in the fibrous structure, the figure $p_f/\bar{p} = 1.5$ could easily be reached.

Finally, it seems feasible to take into account shapes other than circular in a structural model similar to the one discussed here, for example, by considering an orthogonal system of cylindrical (but not circular) walls and radial links. This would incorporate the particular geometry of the disk more accurately.

7 POSSIBLE FAILURE MECHANISMS OF THE ANNULUS FIBROSUS

The intention is here to discuss the previously described injuries to the fibrous structure of the disk, i.e., concentric fissures and radiating tears, in terms of the analyses presented. As mentioned, complete failure of the annulus seldom occurs by compression. This is understandable in light of the structural analysis, since obviously the strains are rather evenly distributed in compression, and all of the fibrous structure is significantly load bearing. As regards the cartilage end plates, on the other hand, the fluid pressure will act mainly on their central area, since peripherally the fibers are densely attached to these plates, leaving less free surface area for the fluid pressure to act on. This creates a load peak in the center of the plates, which often breaks them at a far lower load than would be necessary to rupture the layers of the annulus fibrosus. Again referring to the strain situation in the disk, it is, however, plausible that compression can produce damage to the radial connections (radial links in the structural model) between the layers of the annulus. The positive radial strain, developing in all situations of compression according to the structural model, means, in effect, that these layers are separated and a tensile stress probably created radially. This might produce minute fractures of radial links and initiate the concentric fissures observed in degenerated disks.

In torsion experiments, as mentioned, Farfan et al. [7] were able to produce visible damage of this kind to the annulus. Even then, however, no complete communication between the nucleus and the outside, i.e., radiating tear, developed when the disks were loaded to failure. As already pointed out, the strain situation in torsion is quite different. The strains increase radially from the axis of rotation, with maximum values on the peripheral boundary of the disk. Further, as a result of the geometric arrangement of the fibrous structure (cf. Fig. 1 and the description of the structure of the disk), only about every second layer of the annulus fibrosus will take active part in carrying the load. On combining these two observations, it is not surprising to note that local damage to the peripheral layers of the annulus is seen as a result of torsional loads (Farfan et al. [7]). If a certain peripheral layer partly fractures, it is likely that the radial linking between adjacent layers in the fracture region is also partly destroyed. The compression induced by the obliquely running fiber bundles of the load-bearing layers (Fig. 31) will then tend to separate the layers in the fracture region permanently, thus producing the observed circumferential splits in the annulus. Farfan et al. conclude that these injuries are the forerunners of the clinically frequent radiating ruptures of the annulus fibrosus.

8 DISCUSSION

It has been shown how the structural characteristics of the intact intervertebral disk could be taken into account, at different levels of approximation, in the theoretical mechanical analysis and in the interpretation of experimental results and clinical observations. The structural analysis offers qualitative explanations for the mechanical response and for some of the features of failure of the disk. To arrive at a more quantitative description, however, more experimental data are necessary. In particular, continuous recordings of the fluid pressure in the disk under transient conditions, such as creep and relaxation, and measurements of fluid flow through the disk boundaries are of importance in assigning relevant properties to the elements of structural models of the disk.

Also, the mechanical properties of the disk material need to be studied more closely, although this presents a more difficult experimental problem. Some of the rate dependency of the disk, for instance, probably originates in viscous properties of the ground substance. In the structural analysis presented here, all such effects are pictured through the permeability of the layers of the annulus fibrosus.

GLOSSARY

Anisotropy: variation of mechanical properties of a material with direction in the material.

Annulus fibrosus: peripheral fibrous part of intervertebral disk.

Collagen fibers: load-bearing fibers of the connective tissues.

Creep: increasing strain (deformation) in structure under fixed external loads.

Ground substance: amorphous material (gel) forming matrix for the fibrous structure of connective tissues.

Inhomogeneity: variation of mechanical properties of a material with position in the material.

Intervertebral joint: joint between two adjacent vertebrae.

Intervertebral disk: flexible, fibrous connection between two adjacent vertebral bodies.

Intradiskal pressure: pressure in fluidlike components of the intervertebral disk.

Lumbar spine: lowest portion of the spine comprising five vertebrae above the pelvis.

Nucleus pulposus: central part of intervertebral disk.

Permeability: property of a porous material that allows fluid flow through it.

Stress: load per unit cross-sectional area (force/length^2)

Stress (load) relaxation: diminishing stress (load) in structure kept at a fixed external state of deformation.

Strain: Elongation per unit length (%).

Stiffness: slope of stress (load)-strain (deformation) curve for a material (structure).

APPENDIX A SOLUTION OF EQS. (1) TO (5)

A straightforward elimination among Eqs. (1) to (3), together with the boundary condition $\sigma_z = -p_z$, yields the differential equation

$$\frac{3\, d\sigma_r/dr}{2\psi} + \frac{d}{dr}\left[\frac{d(r\sigma_r)/dr - \frac{1}{2}(\sigma_r - p_z)}{\psi}\right] = 0 \tag{A1}$$

To obtain this equation in a suitable form for numerical evaluation, new dimensionless variables, functions, and parameters are introduced according to the expressions

$$x = \frac{r-a}{b-a} \qquad y = \frac{\sigma_r}{p_m} + 1$$

$$g(x) = \frac{d(1/\psi)/dx}{1/\psi}$$

$$h(x) = \frac{p_z}{p_m}$$

$$p_m = \frac{2\displaystyle\int_a^b p_z\, r\, dr}{b^2 - a^2} \tag{A2}$$

$$k = \frac{a}{b-a}$$

Rewritten, Eq. (A1) then becomes

$$x^2 y'' + \left[\frac{3}{x+k} + g(x)\right] xxy' + \frac{x^2}{2(x+k)} g(x)y$$

$$= \{[1 - h(x)]g(x) - h'(x)\}\, \frac{x^2}{2(x+k)}$$

Introduce, for convenience, the notation

$$P(x) = \left[\frac{3}{x+k} + g(x)\right] x$$

$$Q(x) = \frac{x^2}{2(x+k)} g(x)$$

$$F(x) = {}_1[1 - h(x)]g(x) - h'(x)\} \frac{x^2}{2(x+k)}$$

Equation (A1) then assumes the form

$$x^2 y'' + xP(x)y' + Q(x)y = F(x) \tag{A3}$$

The solution of this linear second-order differential equation consists of the sum of two parts:

$$y(x) = y_c(x) + y_p(x)$$

where y_c is the general solution of the homogeneous equation

$$x^2 y'' + xP(x)y' + Q(x)y = 0$$

and y_p is a particular solution of the complete equation (A3).

According to the method of Frobenius, the complementary solution y_c could be obtained in the form of a linear combination of two power series of the type

$$y = x^s \sum_{\nu=0}^{\infty} a_\nu x^\nu \tag{A4}$$

provided the coefficients $P(x)$ and $Q(x)$ are expressible in Taylor-series form about $x = 0$. Obviously, this is the case when $g(x)$ could be expanded in a Taylor series about $x = 0$. For all such functions $g(x)$, the full complementary solution is

$$y_c = Ay_1 + By_2$$

where A and B are independent arbitrary constants to be determined from the boundary conditions of the problem, and y_1 and y_2 are solutions of the form (A4).

The particular solution y_p could, in the general case, be obtained by the method of variation of parameters. For special simple forms of $F(x)$ (rational expressions), however, pure inspection of Eq. (A3) leads to a particular solution in polynomial form.

Given the stiffness ψ according to Eq. (4) and the lateral pressure p_z according to Eq. (7), a simple situation of the kind discussed arises. The complete solution of Eq. (A3) then becomes

$$y_c = A \sum_{\nu=0}^{\infty} \alpha_\nu x^\nu + B \sum_{\nu=0}^{\infty} \beta_\nu x^\nu$$

$$y_p = C\left[x_m + k - \frac{2b}{6\mu(b-a)} - \frac{2(x+k)}{9}\right] \tag{A5}$$

where the coefficients α_ν and β_ν are given by recurrence relations

$$\alpha_\nu = M_\nu \alpha_{\nu-2} - N_\nu \alpha_{\nu-1} \qquad \beta_\nu = M_\nu \beta_{\nu-2} - N_\nu \beta_{\nu-1}$$

where

$$\alpha_0 = 1 \qquad \alpha_1 = 0 \qquad \beta_0 = 0 \qquad \beta_1 = 1$$

and

$$M_\nu = \frac{\mu(b-a)^2}{2a(b-\mu a)} \frac{2(\nu-2)(\nu+1)+1}{\nu(\nu-1)}$$

$$N_\nu = \frac{(b-a)(b-2\mu a + b/\nu)}{a(b-\mu a)} \qquad \text{for } \nu \geqslant 2$$

Solution with Eq. (1) replaced by Eq. (8)

In this case the shear-stress gradient $(\partial \tau_{zr}/\partial z)_{z=0}$ is assumed to be a known function of r. Then Eq. (8), together with Eqs. (2) to (5), yield a differential equation similar to Eq. (A1), which, after transformation by expressions (A2), takes exactly the form (A3) with the same expressions for the coefficients $P(x)$ and $Q(x)$ but with a different function $F(x)$, determined not only by $g(x)$ and $h(x)$ but also by the function $(\partial \tau_{zr}/\partial z)_{z=0}$. The new $F(x)$ takes the form

$$F(x) = \{[1 - h(x)]g(x) - h'(x)\} \frac{x^2}{2(x+k)}$$

$$- x^2 \left\{ \left[\frac{5}{2(x+k)} + g(x) \right] f(x) + f'(x) \right\}$$

where

$$f(x) = \frac{b-a}{p_m} \left(\frac{\partial \tau_{zr}}{\partial z} \right)_{z=0}$$

Thus the complementary solution y_c is unaltered, and the particular solution y_p becomes modified by $f(x)$. By ignoring the boundary conditions $f(0) = f(1) = 0$ (Fig. 23) and assuming as a simple estimation $(\partial \tau_{zr}/\partial z)_{z=0} = -K$, the particular solution is found [$h(x)$ according to Eq. (7)] as

$$y_p = (C-D) \left[x_m + k - \frac{2b}{6\mu(b-a)} - \frac{2(x+k)}{9} \right] + D \left[x_m + k - \frac{6b}{14\mu(b-a)} \right]$$

$$\tag{A6}$$

where

$$D = \frac{7K(b-a)}{2p_m}$$

APPENDIX B

Solution of Eqs. (10) to (16)

Assume that the model is given a time-dependent compression $\epsilon_z = -\delta(t)$. At time $t = 0$, the compressive strain $\epsilon_z = -\delta(0)$ is imposed instantaneously, thus constituting the initial condition for the transient state.

The compatibility equations (15) are concerned with the fibrous structure of the model. To treat the transient state, however, additional relations for the rate of volume change of each annular interspace are required. Consider, therefore, the geometry at times t and $t + dt$ according to Fig. 28. The deformation quantities at times t and $t + dt$ are

$$u_\nu \qquad u_{\nu+1} \qquad \delta$$

and

$$u_\nu + du_\nu \qquad u_{\nu+1} + du_{\nu+1} \qquad \delta + d\delta$$

The increase in volume of the space between walls ν and $\nu + 1$ (space $\nu + 1$) from time t to time $t + dt$, expressed in these quantities, is

$$dV = \pi[2(r_{\nu+1} \, du_{\nu+1} - r_\nu \, du_\nu) - (r_{\nu+1}^2 - r_\nu^2) \, d\delta] \tag{B1}$$

The volume of fluid passing through wall ν per unit height and time in the radial direction (Fig. 28) is obtained from Eq. (12) as

$$V_\nu = -\kappa_\nu \, \Delta p_\nu \, 2\pi r_\nu$$

and hence, if no flow occurs through the end plates, the increase in fluid volume of space $\nu + 1$ during the time interval dt becomes

$$dV = (V_\nu - V_{\nu+1}) \, dt = 2\pi(\kappa_{\nu+1} \, \Delta p_{\nu+1} \, r_{\nu+1} - \kappa_\nu \Delta p_\nu r_\nu) \, dt \tag{B2}$$

Combining Eqs. (B1) and (B2) yields

$$\kappa_{\nu+1} \Delta p_{\nu+1} r_{\nu+1} - \kappa_\nu \Delta p_\nu r_\nu = r_{\nu+1} \dot{u}_{\nu+1} - r_\nu \dot{u}_\nu - \frac{(r_{\nu+1}^2 - r_\nu^2) \dot{\delta}}{2} \tag{B3}$$

where the dot denotes a time derivative. Using the formula

$$\sum_{i=0}^{\nu-1} (a_{i+1} - a_i) = a_\nu - a_0$$

on the right- and left-hand members of Eq. (B3) and observing that the equation is valid for $\nu = 0$ with $r_0 = 0$ give [replace ν with i in Eq. (B3) and sum]

$$\kappa_\nu \Delta p_\nu = \dot{u}_\nu - \frac{r_\nu \dot{\delta}}{2} \qquad \nu = 1, 2, \dots, n \tag{B4}$$

This relation could also be obtained directly by considering, in the manner above, the total volume inside the wall ν.

Now express Δp_ν in terms of u_ν through the use of Eqs. (13), (10), (11), and (15):

$$\Delta p_\nu r_\nu = E\left(\frac{k_{\nu+1}\,\Delta u_\nu/\Delta r_\nu - k_\nu\,\Delta u_{\nu-1}/\Delta r_{\nu-1}}{2\pi} - \frac{c_{22}u_\nu/r_\nu - c\delta}{\det C}\right) \quad (B5)$$

Insert Eq. (B4) in Eq. (B5):

$$r_\nu^2\left(\frac{\dot u_\nu}{r_\nu} - \frac{\dot\delta}{2}\right) = \kappa_\nu E\left(\frac{k_{\nu+1}\,\Delta u_\nu/\Delta r_\nu - k_\nu\,\Delta u_{\nu-1}/\Delta r_{\nu-1}}{2\pi} - \frac{c_{22}u_\nu/r_\nu - c\delta}{\det C}\right) \quad (B6)$$

Equations (B6) form a set of n linear first-order differential equations governing the motion of the n cylindrical walls of the model. For the case of a sealed disk boundary, the coefficient κ_n is zero, and Eq. (B6) with $\nu = n$ expresses the overall volume constancy.

The initial-state pressure distribution (17) is obtained from Eq. (B5) with $u_\nu/r_\nu = \Delta u_\nu/\Delta r_\nu = \delta(0)/2$ for the volume constancy of each interspace, a relation implicit from Eq. (B1) with $dV = 0$ for all values of ν.

The final-state equations (18) for the case of a sealed boundary ($\kappa_n = 0$) are obtained from Eqs. (B6) with $\dot u_\nu = \dot\delta = 0$ for stationary conditions in the structure.

The solution of the system (B6) is performed in steps, by starting with the equation for $\nu = 1$ and observing the boundary conditions (16) together with the initial-state displacements $u_\nu(0)/r_\nu = \delta(0)/2$.

REFERENCES

1. D. Orne and Y. K. Liu, A Mathematical Model of Spinal Response to Impact, *J. Biomech.*, vol. 4, no. 1, pp. 49–71, 1971.
2. O. A. Beadle, The Intervertebral Discs, *Special Report Series*, no. 161, H. M. Stationary Office, London, 1931.
3. A. B. Schultz and J. O. Galante, A Mathematical Model for the Study of the Mechanics of the Human Vertebral Column, *J. Biomech.*, vol. 3, no. 4, pp. 404–416, 1970.
4. M. Panjabi and A. A. White III, A Mathematical Approach for Three-Dimensional Analysis of the Mechanics of the Spine, *J. Biomech.*, vol. 4, no. 3, pp. 203–212, 1971.
5. A. A. White III, Kinematics of the Normal Spine as Related to Scoliosis, *J. Biomech.*, vol. 4, no. 5, pp. 405–412, 1971.
6. A. B. Schultz, H. Larocca, J. O. Galante, and T. P. Andriacchi, A Study of Geometrical Relationships in Scoliotic Spines, *J. Biomech.*, vol. 5, no. 4, pp. 409–420, 1972.
7. H. F. Farfan, J. W. Cossette, G. H. Robertson, R. V. Wells, and H. Kraus, The Effects of Torsion on the Lumbar Intervertebral Joints: The Role of Torsion in the Production of Disc Degeneration, *J. Bone Jt. Surg.*, vol. 52A, no. 3, pp. 468–497, 1970.
8. H. F. Farfan, R. M. Huberdeau, and H. I. Dubow, Lumbar Intervertebral Disc Degeneration, *J. Bone Jt. Surg.*, vol. 54A, no. 3, pp. 492–510, 1972.
9. A. Viidik, Functional Properties of Collagenous Tissues, *Int. Rev. Connect. Tissue Res.*, vol. 6, 1973.
10. W. J. Virgin, Experimental Investigations into the Physical Properties of the Intervertebral Disc, *J. Bone Jt. Surg.*, vol. 33B, no. 4, pp. 607–611, 1951.
11. T. Brown, R. J. Hansen, and A. J. Yorra, Some Mechanical Tests on the Lumbosacral Spine with Particular Reference to the Intervertebral Discs, *J. Bone Jt. Surg.*, vol. 39A, no. 5, pp. 1135–1164, 1957.
12. K. L. Markolf and R. F. Steidel, The Dynamic Characteristics of the Human Intervertebral Joint, *ASME Winter Ann. Meeting, Biomech. and Hum. Factors Div.*, New York, 1970.

13. E. R. Fitzgerald and A. E. Freeland, Viscoelastic Response of Intervertebral Disks at Audio-frequencies, *Med. Bio. Eng.*, vol. 9, pp. 459–478, 1970.
14. K. L. Markolf, Deformation of the Thoracolumbar Intervertebral Joints in Response to External Loads, *J. Bone Jt. Surg.*, vol. 54A, no. 3, pp. 511–533, 1972.
15. B. Moont, Biomechanics Unit, Dept. Mech. Eng., Imperial College, London, personal communication, 1973.
16. A. Nachemson, Lumbar Intradiscal Pressure, *Acta Orthop. Scand.*, Suppl. 43, 1960.
17. M. Frisén, M. Mägi, L. Sonnerup, and A. Viidik, Rheological Analysis of Soft Collagenous Tissue, *J. Biomech.*, vol. 2, no. 1, pp. 13–28, 1969.
18. L. Sonnerup, Comments on Load-Deformation Characteristics of Soft Connective Tissue Structures, internal report, Div. Solid Mech., Dept. Mech. Eng., Chalmers Institute of Technology, Göteborg, Sweden, 1973.
19. J. O. Galante, Tensile Properties of the Human Lumbar Annulus Fibrosus, *Acta Orthop. Scand.*, Suppl. 100, 1967.
20. L. Sonnerup, Mechanical Analysis of the Human Intervertebral Disc, *Dig. 8th ICMBE*, session 18-2, Chicago, 1969.
21. L. Sonnerup, A Semi-experimental Stress Analysis of the Human Intervertebral Disk in Compression, *Exp. Mech.*, vol. 12, no. 3, pp. 142–147, 1972.
22. T. Belytschko, R. F. Kulak, A. B. Schultz, and J. O. Galante, Finite Element Stress Analysis of an Intervertebral Disc, *J. Biomech.*, vol. 7, no. 3, pp. 277–285, 1974.
23. H. Kraus, Stress Analysis, in H. F. Farfan, "Mechanical Disorders of the Low Back," Lea and Febiger, Philadelphia, 1973.
24. J. W. Dally and W. F. Riley, "Experimental Stress Analysis," McGraw-Hill, New York, 1965.
25. L. Sonnerup, A Structural Analysis of Stress, Strain and Fluid Flow in the Human Intervertebral Disk, internal report, Div. Solid Mech., Dept. Mech. Eng., Chalmers Institute of Technology, Göteborg, Sweden, 1973.
26. A. Nachemson and G. Elfström, Intravital Dynamic Pressure Measurements in Lumbar Discs, *Scand. J. Rehabil. Med.*, suppl. 1, 1970.

THE BIOMECHANICS OF THORACIC AND LUMBAR SPINE FRACTURES: THEIR FIXATION AND STABILIZATION

Gordon C. Robin and Zvi Yosipovitch

The incidence of vertebral fractures and related spinal cord injuries varies with time and place, as does the frequency of involvement of specific vertebrae in the spine. These variations may result from anatomic, pathologic, geographic, historic, or culturo-economic factors. There have been attempts to classify types of spinal fractures and to relate the stability or lack of it to a specific injury. The authors have devised a new classification that relates the mechanics of the fracture to the pathological effect and takes into account the stability of the spine. Most vertebral fractures require little specific treatment; but displaced unstable injuries with actual or potential neurologic involvement usually demand reduction and stabilization. To reduce a displaced fracture requires much smaller forces than those involved in its genesis. This difference results from energy dispersal within the body at the moment of application of the fracturing force, removal of anatomical restraints as a result of the injury and the fracture, and use of anaesthesia and muscle relaxation at the time of surgery. Traction forces of approximately one-half body-weight combined with hyperextension are usually enough to reduce the common fracture dislocation at the thoracolumbar junction; forces larger than this might endanger the spinal cord. Internal fixation techniques have been introduced in the treatment of unstable displaced vertebral injuries in order to reduce and stabilize the spine. These techniques vary from simple wire fixation of vertebral processes, through the use of plates and bolts, to the use of Harrington instrumentation and its modifications. The biomechanical factors involved vary with type and site of injury and with the design of the fixation appliance and its site of purchase on the fractured vertebral column. Modified Harrington instrumentation appears to be the best system thus far available; it affords reduction of the fracture, decompression of the spinal canal, and stabilization until union is achieved. Although much knowledge of tissue and organ biomechanics has been gained in the past few years, this information is of limited clinical value because so many greater variables, such as muscle action, the effect of static or dynamic posture, or the presence of normal or pathological structure in the bone, still cannot be measured in the clinical situation. Therefore, detailed clinical evaluation together with adequate roentgenographic examination must still provide the best basis for choosing among treatment options.

1 INTRODUCTION

As the new epidemic disease "trauma" claims its increasing toll of death and disablement in all parts of the world, the number of fractures demanding treatment by orthopedic surgeons gets larger every day. Among them, the rising number of fractures of the vertebral column constitutes one facet of the surgeon's work that calls for deeper knowledge and understanding, in order to treat the patients involved more effectively. Such knowledge and understanding may also be applied to the prevention of spinal fractures, to help bring to this new epidemic the techniques that have so successfully fought the decimating infectious epidemic diseases of the past.

Vertebral fractures constitute up to 6 percent of all bony injuries [1,2], while fractures of the thoracic and lumbar regions of the spine account for three-fifths of all vertebral fractures [1, 3]. It is accepted that most injuries affect one vertebra only, although in at least one-sixth of the patients, and maybe more, two or more are damaged [2, 4, 5] with varying degrees of severity. These damaged vertebrae may be contiguous or at separate levels, possibly indicating the end results of different types and sites of stress concentration [1, 2, 4, 5].

The great majority of spinal injuries in the thoracic and lumbar regions have a relatively benign course, with no neurological complications and with good long-term results [6]. Nevertheless, the incidence of spinal-cord injury in patients with vertebral fractures is not inconsiderable and varies from 5 to 14 percent in different series [1, 2]. The number of new patients with traumatic spinal-cord injuries in the United States has been estimated at 6000 to 11,000 per annum [7 to 9]; comparison among different regions of the world shows a wide geographical variation, with figures such as 13 per million in Switzerland and 53 per million in California [8, 9].

In fractures of the thoracic and lumbar regions of the spine in one series of cases [10], 17 percent of the patients were found to have spinal neurological involvement. The majority of the patients with such neurological complications suffered from fractures in the thoracic spine down to the tenth thoracic vertebra. Injuries at the thoracolumbar junction accounted for 4 percent of the neurological complications, while only 3 percent were found in patients with pure lumbar injuries [10]. The reason for all these differences is complex and may be related to anatomical, pathological, geographical, cultural, and even economic factors, as will be discussed later.

The most common cause of spinal injuries is road traffic accidents, which account for over 50 percent of all the cases [1, 8]. Other causative factors include falling from heights, falling objects, sports injuries, gunshot wounds and other violent encounters. Spinal-cord injuries occur more often in men than in women and are most frequent in the third decade of life. Factors such as the relative number of vehicles on the roads, the presence of a local mining industry, the average age of a given population, and the local political and international situation can alter the incidence of spinal fractures and their severity, and therefore the frequency of spinal-cord injury resulting from the vertebral lesions [7].

Spinal injuries, though usually benign as far as the health and longevity of the patient are concerned, are, however, a frequent cause of prolonged loss of work, especially in societies where compensation for injury is the way of life; such an injury may cause a heavy economic burden as well as physical and mental suffering for the patient, the patient's family, and the society in which the patient lives. Further study of the mechanisms involved in spinal injuries, their prevention, and their treatment is obviously needed, to improve understanding of the condition, enhance the techniques of treatment, and increase the chances of reconstituting the structure and function of the spine, thus enabling the more rapid and complete return of the patient to a productive role in society, the aim of rehabilitation teams the world over.

2 SITE OF FRACTURE IN THE THORACIC AND LUMBAR SPINE

An extensive review of the literature has shown to the authors that considerable differences of opinion exist among workers with regard to the frequency of vertebral fractures in different parts of the spine. Table 1 shows that some authors have clearly found that the thoracolumbar junction is the most vulnerable part of the spine, while others [1, 11] have found in their particular series that there are two levels of peak frequency, one at the T5-6 level and the other at the thoracolumbar junction. It has been suggested that these regions of maximal incidence of vertebral fractures may correspond to two areas of stress concentration, related to two different mechanical parameters. The anatomical configuration of the vertebral column changes greatly between the cervical and thoracic regions of the spine, and again at the thoracolumbar junction. In the sacrum, individual cylindrical vertebral bodies are replaced by a flat curved plate of bone, perforated in various directions by canals and foramina. The size, position, and shape of the facet joint articulations are but several of the anatomical factors that determine the mechanical stiffness of the spine at the various levels.

The presence of the physiological kyphotic or lordotic curvature and the state of the intervertebral disks also change the resistance of the vertebral column to applied forces. Anatomical variations among vertebrae account in great part for the changes in mechanical reaction found at different levels of the spine. Among others, the presence of the rib cage, connecting the thoracic vertebral body through the curved struts of the ribs to the sternum in front, greatly increases the stiffness of the spine in the thoracic region [12]. This increased stiffness is of course slightly

Table 1   Frequency of injury at various spinal sites

Authors	Number of patients	Site of injury	Percent injuries at site
Nicoll, 1949 [17]	152	T1–T10	4
		T11–T12–L1	58 (L1:30%)
		L2–L5	38
Westerborn and Olson, 1952 [63]	104	T12–L2	64 (L1:35%)
D'Aubigné and Bénassy, 1960 [11]	69	T3–T11	T4–T5 majority
Savastano and Pierik, 1960 [64]	159	T11–L1	73
Griffith et al., 1966 [1]	155	T5–T6	50
		T11–L1	
Wong, 1966 [65]	255	T12–L2	66 (L1 majority)
Andersen and Hørlyck, 1969 [66]	104	T1–T7	14
		T8–T12	43
		L1–L5	43
Frankel et al., 1969 [3]	394	T1–T10	42
		T11–L1	52
		L2–L5	6
Young, 1973 [6]	116	T12–L2	60 (L1 majority)
Meyers, 1978 [7]	109	T1–T9	42.3
		T10–L1	46.8 (T12 majority)
		L2–L5	10.9

altered in the T9–10 region where the anterior connection between rib and sternum is not direct, and even more so at the T11–12 level where the ribs are free in front and can add little to spinal stiffness.

The presence of multisystem injury in patients with spinal fractures is not uncommon. In particular, intrathoracic hemorrhage is frequently associated with thoracic spine fracture, especially where there is neurological involvement. Such additional pathology not only emphasizes the magnitude of the forces involved in the genesis of the fracture, but also (possibly) illustrates the importance of the rib cage in thoracic spinal stability. When the chest wall is violated, force can more easily affect the spine, greater displacement may occur, and the danger of spinal-cord involvement may increase. In our own clinical experience, and in that of others [13, 14], intrathoracic traumatic pathology is common in severe thoracic spine injuries (40 percent or more) and almost nonexistent in minor stable fractures.

The apex of the normal thoracic kyphosis at the T5–6 level may be another of the factors involved in determining the site of fracture after injury, while the abrupt alteration in stiffness at the thoracolumbar junction may be another reason for stress concentration and the increased frequency of fracture at this level [1].

Other authors again have found only one level of peak frequency of spinal fractures, either at the midthoracic level [1] or at the thoracolumbar junction (Table 1). This diversity with regard to the sites of peak frequency, and in relation to the incidence of neurological complications of spinal injuries, is also connected to historical, geographic, and culturoeconomic factors. Series of cases collected in the 1950s and 1960s in various parts of the world differ widely as to the contributory effect of road accidents, which are, as we have noted above, a major causative factor in spinal injuries. The effects of a road accident involving small European cars 20 years ago are obviously different biomechanically from those involving the bigger, heavier, and often faster vehicles that fill the roads of the United States today. The design of the automobile seat, the use of safety belts of various kinds, and the presence or absence of a headrest may all directly affect the end results of an accident. Yet such factors vary considerably by time and place. The height of a coal seam in Pennsylvania may be several times greater than that of some of the seams worked in Southern Scotland in the 1940s. The mechanics of the fracturing force in road and mining accidents may thus be entirely different, and therefore the end result in the patient may be totally dissimilar. There is then no real reason to expect identity in statistics from different places at different times.

Moreover, diverse populations may have dissimilar frequencies of localizing and predisposing features within the skeleton. Geographic and ethnic differences in the frequency of postmenopausal osteoporosis [15] and Paget's disease [16] are well recognized, while other bone diseases such as rickets and osteomalacia vary widely in incidence in different parts of the world. Other factors affecting spinal mobility, such as degenerative spondylosis, congenital spinal defects, inflammatory disease of the spine, and even metastatic tumors, may also greatly differ in geographic and ethnic frequency. Yet, such factors in the individual may be of paramount importance in the location and even occurrence of a fracture in the spine after injury. Such differences may have a considerable effect on epidemiological studies of the problems of vertebral injury and must always be carefully considered. Only from a combination of biological, statistical, cultural, and economic studies, as well as from a deeper realization of the biomechanics involved, can full understanding eventually be obtained.

3 SPINAL FRACTURES AND THEIR CLASSIFICATION

Several authors have attempted to classify vertebral fractures [17, 18], to help clinicians understand the mechanics of injury involved and to aid them in accurate diagnosis of the type of fracture. This is obviously essential in planning optimal treatment aimed at reduction of the fracture and stabilization of the spine, achieving decompression of the spinal cord and roots in cases complicated by neurological defects, and preventing late complications such as deformity and pain.

Detailed clinical examination, accurate history taking, and a complete x-ray study are a *sine qua non* in providing the information crucial to accurate diagnosis. However, the frequent coexistence of other injuries, possibly of a more urgent nature, may make a complete physical examination impossible to perform, while the effects of unconsciousness or the absence of witnesses may make it difficult to obtain accurate information as to how, where, and when the injury was inflicted. Moreover, it should always be recognized that plain x-rays, even if taken in two, three, or four different projections, and even laminography, provide a two-plane visualization of the injury. The integration of different views is far from an accurate method for determining the true spatial relationships of the various fragments of the damaged vertebrae.

During the past few years, computerized axial tomography (CAT) has been introduced as a new technique in the diagnosis of spinal lesions [19], traumatic as well as others. This technique shows great promise as an important tool in furthering our knowledge of the end results of spatial displacement of fracture fragments and possibly allowing reevaluation of routine roentgenographic studies. CAT scanning would appear to be particularly valuable in patients with neural damage, affording visualization of a cross section of the spinal canal at various levels and facilitating the localization of displaced fragments that might be causing mechanical pressure on the spinal cord or root. CAT scanning may even prove the truth of the clinical impression held by many surgeons experienced in the field, that pressure by bony fragments is not the usual cause of neurological involvement in spinal fractures, but that direct damage to the neural elements with hemorrhage, edema, and vascular impairment are the problems that need to be faced by the treating physician. However, CAT scanning is still not generally available, and for practical purposes the average treating physician must, as yet, depend on routine x-ray views to determine whether a spinal injury is "stable" or not.

One of the problems involved lies in the great variety of definitions of stability that are used by different authors. It should be admitted that there is, so far, no definition that correlates the biomechanical situation with the clinical and radiological classifications of fractures of the spine. The criteria for stability defined until now have been very diverse and are often confusing.

Nicoll [17] understood that an injury of the spine was stable when there was no likelihood of an increase in deformity or in the neural defect, but gave no definite prescription as to how the physician at the time of initial treatment could decide whether such a likelihood indeed existed. Holdsworth [18] considered that stability depended on the integrity of the "posterior ligament complex," which includes the capsules of the facet joints, the ligamentum flavum, the interspinous and supraspinous ligament, and the posterior longitudinal ligament of the spine. Again, no help was given as to ways of determining the integrity of these ligaments and structures, except in cases where they are totally disrupted.

Bedbrook [20], on the other hand, considered that it was impossible to define stability or instability of a fracture dislocation of the spine until 8 to 12 weeks had passed after the injury, by which time 90 percent of the injuries had become stable. Obviously, such an approach precludes considering early surgical stabilization as one of the available therapeutic modalities.

Kaufer [21] offered a definition of stability in a spinal fracture as a situation in which the spinal fragments are unlikely to move during the period of healing. In the unstable fracture the fragments might displace prior to final healing, resulting in progress of the deformity or even aggravation of the neural defect. This definition really takes us back to that of Nicoll of 30 years ago, and it suffers from the same limitations.

White and Panjabi [22] came to the conclusion that there is no satisfactory and comprehensive definition for stability in spinal fractures and introduced the concept of "clinical stability," to be differentiated from mechanical stability. This concept not only includes the ability of the spine to sustain so-called physiological loads without neurological involvement being affected or aggravated, but also considers time-related factors such as the development or lack of development of deformity and incapacitating pain. Once more, however, clinical stability as defined by these authors cannot be determined at the initial postinjury and pretreatment examination. At best, a specific injury can be described as "likely to be clinically stable." The value of their concept is as limited, therefore, as the definitions of their predecessors.

In our opinion, the most useful definition for clinical use is that of Kaufer [21]. Admittedly nonspecific and based on expectation, it is at least simple and direct. Moreover, it appears to be a definition whose accuracy and value are likely to grow with time and the increasing experience of the physician. As such, it would seem to be a most useful guide on which the physician can base immediate therapeutic decisions.

Apart from those who sought to classify spinal fractures as stable or unstable, other authors have attempted more graphic classifications [23], although even these have often tried to combine a geometric descriptive diagnosis with thoughts on the mechanical genesis of the fracture that are often not completely accurate. For example, Roberts and Curtis [24] divided thoracolumbar fractures into three groups:

1. Wedge compression fractures with or without posterior element involvement (descriptive)
2. Burst compression fracture (descriptive)
3. Rotational fracture dislocation (descriptive and mechanical)

Wedge compression fractures are said to be the most common type of thoracolumbar injury. They may occur at any level, but as we have pointed out above, they are probably most common at the T5-6 and T10-L1 levels. However, there is another type of fracture of the spine that may be no less frequent, although often missed on x-ray examination and evaluation after trauma. Vertebral end-plate fractures, described in detail by Perey [25] and Rolander and Blair [26], often demonstrate only minimal x-ray deformity and are usually not recognized, although there is an increasing awareness of this kind of fracture, leading to more frequent diagnosis of these injuries. The wider use of bone scanning would certainly facilitate diagnosis, especially in those cases where radiological change is minimal [27] or where there is doubt about whether a particular radiological change in the a vertebra is due to present injury or past pathology. Increased upta isotope would indicate the presence of fresh bone injury at a specifi concentrate the examination of the x-ray plate at this point.

End-plate fractures are caused by lesser degrees of axial compression or angular forces and are the result of the application of forces too great for the bone to withstand but not great enough to produce obvious displacement and compression. Perey [25] has described three different types of end-plate fracture:

1. Fracture in the center of the end plate
2. Fracture in the peripheral area of the end plate
3. Transverse fissures in the end plate

These injuries may result from minimal trauma, or even from physiological loads with no true traumatic incident in the pathological vertebrae of the patient with severe osteoporosis. Their frequency in the latter condition is such that some classifications of the degree of osteoporosis in the spine depend on the occurrence and frequency of these fractures, as well as the more commonly recognized wedge compression fractures.

Experimental data [26], as well as clinical impression, have clearly demonstrated that the end-plate fracture, if central, results from axial compression, and, if peripheral, from angular compressive forces acting on the vertebra in the presence of an intact annulus fibrosus. The superior end plate and the spongy bone beneath it are crushed by the inferior part of the vertebra above. The disk usually remains unchanged, although in the rare cases in which the intervertebral disk is also affected, the inferior plate of the vertebra above may also fail, resulting in narrowing of the disk space and even wedging of contiguous vertebrae. Greater forces may lead to herniation of the disk through the fractured end plate into the cancellous bone of the vertebral body, giving rise to typical "Schmorl's nodes." In other cases, the disk might displace into the neural canal. This phenomenon is very rare, but when it does occur it usually happens in the midthoracic spine and is often complicated by serious neurological deficit.

Similar forces, axial or angular, may cause failure of several vertebrae, and it is not uncommon, once experience in the diagnosis of this type of fracture has been gained, to find several affected vertebrae in the same patient, all resulting from a single fracturing force. Such multiple fractures may be contiguous or separate, or may coexist with a more serious type of fracture at another level (Figs. 1 and 2).

The type of injury that usually causes end-plate fractures is a craniocaudally or caudocranially directed axial force. Because of the physiological curves of the spine and the fact that almost none of the end plates of the vertebral bodies are parallel to the ground (or perpendicular to the craniocaudal axis), such forces are usually a combination of axial and angular forces, the direction of angulation being related to the degree and direction of the tilt of the end plate of the affected vertebra to the horizontal. True axial compression would give rise to a biconcave central compression of the vertebral body, while angular forces would add a wedge compression element.

It is interesting to note that in the spines of children with osteogenesis imperfecta, multiple biconcave vertebral compressions are often seen. Could it be that these fractures, due to physiological loading of grossly abnormal vertebrae,

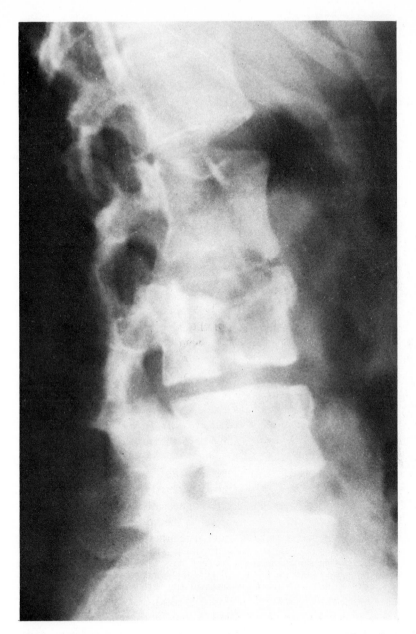

Figure 1 Lateral x-ray showing two continguous vertebral fractures. L3 displays a typical burst fracture, while L4 shows a superior end-plate fracture with minimal deformity. Note the narrowing of the L3–4 disk space.

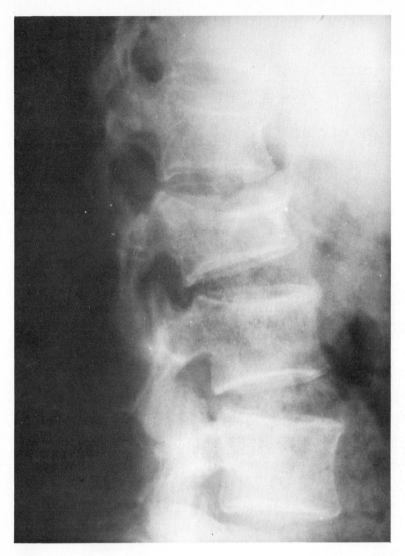

Figure 2 Lateral x-ray showing three contiguous vertebral fractures. L1 and L3 show minimal superior end-plate deformation, while the intervening L2 vertebra demonstrates a wedge compression type of injury.

show that the direction of normal physiological loading on the spine is more or less in the vertical axis? A similar picture may be seen in the severely osteoporotic spine of the steroid-treated child with rheumatoid arthritis. Again, such patients with their grossly limited activity and mobility seldom suffer from the external forces that give rise to fracture of the spine under normal circumstances. The "fish vertebrae" seen in such patients are due to so-called normal forces of body weight, muscle action, etc., acting on the greatly weakened vertebrae that result from the disease or from its treatment.

Compressive forces of greater magnitude acting in the same axial direction (in normal vertebrae) would cause a bursting type of fracture (Fig. 1), the centrally acting compression force, probably transmitted by the disk in a hydrodynamic manner, causing failure in all directions. The different physical properties of the vertebrae under compression, tension, and shear loading may determine at what stage an axial compression end-plate fracture would turn into a burst fracture of the vertebra.

On the other hand, eccentric nonaxial loading must always confer, onto the vertebra, an angular force that will cause a wedge compression fracture when failure occurs (Fig. 2). Forces of this type, of extreme violence, may cause wedging severe enough to impart an excessive bending moment on the posterior osseous-ligamentous-muscular complex. Failure of this part of the vertebral structure markedly increases the degree of immediate mechanical instability as well as the likelihood of the occurrence of late progressive deformity while the body fracture is healing (Fig. 3). The presence of posterior element disruption is thus of utmost importance in determining prognosis and, therefore, treatment modalities [18, 21, 28].

The addition of horizontal plane forces—shearing, translatory, or rotatory—complicates the mechanics of injury even more. In clinical practice it is doubtful if a trauma-induced fracture can occur without such forces, except in the relatively rare case when a weight drops from a height onto the head of an upright subject, or

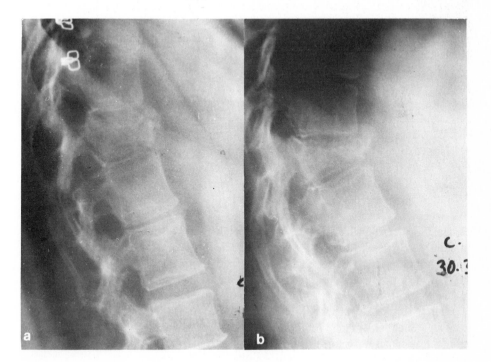

Figure 3 (*a*) Lateral x-ray of the spine showing a fresh wedge compression fracture of L1. (*b*) Three months later: Marked increase in deformity has occurred, while the fracture has united.

possibly in some cases of a fall from a height onto extended lower limbs, the type of injury that classically causes a fracture of the os calcis, the thoracolumbar junction, and even the base of the skull. In most clinical situations, the direction of the fracturing force, the dynamic state of the patient at the moment of injury, and even the patient's posture at rest must nearly always produce a situation in which some horizontal forces are involved. The commonest may be a rotational force determined by the sagittal asymmetry of the fracturing force. A weight falling on the left scapular region of a patient walking with slight flexion of the trunk will obviously cause an axial and an angular force that may lead to a wedge compression fracture at the thoracolumbar junction, while the sagittal asymmetry of the blow will cause a rotational element that may give rise to a translatory deformity at the fracture level. The shearing injury described by Oliveira [29] may be due entirely to horizontally acting forces, while the hyperflexion and distraction mechanics claimed for the Chance fracture [30] has almost certainly a shearing element involved, as demonstrated by horizontal displacement on x-ray.

The complexity of the mechanisms of injury, and the great variation in the end-result picture of the actual fracture and its displacement, account in many ways for the many different attempts at classification of spinal fractures that may be found in the literature, as well as for the failure of the medical profession to arrive at a simple all-inclusive classification and nomenclature for these injuries. White's plea [22] for a unified system has, so far, fallen on deaf ears, as did Roaf's [23] before him, possibly because their engineering mathematical terminology is foreign to most physicians, or possibly because oversimplification leads to too many possibilities for error in assessment of the individual case—the type of error that can invalidate the entire system.

Moreover, the clinical problem of stability of the fracture or its absence, so important to the physician's choice of treatment, must somehow be reflected in the classification of injuries. This, as we have noted above, has so far not been successfully done.

With regard to other authors' attempts at classification, it can be seen that Holdsworth [18] attempted to define fractures as stable or unstable, and that in each category he placed three different types of fracture. Kaufer [21] described the forces involved in each fracture without really determining how an accurate definition could be made from the clinical and radiological findings. Moe and his colleagues [28] used a similar classification but, again, did not clarify how the clinical and radiological picture could be correlated with the direction of the injuring force. Bedbrook [20] tried to relate different mechanical evaluations of fractures to the pathological change found in the spinal cord, but in so doing added little to the understanding of spinal injuries and their neurological complications.

Not to be outdone by other authors, we feel it worthwhile to attempt yet another schema that purports to relate spinal-column injuries to the causative force involved. Such an attempt may simplify the understanding of vertebral fractures until the wider use of three-dimensional evaluation with CAT scanning, and possibly other new techniques, can clarify the problems even more.

In general, the first two injuries in each column of Fig. 4 may be accepted as

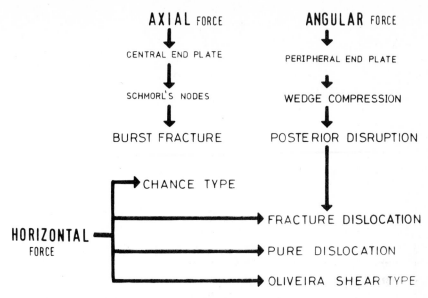

Figure 4 Types of spinal fracture and forces causing them.

stable, while the remainder are a priori unstable, either with regard to the immediate possibility of displacement of the fragments with unguarded movement, or in relation to the danger of the occurrence of late increasing deformity during healing of the fracture. We feel that this is a simple, yet generally applicable, classification, combining geometric description of the fracture, some feeling for the forces involved, and a notion of stability (or otherwise) that may help the surgeon decide *at once* what is the optimal treatment for the individual patient.

4 FORCES REQUIRED FOR THE REDUCTION AND STABILIZATION OF THORACOLUMBAR FRACTURES

Reduction of a fracture dislocation of the spine can be obtained by either open or closed methods, depending on the type of injury, the degree of displacement, the stability or instability of the spinal column, and, probably no less important, the training and experience of the treating surgeon. The vast majority of vertebral fractures show only minimal displacement and are quite stable. Such injuries are best treated by short periods of rest until the acute pain of the fresh injury subsides and then as rapid a return to normal activity as is possible. Union of an end-plate fracture is never a problem, and neither is that of a minor wedge compression fracture. Such fractures are in pure cancellous bone, with a large biologically active surface area of trabeculae in close apposition. The mechanical strength of the compressed vertebra has been shown to be no less than normal [31], since there is no loss of bone and the displaced trabeculae are compressed into a smaller volume than usual. There is therefore almost no danger of instability following even an early return to function.

Although there is a growing body of knowledge about the mechanical properties of single vertebrae, of "motion segments" comprising two adjacent vertebrae and their intervening intervertebral disk, and even of partial and complete cadaveric spines, there is so far little or no accurate knowledge available about the forces required to reduce and stabilize them. In the authors' experience in the operative reduction of thoracolumbar dislocation using Harrington instrumentation, a specially instrumented distraction spreader was used in several cases [32] and the force required for reduction measured. In no case was a force of more than 30 Kp required. Such a force is minute when compared with the impact force of a 70-kg man falling from a four-story building, or the forces involved in a head-on collision of two automobiles traveling at high speed. Yet these are the types of accidents and the orders of magnitude of the forces usually involved in the clinical problem of the fractured spine. Some of the difference between the magnitude of the fracturing force and the force required for reduction obviously lies in the dispersion of energy in soft tissue and bone of the injured person. Some lies in the change in anatomical constraints related to the occurrence of the fracture per se and of ligamentous injury in the region of the fracture. For example, horizontal translation back to the reduced anatomical position is easier after fracture of the articular processes than before, as is evidenced by the relative difficulty that is experienced in reducing the type of dislocation with so-called "locked facets." Moreover, other factors, such as the use of general anesthesia and muscle relaxation in the operative reduction of the spinal fracture, must also play a role. The relatively low force required for reduction also allows overreduction to be obtained more easily and may perpetuate a deformity after treatment that is less than optimal (Fig. 5).

These low forces also explain the success of closed methods of treatment. Bohler [33] has promoted closed reduction under local anesthesia in the treatment of thoracolumbar wedge compression fractures in the area T10–L5 when there is a kyphosis of more than $10°$ and when there is no neurological defect. To limit unnecessary and possibly dangerous treatment in the elderly osteoporotic patient, he also limits his indications to subjects below the age of 60. Since nearly all thoracolumbar fractures are due to a flexion angulatory force, reduction is obtained by hyperextension, raising the upper trunk and/or the extended lower limbs in the prone lying patient, or by dorsal suspension by sling and pulley. According to Bohler, there is no danger of overreduction with this technique of manipulation, since the strong but undamaged anterior longitudinal ligament prevents excessive hyperextension of the vertebral bodies. Because of the possible danger to the spinal cord in closed reduction in midthoracic injuries, he has suggested that in fracture dislocation in the region T1–T9, operative reduction of the fracture be carried out through an anterior transthoracic approach [33].

Louis et al. [34] also have described a technique of closed reduction with the patient supine and under general anesthesia. Axial traction is first applied while the fracture is still in its deformed kyphotic position, and then a hyperextension force is applied directly to the gibbus using a block and tackle. Reduction in lordosis is

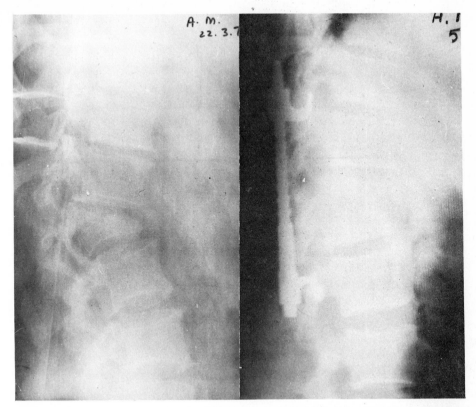

Figure 5 Fracture dislocation of D12–L1 was reduced and stabilized by Harrington instrumentation. Note the increased height of the posterior part of the body of D12 due to overdistraction during reduction.

followed by immobilization using the same type of three-point fixation in a plaster cast that Bohler used after his method of closed reduction. The traction force used by Louis did not exceed 50 percent of the patient's weight, which is similar in order of magnitude to the forces used by the authors during surgical reduction. Immobilization is required for varying periods of time, depending on the degree of initial displacement of the fracture.

Watson-Jones [35] used a similar technique of hyperextension of the spine without anaesthesia, the patient being supported during application of the cast on two tables of different heights. Dunlop and Parks [36], on the other hand, performed manipulative reduction of the spinal fracture under general anesthesia before applying a closely fitting plaster jacket on a Goldthwait frame. Parenthetically, it might be added that there is little difference between this technique and that described by Hippocrates or illustrated by Vidius (Fig. 6), although since many of us still use the Hippocratic method of reduction of dislocated shoulders, perhaps the comparison is not too denigratory!

In spite of the widespread use of these techniques, it is not at all certain that the anatomical reduction of stable fractures is essential for either posture or

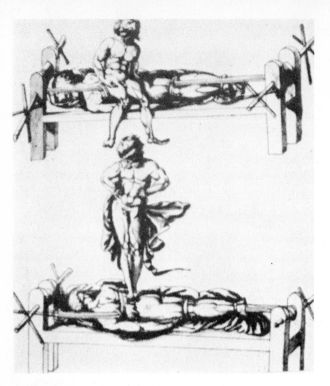

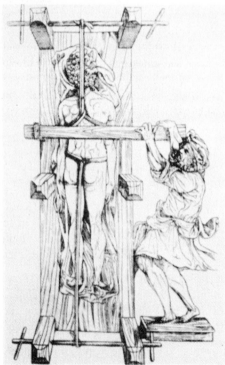

Figure 6 From Vidus Vidius manuscript. *(Courtesy Bibliotheque Nationale, Paris. By permission.)*

function. The deformity resulting even from a markedly wedged vertebra can be easily compensated for by minimal change at other intervertebral segmental levels, while any loss of movement at the injured motion segment resulting from deformity has little or no effect on the total clinical range of movement of the spine. However, unstable fractures that may move or increase in deformity during the healing process, or in patients in whom neurological deficit exists or is a present danger, logically demand reduction while healing is achieved.

Both Nicoll [17] some 30 years ago and Young [6] more recently have suggested that patients treated by closed reduction and plaster immobilization may have more pain and stiffness in the back than those treated by early mobilization with no attempt at reduction of the fracture. Guttmann [37], with his extensive experience in the treatment of traumatic paraplegia, also felt that surgical or manipulative reduction of the vertebral fracture added more complications than warranted by the possible gain of accurate replacement of the spinal fragments. He therefore preferred simple postural methods of achieving vertebral realignment, with no formal manipulative treatment and, more important, no prolonged period of cast immobilization that might cause loss of movement and even pain in parts of the spine left undamaged by the original injury. Such end results of treatment, in his opinion, could interfere with rehabilitation even more than persistent deformity and segmental loss of movement at the site of injury.

In those cases in whom open reduction is considered indicated, a maneuver similar to that described by Bohler may also be used [21], although in the past few years the use of the Harrington outrigger has simplified the technical aspects of spinal distraction, especially in unstable fracture dislocation and in cases with locked facet joints. With the outrigger [13], distraction forces are easily and progressively applied until optimal length is obtained (Fig. 7), and then direct pressure on the spine in the prone patient applies the hyperextension force required. The use of an instrumented distraction apparatus, with which the applied force can be monitored, may be a useful safety precaution. In the severely damaged vertebral column the normal constraints to overdistraction and lengthening, mainly the anterior and posterior longitudinal ligaments, the ligamenta flava, and the obliquely running fibers of the annulus fibrosus, may be ruptured and allow direct distraction of the spinal cord and roots. The forces used in fracture reduction in our experience are very close to those measured by Breig [38] at tension failure of the spinal cord. Great care must be taken, therefore, not to surpass the limits of cord strength in an attempt at better reduction of the fracture. The limits of stretch of the blood vessels that supply the cord are completely unknown, although clinical experience suggests that they are of the same order of magnitude.

If direct hyperextension force cannot be applied, for instance, in the presence of gross comminution of the posterior elements of the spine at the level of injury, hyperextension can be achieved by raising the upper or lower end of the operating table to apply the desired moment. In the special case of locked facets at the lumbosacral level, Samberg [39] used a lamina spreader to apply the required distraction force. White et al. [40] have suggested the use of two crossed Harrington rods to apply the necessary hyperextension force. Once more, no

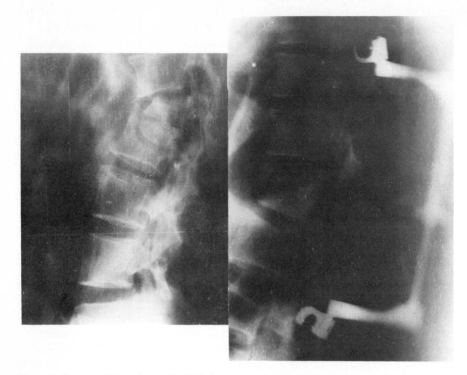

Figure 7 Fracture dislocation at L1–L2 being corrected with the Harrington outrigger.

measurements are available of the order of magnitude of the forces required to reduce fractures and dislocations of the spine with these various techniques.

5 SURGICAL PROCEDURES AND DEVICES

In the past few years surgical treatment for unstable thoracolumbar vertebral injuries has again become widely accepted as the treatment of choice. The treatment includes open reduction of the fracture and internal fixation with various metallic implants. Usually, concomitant spinal fusion is carried out over the segments adjacent to and including the fractured segment, and immobilization is obtained in a spinal brace or cast until fusion of the fracture and/or of the fusion mass is achieved. Together with this, early mobilization of the patient is initiated as soon as the general and neurological status of the patient permits, to facilitate and accelerate rehabilitation.

Operations of this type are usually performed through a posterior approach, although in certain specific cases an anterior or anterolateral approach may be specially indicated. This is particularly so if it is considered that decompression of the spinal canal from posteriorly projecting vertebral body elements is required.

Such cases may be most frequently encountered in the thoracic spine where retraction of the spinal cord to demonstrate and relieve posterior compression by the damaged vertebral body may be technically difficult and fraught with additional danger to the spinal cord and its blood supply. Kelly and Whiteside [41] have suggested that transthoracic decompression is the treatment of choice in these cases. Usually, however, the posterior approach is the easiest, most familiar, and quickest; it allows rapid demonstration of the unstable posterior elements of the spine that determine to so large an extent the total stability of the injured vertebral complex.

In those cases where anterior decompression is indicated, a second-stage posterior instrumentation and spinal fusion is usually mandatory to ensure stability and maintenance of reduction throughout the healing period. Although there is little experience of the anterior approach to the spine in the treatment of thoracic and lumbar fractures, enough knowledge has been gained in the cervical spine to show that anterior surgery carried out to stabilize fracture dislocation, in the presence of posterior bony or ligamentous damage, is often complicated by total loss of stability and marked increase in deformity [42]. The anatomical situation in the trunk is basically very similar to that of the neck, and the dangers of increased instability after anterior surgery are not small. Flesh and his colleagues [43] attempted to overcome these problems by carrying out posterolateral decompression of thoraco-lumbar fractures with neurological involvement and performing spine fusion with Harrington instrumentation, all at one stage.

When posterior open reduction is performed, laminectomy is not required, since reduction of the fracture with Harrington instruments restores the spinal canal to its anatomical size and shape. Any residual compression from a fractured vertebral body is anterior to the cord and nerve roots and thus cannot be relieved by laminectomy. Often the vertebral body lies free in front of the spinal canal, being separated from the posterior elements through bilateral pedicle fractures. In many cases, moreover, the neurological problem is not one of true mechanical pressure but rather a traction lesion of the neural elements over the projecting displaced fragment, with or without vascular compromise as a result of the stretch. Laminectomy cannot relieve this problem.

If posterior reduction does not achieve complete release of the neural stretching, then only anterior decompression can alter the mechanical arrangement. Yet, still today, many orthopedists faced with the problem of stabilizing the fractured spine find only too frequently that laminectomy has already been performed; to the instability of the fracture has been added the additional destabilizing effect of excision of the spinous processes and parts of the lamina and the intersegmental ligaments, supraspinous, interspinous, and ligamenta flava, all removed in a usually vain attempt to improve neurological function [43]. Most of the recent series of spinal fractures treated by stabilization with Harrington instruments have included a large number of cases in which so-called decompression has already been carried out [43, 44].

Several devices have been advocated over the years to achieve immobilization and internal fixation of the spine after open reduction. Different appliances are applied to various parts of the vertebral column—the spinous processes, laminae, pedicles, facet joints, and vertebral bodies being variously used with different surgical implants.

Spinous processes: wiring; Wilson plates; Meurig-Williams plates; Crawford-Adams
    plates
Lamina and facets: Harrington instrumentation (distraction and compression);
    Knodt rods; Kempf rods; Harrington instrumentation with cement; Weiss springs
Pedicles: Roy-Camille plate and screws
Vertebral bodies: plates; cortical bone grafts; cement

Failure of fixation of implants of various types can relate to the device itself, to the bone-implant interface, to the structure and material properties of the bone, or to failure to use the postoperative external fixation cast or brace, that has been found essential with almost all the techniques. The moments and torques applied to a 3-mm-diameter bolt, inserted through a spinous process to fix a pair of Meurig-Willams plates on each side of the bone, by the unrestrained movement of a patient bending, twisting, or even turning in bed are very great and rapidly obviate solid fixation and delay or prevent healing and the achievement of the solid fusion required. Moreover, the spinous processes, commonly used as the *point d'appuy* of the fixation apparatus in the earlier techniques, are frequently damaged by the original injury and, at best, are a mechanically weak part of the vertebra with thin cortices not capable of withstanding significant stress. Thoracic spinous processes are also small and must be further weakened when a hole is drilled through them for the transfixion bolt. If nothing else, the hole acts as a stress raiser with frequent eventual failure.

Fixation techniques dependent on the spinous processes are therefore in general less successful than those using other parts of the vertebra for fixation. In addition to the biological reasons for failure of fixation of appliances attached to the spinous processes, purely mechanical factors may play a part. The horizontal distance of the spinous process from the axis of rotation of the vertebral body is much greater than the distance from lamina, facet joint, or pedicle. Smaller moments are applied to appliances based on these latter anatomical structures than to those fixed to the spinous process. The failure of appliances fixed to spinal processes is frequent, and is one of the reasons for the condemnation pronounced by followers of Guttmann and the conservative school [37, 45]. It is of interest to note that in spite of the widespread poor results seen, no formal study of the forces involved has ever been carried out, as far as we can ascertain. Failure of these appliances usually results from loosening of fixation and/or fracture of the spinous process, either during application of the appliance or later. Loss of fixation brings in its wake recurrent displacement or angulation, gibbus formation, pressure sores, infection, and exposure of the metal. What cogent arguments for the supporters of the postural methods of reduction!

Wire fixation, on the other hand, can be of value [21], especially if reinforced with cement [46]. However, external immobilization with a cast is obligatory if such fixation is used. It is possible that single-wire fixation is even better than the plates and bolts of the Wilson and Meurig-Williams devices, especially when the transfixion bolts of the latter pass between the spinous processes, either because of damage to the bony structure or because the anatomical configuration of the spinous processes is not in alignment with the screw holes in the plates. Wire sutures fixed around intact cortices of the spinous processes in the thoracolumbar region may well give better mechanical fixation, although this again has never been tested in the laboratory, as far as we can discover. Study of a wire-cement construct in the cervicodorsal area showed that failure occurred with forces equal to the weight of the head [44], so that little reserve is available and rigid external fixation is essential. It is possible that the strength of fixation can be improved by increasing the number of turns of the wire (Fig. 8) around the processes, or even by altering the gauge of the wire, although even this has not yet been tested, and no optimal figures are available in the literature. Kaufer [21], after experience with several techniques of internal fixation of the spine, preferred wiring even to Harrington instrumentation, unless wiring is unfeasible because of spinous process fracture or in the area of the thoracic spine. In the thoracic region the slope of the spinous process almost completely obviates the use of the wiring technique, unless the wire is passed through the spinous process in its cephalad part. But this entails drilling a hole through the bone and thus further weakening the mechanical assembly.

Wire fixation does have other advantages. It is simple, rapid, and cheap and

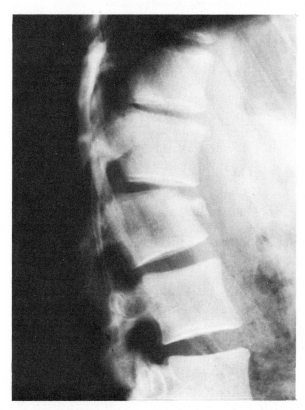

Figure 8 Fracture dislocation at D10–L1 reduced and held with single wire fixation around the undamaged spinal processes.

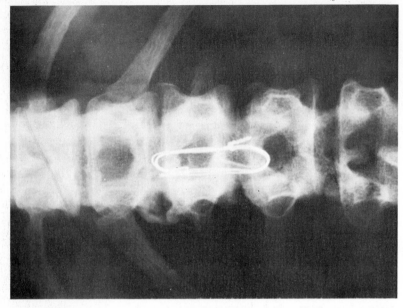

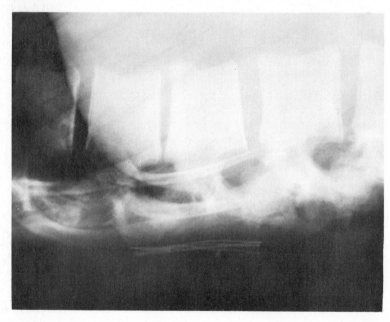

Figure 8 Fracture dislocation at D10–L1 reduced and held with single wire fixation around the undamaged spinal processes. (*Continued*)

requires little surgical expertise. Fixation of two to three vertebrae around the level of injury should suffice, and thus there is little danger of widespread interference with spinal mobility. The amount of surgical exposure, dissection, and retraction of tissues in the region of the fracture is minimal, and thus the danger of infection and other surgical complications is low. In general, with this technique the possibility of grossly affecting movement of the spine as a whole is of no significance. Rehabilitation potential is thus little affected in an adverse way, while the fixation, if adequate, may accelerate the patient's return to function.

6 HARRINGTON INSTRUMENTATION

The treatment of spinal deformity, especially scoliosis, was revolutionized when Harrington [47] first introduced his technique in the early 1960s. Since then, a large number of patients have undergone successful instrumentation for scoliosis and kyphosis, usually together with fusion of the involved segment of the spine. Several years after his first use of the appliances for spinal deformity, Harrington applied the system to the reduction and fixation of spinal fractures [48, 49], as did several other surgeons who had already gained experience with the system in the treatment of spinal deformity. By now, an increasing experience has been gained in many centers of the world. Today, Harrington instruments are probably the most commonly used devices in the surgical treatment of fractures in the thoracolumbar region of the spine, and they have all but replaced the plates and bolts of the previous generation. As has already been pointed out, the point of application of the system is the lamina or facet joint with its relatively thick cortical layers, or over the thick lower thoracic transverse process at its base, close to the pedicle— areas of bone which appear to be much "stronger" than the spinous processes. Reduction of the fracture is usually obtained by using the outrigger device inserted into Harrington hooks placed below and above laminae separated by one vertebral segment from the level of injury. Gradual progressive distraction, preferably under x-ray control, allows extension of the spine to its full length, and the application of a hyperextension force directly to the spine at the level of the injured segment facilitates correction of the wedge compression element of the fracture.

As mentioned above, the hyperextension force can be applied as described by White [49], two Harrington distraction rods being used as crossed levers to correct the deformity. Most surgeons replace the outrigger with a distraction rod, insert another distraction rod on the other side of the midline, and carry out a posterior spine fusion of the instrumented segments, usually four in number. Taylor [50] and Jacobs et al. [51] perform fusion only of the vertebrae directly involved in the injury. This usually demands removal of the Harrington rods once fusion is attained, since without arthrodesis of the additional segments there is almost always failure of the instrument-bone interface, or spontaneous fracture of the rods with subsequent loosening, pain, and even loss of reduction. Other techniques that have been tried include the use of interspinous wiring of the fractured vertebral segments, together with two distraction rods spanning two vertebrae above and below the fracture [52]

(Fig. 9). The posterior fixation applied by the wire limits the possibility of overdistraction in the presence of anterior longitudinal ligament relaxation or injury and applies a moment to correct the kyphotic anterior wedging seen in most compression injuries of the thoracolumbar vertebrae. This combination is similar to the technique used by Leatherman [53], in which a distraction rod is applied on one side of the spine and a compression rod on the other side of the midline. In the presence of lateral scoliotic angulation, the Leatherman technique seems mechanically logical, though more difficult technically than the wire and distraction rod combination.

Other authors have described the technique of using two compression systems [43, 44], once reduction is achieved by elongation and hyperextension of the spine. The compression assemblies are usually applied around the inferior laminar edge of the lowest vertebra to be instrumented and above the transverse process of the uppermost vertebra, although the upper hooks can also be placed above the lamina of the superior vertebra into the spinal canal in the epidural space. This usually necessitates partial laminectomy of the next vertebra above the one instrumented, to clear the way for the insertion of the hook, if the vertebrae are in the thoracic region of the spine.

The corrective forces are applied to the spine in various ways when the different Harrington systems are used. The distraction rods correct and hold the deformity by elongation sufficient to restore full length to the ligamentous structures of the spine, especially the anterior longitudinal ligament, which is reported to be intact in the vast majority of compression injuries of the spine [48, 49]. The intact ligaments are throught to "guide" the fracture fragments back to anatomical position, once they are stretched to the full, aided by the three-point pressure effect asserted by the rod to correct the kyphosis. The compression system reduces and stabilizes the anterior wedging of the compressed vertebra by its action well behind the axis of rotation of the vertebral body (Fig. 10).

Biomechanical studies of the effectiveness of the two systems have been published. Stauffer and Neil [54] reported on the structural stability of Harrington instruments in flexion-rotation fractures of the thoracolumbar spine in cadavers. They compared strength, mode of failure, and ease of application of the distraction and compression systems. The compression assembly was found more difficult to apply (as any experienced scoliosis surgeon could have testified without the laboratory testing) and, as mentioned above, frequently requiring partial laminectomy of an additional cephalad vertebra to facilitate insertion of the upper hook. However, double compression rods apparently give best strength of fixation in comminuted fracture-dislocations of the spine. Distraction rods were found easier to apply, facilitated reduction in displaced fractures, and were mechanically more stable after insertion. Dickson and Harrington [49] preferred the distraction system provided that the anterior longitudinal ligament was intact (though there is no way of knowing this in most injuries when the approach for surgery is posterior).

Kempf et al. [55, 56] concluded that the compression system is preferable,

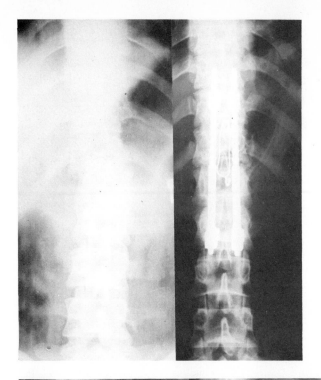

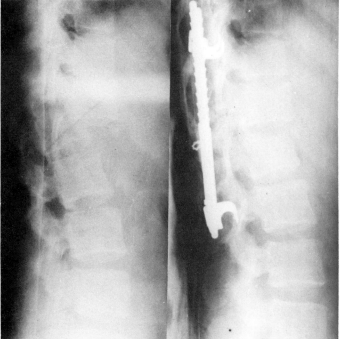

Figure 9 Fracture dislocation at D12–L1 treated by dual Harrington distraction rods with interspinous wiring at the fracture level.

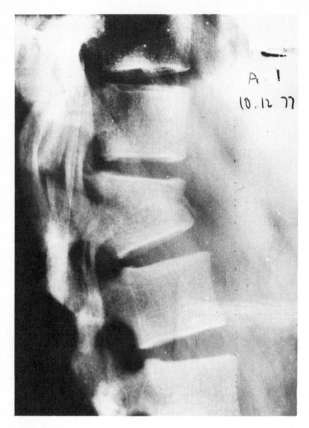

Figure 10 Compression fixation used to correct a compression fracture dislocation at D12–L1.

especially in unstable fracture-dislocations when the posterior cortex of the body is intact and stable, although in the presence of damage to the posterior cortex, distraction fixation must be used. These authors have devised a compression rod that appears much simpler to use than the Harrington compression system. This rod is basically a Harrington distraction rod with a reversed ratchet. Flesh et al. [43] also used both systems and concluded that the distraction rod is better in stabilizing thoracolumbar dislocations. Our own experience [13] suggests that the distraction rod is best applied in the thoracic spine, but in the lumbar spine, especially in flexion-rotation injuries with severe ligamentous disruption in the posterior elements, overdistraction is not uncommon. In these cases, distraction and wiring (Fig. 8) or distraction and compression rodding may be preferrable.

In the lumbar spine, compression rods may be indicated to correct fully the kyphotic deformity and restore the physiological lordosis. In this region of the spine, the relatively rigid distraction rod cannot apply three-point pressure with its corrective moment against the kyphotic deformed vertebra, at least not sufficiently to achieve full reduction. The use of the distraction rod may perpetuate a residual kyphotic deformity after healing of the fracture and the fusion mass over the instrumented segments. This deformity may have significant functional effects, as

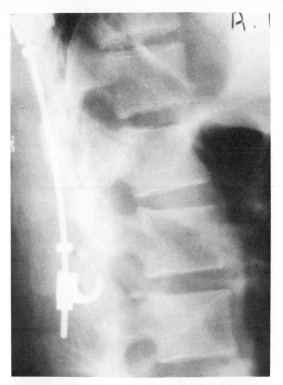

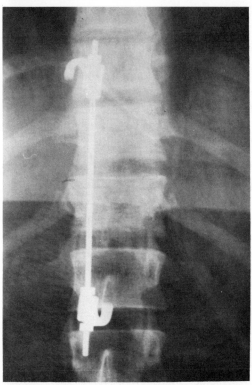

Figure 10 Compression fixation used to correct a compression fracture dislocation at D12–L1. (*Continued*)

has been shown in those cases where a similar problem was caused in the treatment of scoliosis. Compression rods, being much more flexible, allow full restoration of the lumbar curve once reduction and full length are achieved by distraction (Fig. 9). A similar end result may also be achieved by interspinous wiring or possibly by using prebent Moe-type distraction rods.

Weiss springs, modified from implants originally introduced for the treatment of scoliosis [57], have also been used in the stabilization of thoracolumbar spinal injuries. Good results have been claimed in Poland [57], but a multicenter study carried out in the United States [58] showed less convincing results. The work of Stauffer and Neil [54] on the biomechanical value of this type of instrumentation proved it significantly less effective than the Harrington system of either type.

Experience with pedicle fixation using Roy-Camille's plates [59, 60] has been limited, and little comparative information is available. These plates are fixed by screws inserted through the pedicles into the vertebral body, and by shorter screws that transfix the facet joints. They cannot reduce a displaced fracture, however, and full correction of the deformity must be obtained by open or closed methods before fixation is attempted. There have been reports of considerable loss of correction during the healing process [55, 60], even when immediate fixation seemed adequate. This is not surprising, since ordinary bone screws seldom remain rigidly fixed in cancellous bone unless they pass through solid cortical bone on each side. This cannot be done with the Roy-Camille system. Experience with the fixation of even specially designed cancellous bone screws for vertebral bodies, such as in the Dwyer system used in the treatment of scoliosis, shows that failure of fixation is not uncommon, especially in the presence of osteoporosis from any cause.

Anterior interbody fixation with bone grafts demands biological union, and no mechanical testing in the laboratory is really possible. Methyl methacrylate cement has been used, mainly in patients with pathological fractures, and again no mechanical testing has been carried out. Some studies have been performed on the mechanical aspects of combinations of methyl methacrylate with Harrington rods [61], although not with regard to fracture fixation.

7 SUMMARY AND CONCLUSIONS

This chapter is being written several years before its time. Although considerable information exists about the material properties of bone, disk, articular cartilage, and the various ligamentous tissues that make up the vertebral column, accurate information about the interplay among these different tissues is limited to that obtained from a few experiments carried out on cadaveric specimens after sequential removal of various bony and ligamentous structures. Even these experiments have been largely performed on the so-called motion segments of two vertebrae and their intervertebral disk. The effect of muscle tone, and in particular of actively contracting muscle, cannot yet be taken into account. There is really no method presently available for measuring the force of contraction of muscles, especially of trunk muscles. Electromyographic monitoring may give some idea of the degree and timing of contraction of particular muscles in specific activity, but so far no experiments have been carried out, even in animals, to trace the effects on trauma of muscle contraction at the moment of injury. Nevertheless, the part played by muscle in the posture and dynamics of the human spine are considerable, as evidenced by the clinical pictures seen when paralysis, overaction, and disease change the physiological relationships among the various parts of the skeletal system. Even the effects on the spine of movement and energy absorption of the head and limbs are barely understood, though the syndrome of "whiplash" injuries of the cervical spine suggests that acceleration of the head in relation to the trunk may cause considerable disruption, at least functionally, of the intricate bone-ligament-muscle system involved.

Even more fundamental are the possible different physical properties of live blood-perfused oxygenated tissue when compared to cadaveric structures, however soon after death they are examined. The fact that defrosted bone specimens, frozen immediately after death, are physically similar to fresh cadaveric samples does not prove that live tissues are also similar to cadaveric ones in their response to force. Any experienced surgeon recognizes the differences between the live ligaments seen at operation to those seen in the anatomy laboratory. The interspinous ligament of a patient undergoing spinal fusion often appears to contain almost fluid fat globules that must have different physical properties from the ligament seen at postmortem examination, when the body temperature has dropped $20°C$ and the fat is no longer fluid. Moreover, even a single tissue is not necessarily isotropic in its mechanical behavior. As far as bone is concerned, it is known that different structural areas have varying physical properties. What is not widely recognized is that, even at the microscopic level, physical properties change from area to area. Such changes appear to be related to fiber orientation within the bone [62]. No knowledge of the distribution and direction of collagen fibers within the vertebrae is available, and therefore another factor essential to so-called scientific study is lacking.

Today, any attempt at interpreting the mathematics of laboratory testing into the pathology of the clinical state is, at best, theoretical and, at worst, possibly confusing. Even the mechanics of the causes of injury is barely understood. High-speed photography of doll-like structures in crashing driverless vehicles may given some rough information on the type of acceleration and deceleration experienced in a head-on collision, but it does not in any way give accurate information concerning the fate of a living human body in the same circumstances. We are still therefore at the stage where clinical impression and retrospective statistical evaluation of clinical results may give as much understanding as the best-equipped bioengineering laboratory when a decision about the best available treatment for a particular patient is required. Much more information is needed at all levels and from all members of the multidisciplinary teams that are involved in the study of spinal injuries. Such knowledge, related to both clinical and engineering sciences, must then be correlated. Our hope is that by the time this book appears in its next edition, we may have advanced to the stage where the results of laboratory studies have become applicable to the clinical situation, to determine the accuracy of diagnosis, the choice of treatment techniques, the prognosis, the rehabilitation potential, and, maybe, as has happened with other epidemic diseases like smallpox and malaria in the past, some ways to prevent injury on the roads, in the factory, and in the home. This should be our final aim.

REFERENCES

1. H. B. Griffith, J. R. W. Cleave, and R. G. Taylor, Changing Patterns of Fracture in the Dorsal and Lumbar Spine, *Br. Med. J.,* vol. 1, pp. 891–894, 1966.
2. G. Schmorl, and H. Junghans, "The Human Spine in Health and in Disease," 2nd ed., translated and edited by E. F. Beseman, pp. 262–283, Grune & Stratton, New York, 1971.
3. H. E. Frankel, D. O. Hancock, J. Hyslop, J. Melzak, L. S. Micaelis, G. H. Ungar, J. D. S. Vernon, and J. J. Salsh, The Value of Postural Reduction in the Initial Management of Closed Injuries of the Spine with Paraplegia and Tetraplegia, *Paraplegia,* vol. 7, pp. 179–192, 1969.
4. C. Hirsch, and A. Nachemson, Clinical Observation on the Spine in Ejected Pilots, *Acta Orthop. Scand.,* vol. 31, pp. 135–145, 1961.
5. Personal observation of the authors (unpublished).
6. M. H. Young, Long Term Consequences of Stable Fractures of the Thoracic and Lumbar Vertebral Bodies, *J. Bone Jt. Surg.,* vol. 55B, pp. 295–300, 1973.
7. P. R. Meyer, Jr., Complications of Treatment of Fractures and Dislocations of the Dorsolumbar Spine, in C. H. Epps, Jr. (ed.), "Complications in Orthopaedic Surgery," vol. II, p. 645, Lippincott, Philadelphia, 1978.
8. J. F. Krauss, C. E. Franti, R. S. Riggins, D. Richards, and N. O. Borhani, Incidence of Traumatic Spinal Cord Lesions, *Chron. Dis.,* vol. 28, pp. 471–492, 1975.
9. J. F. Kurtzke, Epidemiology of Spinal Cord Injury, *Exp. Neurol,* vol. 48, pp. 163–236, 1975.
10. R. A. Riggins and J. F. Krauss, The Risk of Neurologic Damage with Fractures of Vertebrae, *J. Trauma,* vol. 17, pp. 126–133, 1977.
11. R. M. D'Aubigné and J. Bénassy, Pronostic et traitement des paraplégies traumatiques dorsales, *Mem. Acad. Chir.,* vol. 86, pp. 671–676, 1960.
12. A. A. White and M. M. Panjabi, "Clinical Biomechanics of the Spine," p. 45, Lippincott, Philadelphia, 1978.
13. Z. Yosipovitch, G. C. Robin, and M. Makin, Open Reduction of Unstable Thoracolumbar Spinal Injuries and Fixation with Harrington Rods, *J. Bone Jt. Surg.,* vol. 59A, pp. 1003–1015, 1977.
14. J. R. Silver, Chest Injuries and Complications in Early Stages of Spinal Cord Injuries, *Paraplegia,* vol. 5, pp. 226–245, 1968.
15. B. E. G. Nordin, International Patterns of Osteoporis, *Clin. Orthop.,* vol. 45, pp. 17–30, 1966.
16. C. H. G. Price and W. Goldie, Paget's Sarcoma of Bone, *J. Bone Jt. Surg.,* vol. 51B, pp. 205–224, 1969.
17. E. A. Nicoll, Fractures of the Dorso-Lumbar Spine, *J. Bone Jt. Surg.,* vol. 31B, pp. 376–394, 1949.
18. F. Holdsworth, Fractures, Dislocations, and Fracture-Dislocations of the Spine, *J. Bone Jt. Surg.,* vol. 52A, pp. 1534–1551, 1970.
19. P. W. Nykamo, J. M. Levy, F. Cristensen, R. Dunn, and J. Hubbard, Computed Tomography for a Bursting Fracture of the Lumbar Spine, *J. Bone Jt. Surg.,* vol. 60A, pp. 1108–1109, 1978.
20. G. Bedbrook, Treatment of Thoracolumbar Dislocation and Fractures with Paraplegia, *Clin. Orthop.,* vol. 112, pp. 27–43, 1975.

21. H. Kaufer, Fractures and Dislocations of the Spine; Part 2: The Thoracolumbar Spine, in C. A. Rockwood and D. P. Green, Jr. (eds.), "Fractures," pp. 892–898, Lippincott, Philadelphia, 1975.

22. A. A. White and M. M. Panjabi, "Clinical Biomechanics of the Spine," p. 192, Lippincott, Philadelphia, 1978.

23. R. Roaf, International Classification of Spinal Injuries, *Paraplegia*, vol. 10, pp. 78–84, 1972.

24. J. B. Roberts and P. H. Curtis, Stability of the Thoracic and Lumbar Spine in Traumatic Paraplegia Following Fracture or Fracture Dislocation, *J. Bone Jt. Surg.*, vol. 52A, pp. 1115–1130, 1970.

25. O. Perey, Fractures of the Vertebral End Plate in the Lumbar Spine—An Experimental Biomechanical Investigation, *Acta Orthop. Scand.*, vol. 25, p. 34, (suppl.), 1957.

26. S. Rolander and W. E. Blair, Deformation and Fracture of Lumbar End Plate, *Orthop. Clin. North Am.*, vol. 6, pp. 75–81, 1975.

27. W. Lotz, Scintigraphic Demonstration of Roentgenographically Doubtful Vertebral Fractures, *Fortschr. Geb. Roentgenstr. Nuklearmed.*, vol. 129, pp. 228–234, 1978.

28. J. H. Moe, R. B. Winter, D. S. Bradford, and J. E. Lonstein, "Scoliosis and Other Spinal Deformities," pp. 612–624, Saunders, Philadelphia, 1978.

29. J. C. De Oliveira, A New Type of Fracture-Dislocation of the Thoracolumbar Spine, *J. Bone Jt. Surg.*, vol. 60A, pp. 481–488, 1978.

30. W. S. Smith and H. Kaufer, Patterns and Mechanisms of Lumbar Injuries Associated with Lap Seat Belts, *J. Bone Jt. Surg.*, vol. 51A, pp. 239–255, 1969.

31. R. Plaue, Die Mechanik des Wirbelkompressionsbruchs, *Zentralbl. Chirl.*, vol. 98, p. 761, 1973.

32. M. Arcan, G. C. Robin, and A. Simkin, A Photoelastic Force-Indicating Spreader for the Correction of Scoliosis, *Biomed. Eng.*, vol. 10, pp. 451–452, 1975.

33. L. Bohler, General Considerations in the Treatment of Spinal Fractures, in "Treatment of Fractures," pp. 329–387, Grune & Stratton, New York, 1956.

34. R. Louis, C. Maresca, and P. Bel, Fractures instable du rachis. La reduction orthopédique, *Rev. Chir. Orthop.*, vol. 63, pp. 449–451, 1977.

35. R. Watson-Jones, The Results of Postural Reduction of Fractures of the Spine, *J. Bone Jt. Surg.*, vol. 20, pp. 567–586, 1938.

36. J. Dunlop and C. H. Parker, Correction of Compressed Fractures of the Vertebrae, *J. Am. Med. Assoc.*, vol. 94, pp. 89–92, 1930.

37. L. Guttmann, "Spinal Cord Injuries," pp. 125–127, Blackwell, Oxford, 1973.

38. A. Breig, "Biomechanics of the Central Nervous System: Some Basic Normal and Pathological Phenomena," Almquist & Wiksell, Stockholm, 1960.

39. L. C. Samberg, Fracture Dislocation of the Lumbosacral Spine. A Case Report, *J. Bone Jt. Surg.*, vol. 57A, pp. 1007–1008, 1975.

40. A. A. White, M. M. Panjabi, and C. L. Thomas, The Clinical Biomechanics of Kyphotic Deformities, *Clin. Orthop.*, vol. 128, pp. 8–17, 1977.

41. R. P. Kelley and T. E. Whitesides, Jr., Treatment of Lumbodorsal Fracture-Dislocations, *Ann. Surg.*, vol. 167, pp. 705–717, 1968

42. P. K. Van Peterghem and J. F. Schweigel, The Fractured Cervical Spine Rendered Unstable by Anterior Cervical Fusion, *J. Trauma*, vol. 19, pp. 110–114, 1979.

43. J. R. Flesh, L. L. Leider, D. L. Erickson, S. N. Chou, and D. S. Bradford, Harrington Instrumentation and Spine Fusion for Unstable Fractures and Fracture-Dislocations of the Thoracic and Lumbar Spine, *J. Bone Jt. Surg.*, vol. 59A, pp. 143–153, 1977.

44. F. R. Convery, M. A. Minteer, R. W. Smith, and S. M. Emerson, Fracture Dislocation of the Dorsal-Lumbar Spine. Acute Operative Stabilization by Harrington Instrumentation, *Spine*, vol. 3, pp. 160–166, 1978.

45. P. H. Roberts, Internal Metallic Splintage in the Treatment of Traumatic Paraplegia, *Injury*, vol. 1, pp. 4–11, 1969.

46. M. M. Panjabi, W. Hoffa, A. A. White, and K. J. Kegy, Posterior Spine Stabilization with Methyl Methacrylate. Biomechanical Testing of a Surgical Specimen, *Spine*, vol. 2, pp. 241–247, 1977.

47. P. R. Harrington, Treatment of Scoliosis. Correction and Internal Fixation by Spine Instrumentation, *J. Bone Jt. Surg.*, vol. 44A, pp. 591–602, 1962.

48. P. R. Harrington, Instrumentation of Spine Instability Other than Scoliosis, *S. Afr. J. Surg.*, vol. 5, pp. 7–12, 1967.

49. J. H. Dickson, P. R. Harrington, and D. E. Wendell, Results of Reduction and Stabilization fo the Severely Fractured Thoracic and Lumbar Spine, *J. Bone Jt. Surg.*, vol. 60A, pp. 799–805, 1978.

50. T. K. W. Taylor, personal communication, 1977.

51. R. R. Jacobs, M. A. Asher, and R. K. Snider, Dorso-Lumbar Spinal Fractures: Recumbent versus Operative Treatment, *Orthop. Trans.*, vol. 2, p. 198, 1978.

52. Z. Yosipovitch and G. C. Robin, unpublished observations.

53. K. D. Leatherman, cited by Kaufer (21).

54. S. E. Stauffer and J. L. Neil, Biomechanical Analysis of Structural Stability of Internal Fixation in Fractures of Thoraco-Lumbar Spine, *Clin. Orthop.*, vol. 112, pp. 159–164, 1975.

55. I. Kempf, B. Briot, M. Fernandez, A. Grosse, and M. Renard, Le traitement des traumatismes vertebro-médullaires. Intèrêt de la fixation des fractures et fracture luxation du rachis dorso-lumbaire a l'aide du matériel de Harrington en compression, *Rev. Chir. Orthop.*, vol. 59, pp. 477–489, 1973.

56. I. Kempf, J. H. Jaeger, B. Briot, and A. Lemaguet, L'Ostéosynthèse en compression des fractures et fractures-luxations due rachis par le matèriel de Harrington inversé, *Rev. Chir. Orthop.*, vol. 63, pp. 458–462, 1977.

57. M. Weis, Dynamic Spine Alloplasty (Spring Loading Corrective Devices) after Fracture and Spinal Cord Injury, *Clin. Orthop.*, vol. 112, pp. 150–158, 1975.

58. P. R. Meyer, jr, J. S. Rosen, B. B. Hamilton, and W. Hall, Fracture-Dislocation of the Cervical Spine: Transportation, Assessment and Immediate Management, *AAOS Instruct Course Lect.*, vol. 25, p. 171, 1976.

59. R. Roy-Camille, D. Berteaux, and J. Saillant, Synthèse du rachis dorso-lumbaire traumatique par plaque visées dans les pédicules vertebraux, *Rev. Chir. Orthop.*, vol. 63, pp. 452–456, 1977.

60. Y. Choucair, Y. Pellettier, F. Iborra, and R. Denjean, Reduction des fractures fraîches du rachis dorse-lombaire par traction lordosante et osteosynthèse par plaques de Roy-Camille, *Montpellier Chir.*, vol. 21, pp. 333–342, 1975.

61. G. C. Robin, H. Stein, A. Simkin, and I. Siegel, The Effect of Methyl Methacrylate Cement on Loading of Harrington Instruments in the Spine—A Preliminary Experiment, *Med. Biol. Eng.*, vol. 12, pp. 241–245, 1974.

62. A. Simkin and G. C. Robin, Fracture Formation in Different Collagen Fiber Patterns of Compact Bone, *J. Biomech.*, vol. 7, pp. 183–188, 1974.

63. A. Westerborn and O. Olsson, Mechanics, Treatment and Prognosis of Fractures of the Dorso-Lumbar Spine, *Acta Chir. Scand.*, vol. 102, pp. 59–83, 1952.

64. A. A. Savastano and J. Pieril, Traumatic Compression Fractures of the Dorsolumbar portion of the Spine, *J. Int. Coll. Surg.*, vol. 34, pp. 93–101, 1960.

65. P. C. N. Wong, Vertebral Column and Os Calcis Fracture Patterns in a Confined Community (Singapore), *Acta Orthop. Scand.*, vol. 37, pp. 357–366, 1966.

66. P. T. Andersen and E. Hørlyck, Fracture of the Spine, *Acta Orthop. Scand.*, vol. 40, pp. 653–663, 1969.

MECHANICS OF THE DEFORMITY AND TREATMENT IN SCOLIOSIS, KYPHOSIS, AND SPINE FRACTURES

J. E. Lonstein and R. B. Winter

The spinal column forms the longitudinal bony axis of the skeleton, protecting the spinal cord and allowing motion. The normal anatomy and mechanics form a basis for the understanding of spinal pathology. When a spine deformity occurs, there is an alternation in the normal mechanics. This chapter presents current knowledge of the changes in normal spinal mechanics in scoliosis and kyphosis. The principles of treatment, which can be either with a brace or surgery, are described and surgical approaches with different implants are discussed.

Trauma to the spine damages the bony and nervous elements. The types of bone injuries, along with the mechanics and treatment of each type are described.

1 INTRODUCTION

The spinal column developmentally forms the central longitudinal axis of the animal. It protects the spinal cord, and along it run the longitudinal vascular channels. The ribs and limb girdles that give the organism mobility are attached to it. In the human these functions still exist, although the spinal column is no longer central. This chapter reviews some of the normal biomechanics of the spine as well as that of spine deformities and fractures and their treatment.

2 ANATOMY

The spinal column consists of 24 vertebrae articulated with each other. There are 7 cervical, 12 thoracic, and 5 lumbar vertebrae. The sacral and coccygeal vertebrae are fused together, forming the sacrum, which completes the posterior portion of the pelvic ring. Each vertebra is made up of an anterior solid cylinder of bone, the body, and a posterior arch over the spinal cord consisting of the pedicles and laminae (Fig. 1). From this arch extend three processes for muscular attachments—the spinous process in the midline posteriorly and the transverse processes laterally—which arise at the junction of the pedicle and lamina. The articular processes project from the upper and lower surfaces of the lamina, and their articulation forms the intervertebral facet joints. There are variations of this anatomy in the cervical, thoracic, and lumbar regions.

The vertebrae articulate through three joints—the intervertebral disk between the adjacent vertebral bodies and the two facet joints. The ligaments connect and stabilize the vertebral column (Fig. 2). These ligaments are the anterior and posterior longitudinal ligaments, the ligamentum flavum between the laminae, and the interspinous, supraspinous, and intertransverse ligaments [1]. In addition, the capsular ligaments surround the facet joint. These ligaments, together with the long and short spinal muscles and abdominal muscles, stabilize the spine.

The normal spine is straight and symmetrical in the frontal plane. In the sagittal plane there are normal curvatures—a curve convex anteriorly in the lumbar and cervical areas and convex posteriorly in the thoracic and sacrococcygeal areas. An anteriorly convex curve is termed lordosis, and a posteriorly convex curve kyphosis.

3 NORMAL MECHANICS AND KINEMATICS

Certain facts concerning the normal mechanics and kinematics of the spine [2] are important. The vertebral bodies increase in size from above downward. The work of Messerer [3], Perry [4], and Bell et al. [5] has shown that the vertebral bodies increase in compressive strength from above downward.

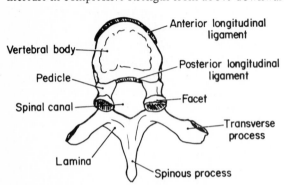

Figure 1 Typical thoracic vertebra as viewed from above.

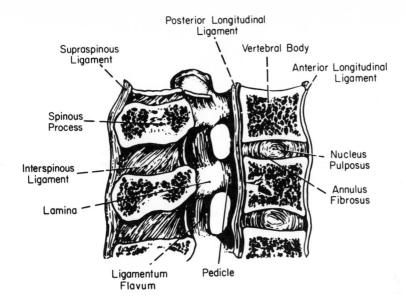

Figure 2 Median view of several vertebrae to illustrate the ligaments of the spinal column. *(From Woodburne [212].)*

The spine ligaments are structures that are most effective in carrying loads in the direction of their fibers. The ligaments allow physiological movement but also restrict movement within well-defined limits. This applies especially to suddenly applied forces in trauma, where the ligaments resist disruptive forces and absorb a large amount of energy before failure. The anterior and posterior longitudinal ligaments and the disks degenerate with age [6]. When samples of the anterior and posterior longitudinal ligament were tested with load deformation curves, the anterior ligament was found to be twice as strong as the posterior longitudinal ligament [7]. Roaf [8] has claimed that it is not possible to disrupt the anterior longitudinal ligament by flexion or extension of the spine, but rotation must be present for disruption. The only other ligament evaluated has been the ligamentum flavum. Nachemson and Evans [7] showed that a resting tension was present in this ligament, this tension decreasing with age.

In studying and describing spinal motions, a motion segment consisting of two vertebral bodies and the connecting intervertebral disk and ligaments is used [9]. A three-dimensional coordinate system (the right-handed Cartesian system) is shown in Fig. 3). Two motions are possible in relation to each axis, namely rotation and translation. This gives six possible motions or degrees of freedom. Rotatory motion normally occurs; about the x axis, this motion is flexion and extension, around the z axis lateral bending, and around the y axis axial rotation. Depending on the specific motion segment with the differing anatomy and orientation of facets, the normal range of rotation about the three axes varies (Fig. 4). Flexion and extension

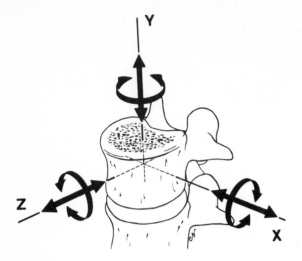

Figure 3 Three-dimensional co-ordinate system (right-handed Cartesian system) placed at the center of the upper vertebra of the motion segment. Rotation and translation are possible in relation to each axis, giving six possible degrees of freedom.

are high in the cervical area, minimal in the thoracic area, and then become greater in the lower portion of the lumbar spine. Lateral bending occurs to some degree at all levels, being slightly higher in the upper cervical and thoracolumbar areas. Axial rotation is highest at the C1–C2 segment and decreases downward to the low thoracic area, being lowest in the lumbar area [10, 11]. Agostini et al. [12] have shown that in the thoracic area the rib cage substantially decreases the motion of

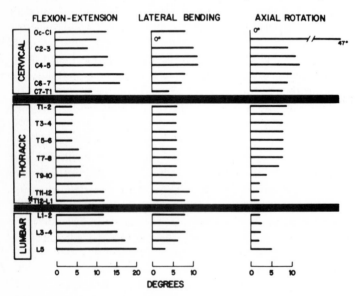

Figure 4 Composite of representative values for rotation at the different levels of the spine in the three planes of motion. *(From White and Panjabi [11].)*

the spine in all physiological ranges. The removal of the sternum was found to negate completely the stiffening effect of the rib cage.

In the intact spinal column the motions that occur are not simple motions as described above but a combination of motions in more than one plane. In addition, coupling of motions occurs. The term coupling is applied when motion in one plane or about one axis is consistently associated with one or more other motions. Coupling of lateral bending and axial rotation in the cervical spine is well described [13]. The motion is such that with the bending of one's head to the left, the vertebrae rotate counterclockwise as viewed from above, the vertebral body rotating into the concavity of the curve. This coupling continues into the upper thoracic area but is less marked; i.e., lateral bending produces less axial rotation. In the mid and low thoracic areas this coupling is not as marked nor as consistently present [10, 11]. In these latter areas the coupling is actually reversed, i.e., lateral bending causing rotation of the vertebral body into the convexity of the curve formed.

The resistance of the motion segment to deformity is important. This is measured as sitffness, which is resistance to the applied force, and as flexibility, which is the ability to deform with the application of the force. The spine segments are stiffer in compression than under tension in the thoracic and lumbar regions [14], and this stiffness increases with higher loads [15, 16]. In the thoracic region, the shear stiffness is the same in all directions in the horizontal plane [14], and slightly higher in the lateral than anteroposterior direction in the lumbar area [17 to 19]. The stiffness in shear is much less than that in axial compression, being 8 percent in the thoracic region [14] and 15 percent in the lumbar region. Thus, the spine is more flexible during shear.

The spine motion segment is more flexible (less stiff) in flexion than in extension by 25 to 30 percent. On removal of the posterior elements the extension flexibility increased to equal that in flexion, with no change in the latter [20, 21]. The stiffness for lateral bending was the same as that for flexion, with no change after removal of the posterior elements.

The stiffness for axial rotation is markedly different from that for the other motions. Torsional stiffness in the upper thoracic spine is constant and is approximately equal to that for flexion or lateral bending. From T7 to L4 there is a gradual increase in torsional stiffness, the value of L3-4 being about nine times the value at T7-8 [20]. The thoracolumbar junction has the highest torsional stiffness, about 11 times that of T7-8. Removal of the posterior elements had little effect on the torsional stiffness in the upper thoracic region, but below T7 the results gave lower values than in the intact spine. In addition, in the lumbar area, the rotation was increased for the same torque [21].

A recent study by Nachemson et al. [22] evaluated the influences of age, sex, disk level, and degeneration on the mechanical behavior of 42 fresh-cadaver lumbar motion segments. The individual differences in the motion segments from different cadavers overshadowed those due to age, sex, disk level, and disk degeneration. In general, females were slightly more flexible than males, and grossly degenerated disks deformed more in compression and less in flexion and extension.

4 SCOLIOSIS [23]

Scoliosis is defined as a lateral curvature of the spine in the erect position, the curvature occurring in the frontal plane. Two important changes are seen with this curvature. First, the lateral curvature is coupled with rotation so that the vertebral body is rotated toward the convexity of the curve. Second, the individual vertebrae in the area of maximal lateral deviation become deformed with a narrow lamina on the concavity and deformation of the pedicles, and the transverse process on the convexity is angulated posteriorly (Fig. 5). As bone is a living tissue, it will respond to stresses placed on it with changes in structure, these changes obeying biological laws. Two of these are important in the discussion of spine deformities. Wolff's law discusses the interdependence of structure and function. It states, "Every change in the form and/or function of bones is followed by changes in their internal structure, and equally definite changes in their external configuration in accordance with mathematical laws" [24]. In addition, forces affect growth, and Heuter [25] and Volkmann [26] proposed the thesis that compression inhibits growth while tension stimulates it.

4.1 Classification

The spinal column is in a delicate balance that is maintained by bony and ligamentous integrity with muscle support. Any alteration in any of these structures can theoretically affect this balance and result in a spinal deformity.

There are numerous known causes of scoliosis, and numerous conditions and diseases are associated with scoliosis. These can be classified etiologically as follows [23]:

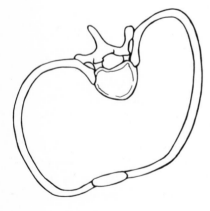

Figure 5 Cross-sectional representation of the apical vertebra of a thoracic scoliosis, the concavity of the curve being on the left. The spinous process is rotated toward the concavity, the lamina on this side is short, and the transverse process on the convexity is angulated posteriorly. The posterior rib prominence on the convexity and anteriorly on the concavity is also shown.

1. Idiopathic
2. Neuromuscular
   a. Neuropathic,
      Upper motor neurone
      Lower motor neurone
   b. Myopathic
3. Congenital
   a. Failure of formation
   b. Failure of segmentation
4. Neurofibromatosis
5. Mesenchymal
6. Rheumatoid disease
7. Trauma
8. Extraspinal contracture
9. Osteochondrodystrophies
10. Bone infection
11. Metabolic disorders
12. Related to lumbosacral joint
13. Tumors
14. Hysterical
15. Nerve-root irritation

A biomechanical classification drawn up by White and Panjabi [10] is the following:

1. Alteration of intrinsic osseous structures
   a. Abnormality of bone structures (osteogenesis imperfecta, infection)
   b. Abnormality of geometry (hemivertebra, fracture, dislocation)
   c. Abnormal kinematics (unsegmented bar, fracture, dislocation)
2. Alterations of intrinsic ligamentous structures (Marfans, myelomeningocoele)
3. Alterations in static or dynamic balance
   a. Neuromuscular static balance (polio, syringomyelia)
   b. Neuromuscular dynamic balance (cerebral palsy, muscular dystrophy)
   c. Postural dynamic balance (leg-length discrepancies)
   d. Thoracic static balance (thoracoplasty)
4. Congenital scoliosis (deformity intrinsic to vertebral body)
5. Miscellaneous
6. Idiopathic scoliosis

The overall prevalence of spinal deformities varies greatly in reported series. Shands and Eisberg [27] found a curve of $10°$ in almost 2 percent of the population they studied, whereas Kane and Moe [28] in a sample population of young adults, found that 1 in every 750 had been referred to a scoliosis clinic for possible treatment. Early detection of spinal deformities by school screening is widespread, and in a review of the results of these programs [29, 30], the prevalence of scoliosis was found to be 3 to 4 percent, the majority of curves being small and not progressive.

In the most common type of scoliosis the etiology is unknown, the cases being classified in the idiopathic group [31]. There is a definite genetic pattern in these cases [32 to 34], and the long-term effects of untreated deformities have been well documented [35 to 37]. As stated, the majority of curves do not progress, and studies have shown that in the United States 1.5 per thousand children [28], in England 4 per thousand children [34, 38], and in Sweden 3 per thousand children [39] will develop progressive curves of 25° or more. Approximately one-third of these will require surgery, and two-thirds will be controlled by a brace [28, 39].

4.2 Experimental Scoliosis

In animal models, numerous experimental studies [40, 41] have been performed to cause scoliosis. These can be classified as transection of muscles and ligaments, denervation of muscles, and procedures on the vertebrae or ribs [42 to 45] and on the central nervous system. Their applicability to understanding scoliosis in humans is variable, but they do point out that the balance maintaining a straight spine is very delicate, and numerous factors can alter that balance.

The etiology of idiopathic scoliosis is still unknown, although more information is being accumulated about this disease. Girls with idiopathic scoliosis have been shown to be taller than their peers [46, 47] and to have a maturer skeletal age [48]. Some evidence has been found that the collagen metabolism is altered in these children [49 to 55], but whether this is the cause or result of the scoliosis is not known. Recent new evidence has thrown light on the possible etiology of idiopathic scoliosis. Several reports have found that the muscles at the apex of the curve have abnormal histochemical staining [56 to 60]. Yarom and Robin [61, 62] have shown electron-microscopic changes in the back and peripheral muscles in idiopathic scoliosis, suggesting a neuromuscular etiology [63 to 65]. Postural equilibrium has been found to be abnormal in patients with idiopathic and not other types of scoliosis by workers in Japan [66 to 68], Sweden [69], and the United States [70]. With sophisticated testing, this dysfunction has been shown to be due to a lesion in the vestibular pathway, the proposed site being the vestibular nucleus [71]. Currently, idiopathic scoliosis is thus thought to be caused by minimal vestibular dysfunction, with a neuromuscular curve resulting.

4.3 Biomechanics

The mechanics and kinematics of scoliosis are as yet ill understood. Any explanation of pathomechanics must cover the complexities of the deformities that naturally occur. Even though there are numerous causes and associated conditions as shown earlier, the presenting deformities are remarkably similar. A commonly found pattern is a thoracic curve convex to the right, associated with a lumbar curve convex to the left. In addition, in idiopathic scoliosis, the vertebral levels are consistent, as shown by Moe and Kettleson [72]. The thoracic curve extends from T5 to T11, and the lumbar curve from T11 to L4. Why are these levels so consistent? As humans are upright and walk with the head in balance over the pelvis, the sum of all the curves to the right approximately equals the sum of all the curves to the left. In each curve the vertebra in the center of the curve is horizontal, the vertebrae on either side tilting in opposite directions away from the horizontal, to a maximal tilt at the end of the curve. This end vertebra is common to two adjacent curves, and the angle formed by the two end vertebrae of a curve can be measured and indicates the magnitude of the curvature, as first described by Cobb [73]. In scoliosis, the vertebrae not only deviate laterally but also rotate, as explained in Sec. 3. The coupling is opposite to that normally found; i.e., the vertebral body deviates toward the convexity of the curve, with the spinous process pointing to the concavity. The vertebral architecture changes, especially at the apex of this curve, perhaps representing the Heuter-Volkmann law. The lamina on the concavity is short, and the spinous process rotated is to the concavity. The transverse process on the convexity is angulated more posteriorly (Fig. 5).

In addition to the vertebral rotation, there is rotation of the rib cage in the thoracic area. This results in a posterior prominence on the convexity of the curve, which is accompanied by an anterior prominence on the concavity. In addition, the ribs become deformed with more angulation at the rib angle, which accentuates the deformity (Fig. 5). Theoretically, the amount of rib prominence should correlate with the amount of vertebral rotation, the latter being related to the magnitude of the curve. This correlation does not exist [74]. This thoracic rotation and lumbar muscle prominence always accompany scoliosis, and they enable early detection of a spinal deformity with school screening [29].

One of the perplexing problems in idiopathic scoliosis is that of curve progression, i.e., increase in curve magnitude with time. Even though it has been found that 3 to 4 percent of school children have a curve, only a small number will progress so that only 1 to 3 per thousand will ever require treatment. It is also known that progression is more common in girls [30] and will occur during the adolescent growth spurt. Why do these specific curves [75] progress? Is it a biomechanical property of the curve in which stability, balance, vertebral size, and vertebral tilt play a role, or are the biochemical properties of the ligaments, muscles, and disks important?

Some studies have been performed on the spinal ligaments in idiopathic scoliosis. Waters and Morris [76] compared the *in vitro* mechanical properties of the interspinous ligaments of patients with idiopathic scoliosis with those of scoliosis of other etiologies. No significant differences were found. Nordwall [77] compared the mechanical properties of the interspinous ligaments and tendons of the erector spinal muscles in patients with idiopathic scoliosis, scoliosis of known cause, and spondylolysthesis. In this study as well, no significant differences were found.

The ligamentum flavum has been credited with playing a role in idiopathic scoliosis. Rolander [16] found that they play an important role in dictating normal spinal motion. This ligament and the facets have been shown experimentally by White [78] to limit the axial rotation in the normal thoracic spine. In addition, if they are removed experimentally, scoliosis results [44].

Because of the lack of data for understanding scoliosis and the difficulty of *in vivo* experimentation, some sort of a model is necessary to investigate the mechanics of the deformity. Animal models are not applicable, as nearly all experimental animals are quadrupeds, and the application of data to humans is invalid given their upright stance and differences in weight distribution and spinal loading.

The simplest models are mechanical in type [79 to 84]. Rogers [85] used flexible rods and investigated the factors related to curve causation. The only positive finding was that imbalance in the posterolateral muscles (erector spinae) would result in a curve. Lindahl and Reader [81] used a mechanical model and showed that the spine can bend without rotation if the ends are not fixed. Rotation occurs if the ends are restrained, with maximal rotation occurring at the center of the curve, this configuration giving the least deformity for the amount of curve. They postulated that idiopathic scoliosis was due to a posterolateral restraint, either owing to a contracture in this area or because the ligaments are slightly tight and a curve occurs with growth on the opposite side.

Mathematical models have become popular, and with the use of high-speed computers this information can be used to analyze the mechanics of the spine and to construct models that can be readily manipulated [86 to 89]. The currently used models show the qualitative behavior of the isolated ligamentous spine and reproduce the effects of treatment on a scoliotic spine.

Schultz et al. [88, 90] used such a model to determine what three-dimensional morphologic changes may be important in the development of scoliosis. They found that a mild scoliotic configuration can be achieved within the normal motion capacity of the spine. Asymmetry of the vertebrae was not required to simulate idiopathic scoliosis. Alterations in length of the anterior soft tissues did not reproduce the geometry of idiopathic scoliosis. Alterations in the posterolateral structures were necessary to produce a scoliotic configuration. Depending on what the alterations were, only a transverse or frontal plane rotation, or a combination of these, was produced. These two rotations did not seem to be kinematically coupled. As these motions seemed to be independent, no simple change in geometry of the column would produce these two important features of scoliosis. Changes in length of the anatomic structures in the region of the transverse processes and deep back muscles appear to be involved in producing the geometric configuration of idiopathic scoliosis. The mathematical computer model of Belytschko [86] measures the response of the vertebral columns to forces and is used in the evaluation of treatment modalities.

An interesting hypothesis has been forwarded by Vercauteren [91]. He states that the vertebral bodies are normally tilted in the sagittal plane, depending on the amount of physiological kyphosis and lordosis. He proposes that the direction of vertebral rotation is, in large part, imposed by their inclination in the sagittal plane. This emphasizes the importance of a three-dimensional concept of the spine and the frustrations of looking at it clinically with two-dimensional x-rays. Perhaps only when the curve can be simply and accurately represented by a three-dimensional value will the biomechanics of scoliosis be understood. Another problem is correlating the clinical, vestibular, and electron-microscopic findings in idiopathic scoliosis with the mathematical models.

4.4 Treatment

The object of treating scoliosis is to prevent curve progression and, with larger curves, to straighten the curve and maintain the spine in this straightened position. With smaller curves a brace will control progression, and with larger curves surgery will provide correction and enable the spine to be stabilized in the corrected position.

Certain biomechanical principles apply to all types of treatment. The spine is a linkage of solid structures (vertebrae) connected by mobile tissue (disks and ligaments) and functions as a biological viscoelastic structure.

Two phenomena occur because of this viscoelastic behavior—creep and relaxation [92]. Creep is defined as the deformation that follows the initial load on a material and occurs as a function of time without further loading. Thus, when a corrective force is applied to a deformity, there is correction with lengthening of the segment of the spine. The subsequent correction that occurs because of the same force over a period of time is due to creep. When a load is applied to a viscoelastic material and the deformation remains constant, the observed subsequent decrease in load with time is relaxation. Clinically, a force is used to correct a spinal deformity, but with time the correction is unchanged and the force decreases.

Different corrective forces can be applied to a scoliotic spine, and simulation and evaluation of the effects require a complex three-dimensional model. White and Panjabi [92] found that certain basic principles can be illustrated with a simplified model. The scoliotic spine is represented by two limbs AC and CB, each limb being of length L. The limbs are connected in this model by a torsional spring and are oriented to simulate a curve of $\theta°$ as measured by the Cobb method (Fig. 6). An axial, transverse, or combined force can be applied to the spine to correct the deformity. The correction obtained is not due to a simple stress in the spine but rather to bending moments at each intervertebral disk level, the combination of these resulting in correction of the angular deformity.

If an axial force F is applied to the two ends of the spine segment at points A and B, elongation and straightening occur. The corrective movement at the apex of the curve is represented by the force F multiplied by its perpendicular distance to the apex of the curve D (Fig. 7b). As the curve increases in magnitude, the distance

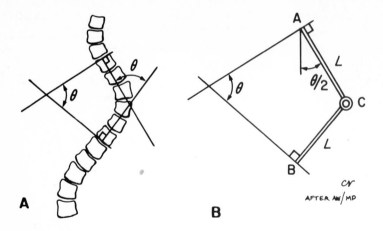

Figure 6 Model for the correction of scoliosis. (*A*) Scoliotic curve of $\theta°$. (*B*) Simplified model with two solid limbs *AC* and *CB* connected by a torsional spring at *C*, a curve of $\theta°$ being shown. *(From White and Panjabi [92].)*

D increases; in addition, the radius of the curve decreases, forming what has been termed a "short-radius" curve. As *D* increases, the correctional ability of the force increases—in other words, the corrective ability of an axial force increases with the severity of the curve.

A transverse load is shown being applied to the apex of the curve in Fig. 8. The

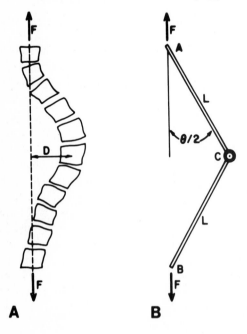

Figure 7 Application of axial force *F* to a scoliosis curve, *D* being the perpendicular distance of the force from apex of the curve. (*A*) Scoliotic spine subjected to an axial force. (*B*) Simplified model of scoliotic spine subjected to an axial force. *(From White and Panjabi [10].)*

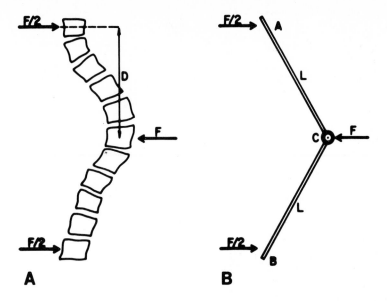

Figure 8 Application of a transverse load F to a scoliotic curve results in a corrective force $F/2$ at the ends of the curve. D is the perpendicular distance of $F/2$ from the apex of the curve. (A) Scoliotic spine subjected to a transverse force. (B) Simplified model of scoliotic spine subjected to a transverse force. *(From White and Panjabi [10].)*

force F results in a corrective moment at the apex of the curve equal to the force at the end of the curve ($F/2$) multiplied by the perpendicular distance D of this end to the apex of the curve. With smaller curves the distance D increases, a "long-radius" curve resulting. The distance D decreases as the deformity increases, the corrective ability of a transverse load thus decreasing with curve increase. An axial force is more efficient for correction of short-radius curves, whereas a transverse force corrects long-radius curves.

These corrective forces can act alone or together, and, in general, a combination of an axial and a transverse force is most beneficial. A comparison of the efficiency of these forces has been made by White and Panjabi [10]. The relative bending moment at the apical disk space was calculated, and more correction was obtained with increased bending moment. Figure 9 shows these results graphically, with the angular deformity measured in degrees by the Cobb method [73]. On the vertical axis the factor M/FL represents the relative corrective moment, where M is the corrective force moment, F is the corrective force, and L the distance AC of Fig. 6; the values of F and L are the same for all three graphs. It is seen that the corrective moment of an axial load *increases* as the angular deformity increases, while that of a transverse load *decreases* as the deformity increases. The two curves cross at an angular deformity of $53°$, indicating that a transverse force is more efficient below this value while an axial force is more efficient above it. The graph also shows that a combined load theoretically has the best relative corrective moment.

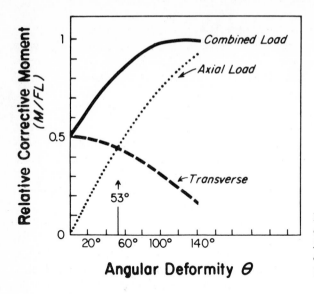

Figure 9 Graphical representation of relative corrective moment M/FL as a function of the angular deformity in degrees. *(From White and Panjabi [92].)*

Another corrective force that can be applied to a spinal curvature is one of axial compression applied on the convexity of the curve. This force can be applied either posteriorly or anteriorly.

The types of treatment for scoliosis are exercises, traction, bracing, casting, and surgery. Each of these will be discussed with the pertinent biomechanical aspects of the treatment. A biological principle is important at this stage. The scoliosis initially is very flexible when examined by axial distraction or by lateral bending in the supine position to the convexity of the curve. Both these evaluations can be performed while an x-ray is being taken, and a measurement of the flexibility obtained. Changes occur in the curve so that the flexibility decreases and the stiffness increases. The curve is said to have become more *structural*. The exact site of the change is unknown—whether it is in the posterior ligaments, inter-transverse ligaments, muscle, or intervertebral disk. With a curve of long standing, disk space and vertebral body wedging occur. The contribution of the abnormal anatomy of the vertebra in scoliosis (Fig. 5) to the change in flexibility is unknown.

Exercises Early theories held that scoliosis was postural in origin and thus exercises were prescribed to "reeducate" the muscles and correct the curve. No evidence exists that there are any beneficial effects of exercise in controlling a progressive curve. As the majority of scoliosis is idiopathic in origin and the majority of these curves do not progress, exercises used for these nonprogressive curves will be "successful." Exercises have been shown not to increase correction over initial side bending values, but exercises have been shown in a study to increase the flexibility of a curve [93].

Traction There are a number of ways of applying an axial corrective force to the spine to try to obtain correction before surgery. The Cotrel method [94, 95] uses a head halter and pelvic straps, the force being applied through the skin. Larger forces can be applied through the bone with a halo on the head (a metal band screwed into the outer table of the skull) and pins in the distal femur just above the knee; this technique is called halo-femoral traction [23]. Weights are applied in these methods, with the patient flat in bed. A halo can be used with a patient sitting in a wheelchair, weights being applied to the halo and the body weight acting as countertraction (halo-wheelchair traction). A halo can be used in conjunction with a pelvic hoop that is attached to the pelvis with transfixing pins. In this method the two hoops are attached via solid rods, with a distracting turnbuckle added to obtain an axial corrective force (halo-hoop traction [96 to 98]).

Experimental work has been done concerning the length of time necessary for maximal correction and the amount of correction obtained. The time/correction factor has been evaluated using halo-femoral traction. Studies [99 to 101] show that the optimal correction is obtained after 10 days using 8 kg of weight at each end. Prolonged traction did not increase the correction obtained [100], and the ideal effect is the transformation of a short-radius curve to a long-radius curve. If the correction in traction is compared to that obtained on an initial side bending flexibility film, no significant difference is found with either Cotrel [93, 102] or halo-femoral [89] traction. Halo-femoral traction has been found useful [103] for the correction of an oblique pelvis or in multiple-stage corrective surgery.

The halo hoop is a powerful correction device, the forces used being up to 360 to 400 N as measured by transducers in the uprights [97]. The complications with its use are many [104], and because of the position of the pelvic pins, fusion to the sacrum and obtaining pelvic bone for the fusion are impossible. Because of its control of both torque and bending, the halo hoop has been shown to be an effective holding device after anterior and posterior osteotomies, where instability is feared. The usefulness of this technique in routine procedures has not been shown.

Spinal orthoses [23, 105 to 107] Mild to moderate scoliotic curves are treated nonoperatively with orthoses (braces). The two main types are the TLSO (thoracolumbar sacral orthosis) and the Milwaukee brace. These are fitted to control progressive curves. The Milwaukee brace was designed 30 yr ago by Blount et al. [108], and the modern brace consists of a molded plastic pelvic section to which three uprights are attached—one anterior and two posterior (Fig. 10a). A neck ring that fits under the occiput and chin stabilizes the uprights, and has two small occipital pads and a throat mold that fits below and within the mandible. The spine is not accessible to a direct lateral force, and the corrective force is applied via the ribs in the thoracic area and the paravertebral muscles in the lumbar area. Pads attached to the uprights for thoracic curves or in the pelvic section for lumbar curves apply these forces [109].

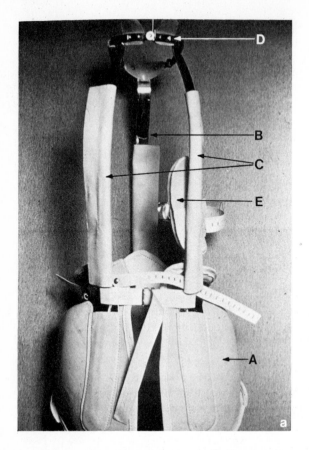

Figure 10 (*a*) Milwaukee brace showing pelvic section *A*. With one anterior (*B*) and two posterior (*C*) uprights, the neck ring *D* has the throat mold anteriorly and occipital pads posteriorly. Pads are attached to the uprights for curve correction, a thoracic pad *E* being shown.

The brace is worn 23 h/day during the active growing years and is gradually removed at the end of spine growth. Clinical studies at the end of the brace wearing show curve correction generally of 18 to 20 percent [72, 110 to 112]. Two recent long-term studies [113, 114] have, however, shown in a follow-up after 10 yr out of the brace, that the curve on an average is the same as the curve at the initiation of bracing—the bracing thus controlling the curve but not correcting it.

The Milwaukee brace biomechanically works on the three-point correction principle (Fig. 10, *b* and *c*) [23]. The pelvic section forms a stable base to support the uprights and is stabilized by three force points, *D, E,* and *F* in Fig. 10*c*. If there is a marked tendency for the spine to list to the convexity of the thoracic curve, the pelvic section is extended over the trochanter at *F* to give greater stability to the pelvic section. To control the thoracic curve through the thoracic pad *C*, the three-point system consists of the axillary sling *B*, the thoracic pad *C*, and the pelvic section *E* on the opposite side. The righting reflex is very powerful, and after a few months the force exerted by the axillary sling is minimal and the sling can be removed. The third point is only theoretical and is made up of the righting reflex, with the side of the neck ring *A* helping induce this reflex.

As the spine deformity is in three dimensions, the exact location of the thoracic pad is important and depends on the amount of thoracic kyphosis present. With marked thoracic kyphosis, the force vector to control the curve must be anterolateral: anterior for the kyphosis and lateral for scoliosis. This is achieved by using a long anterior outrigger to attach the thoracic pad to the anterior upright and placing the pad under the posterior upright to control the kyphosis (Fig. 11a). This combination gives an anterolateral vector. With minimal kyphosis the anterior outrigger is short or absent, and the thoracic pad is placed lateral to the posterior upright. This moves the force vector more laterally (Fig. 11b). In some cases where the anterior rib prominence is large (Fig. 5), a support is placed over the ribs to help "derotate" the thorax.

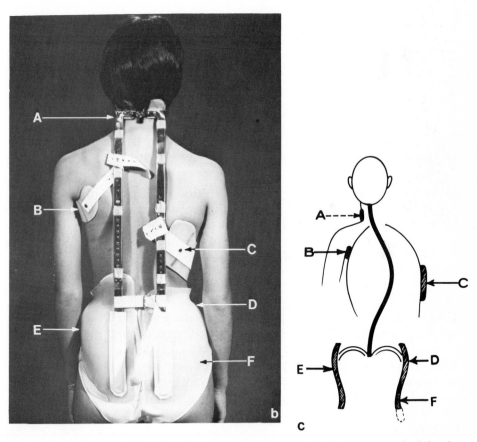

Figure 10 (Cont.) (b) Posterior view of a patient in a Milwaukee brace, the force point being the same as in part c. (c) Three-point correction principle for thoracic scoliosis. The force points D, E, and F stabilize the pelvic section. The three force points to correct the curve are the thoracic pad C, with the axillary sling B and the lateral aspect of the pelvic section E on the opposite side balancing it. The lateral aspect of the neck ring A helps to induce the righting reflex. (Part c from Moe et al. [23].)

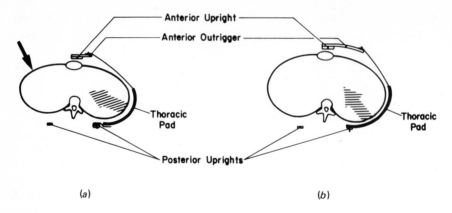

Figure 11 Location of thoracic pad related to the amount of kyphosis present. (*a*) Reduced thoracic kyphosis. The anterior outrigger is short, and the thoracic pad is placed with its medial border lateral to the posterior upright. This combination gives a more lateral corrective force. (*b*) Increased thoracic kyphosis. The anterior outrigger is long, and the thoracic pad is placed with its medial border under the posterior upright. This combination gives an anterolateral corrective force. *(From Winter and Carlson [107].)*

Biomechanical studies [115] have been performed on the brace to evaluate the forces exerted. The areas of interest have been the effect of the pelvic girdle, traction forces, and lateral forces. Nachemson and Morris [116] measured intradiskal pressure *in vivo* in different positions. When an inflated corset was worn the pressure decreased by 25 percent. As the pelvic girdle of the orthosis has a firm abdominal apron, this results in increased intraabdominal and intrathoracic pressure, which decreases the load on the disk. The orthosis passively reduces the lumbar lordosis, and Swedish investigators [117] have shown radiographically that this reduction reduces the magnitudes of both the lumbar and thoracic scoliotic curves, even without additional lateral pads.

Studies [118 to 121] have measured the traction forces with dynamometers placed in the occipital pads and chin rest or throat mold. With a chin rest (used before the advent of the throat mold), the traction force was 11 to 19 N and increased with walking, recumbency, and the supine position (to 49 N). This traction force was so powerful that growth changes in the mandible and face resulted [122 to 126]. With the new throat mold, which does not touch the mandible, the traction force is markedly reduced to 3.8 N standing and 12 N in the supine position. There is a slight increase in the standing position [120] with the thoracic pad removed (to 4.8 N). The force on the thoracic pad was measured with both the old chin rest and the new throat mold. The forces were no different with these two devices, and measured 37 N during stainding. The forces increased with larger curves, measuring 64 N with a 40° to 50° curve. These figures indicate that the distractive force is minimal, the main force in the orthosis being due to the lateral pad. This supporting role of the brace was shown by Nachemson and

Elfstrom [127], who used a Harrington rod with a force gauge. They found that the thoracic pad was the most effective in reducing the load on the Harrington rod, a distractive force being unnecessary.

Andriacchi et al. [128], using a computer-based mathematical model of the spine, evaluated correction of curves with a Milwaukee brace. They used 10 to 20 N of distractive force and 20 to 40 N of lateral force and found that the spine acts as a beam. They confirmed the importance of the lateral pad in scoliosis treatment, and had an 80 percent accurate prediction of brace outcome with their model.

For a lumbar or thoracolumbar curve, the TLSO is used [23]. This is a molded pelvic brace with paravertebral extensions so that the lumbar lordosis can be controlled. A firm pad (Fig. 12a) is built into the orthosis and exerts its forces through the paravertebral muscles. This orthosis also works on the three-point corrective system. The corrective pad B in Fig. 12b is balanced by the midlateral area of the pelvic portion C on the opposite side, and the lower end of the orthosis D on the same side. In many cases there is a tendency for the orthosis to tip owing to the corrective force, and this tendency is controlled by extending the lower

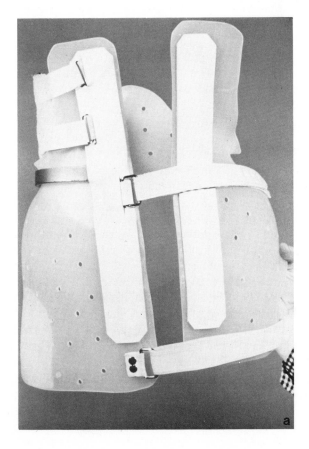

Figure 12 (*a*) Thoracolumbar sacral orthosis (TLSO).

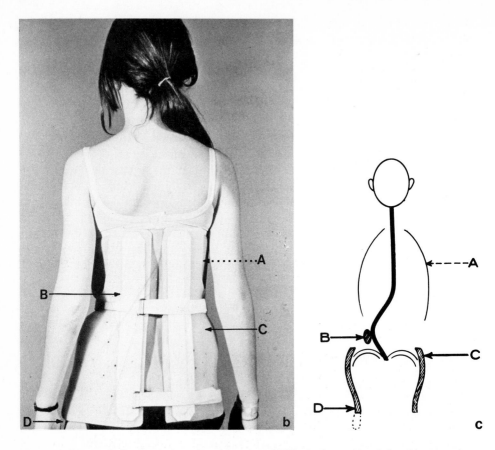

Figure 12 (*Cont.*) (*b*) Posterior view of a patient in a TLSO, the force points being the same as in part *c*. (*c*) Three-point corrective system for lumbar scoliosis. The three force points are lumbar pad *B*, the pelvic brim *C* on the opposite side, and the lower end of the pelvic portion (or trochanteric extension), *D* being the third point. When fitted, the axillary extension *A* induces a righting relfex. *(Part c from Moe et al. [23].)*

portion of the orthosis at *D* over the greater trochanter. Originally, an extension at *A* helped balance the forces by inducing the righting reflex, but this reflex is so powerful that this extension is not usually necessary.

No studies are available on the forces in the TLSO. As with the Milwaukee brace, the control of lumbar lordosis is important for curve control, and the abdominal apron plays a role in this control and in reducing intradiskal pressure [116].

Surgical procedures *Posterior approach* In cases of moderate to severe scoliosis, correction involves major surgery. This procedure involves correcting the lateral curve and fusing the spine in this corrected position [129]. The surgery until the early 1960s involved correction in a body cast with subsequent spinal fusion. Cochran and Waugh [118] evaluated the forces in two types of casts. For the surcingle cast, the lateral force during cast application was 230 N with an average curve of 70°. This force decreased 30 percent within 10 min. In the application of the localizer cast, the average lateral force was 70 N, and 145 N of traction was used.

In the early 1960s Harrington instrumentation [130, 131] replaced cast correction. In this procedure a posterior surgical approach is made, and the posterior elements of the spine (spinous process, laminae, transverse processes, and facet joints) visualized in the area of the lateral curve. Hooks are placed over the laminae at the upper and lower ends of the concave side of the curve, and a Harrington distraction rod (A in Fig. 13) is inserted. One end of the rod has ratchets that allow a gradual distractive force to be applied. The spine is decorticated, and chips of bone are taken from the posterior pelvis and placed along the spine. After 5 to 7 days a cast is applied to help hold the spine; it is removed 6 to 9 mo later, when fusion is achieved and the spine is stabilized [23].

Additional instrumentation is occasionally used. A Harrington compression apparatus (C in Fig. 13) consists of a flexible threaded rod with hooks that are placed around the transverse processes on the convexity of the curve. By positioning

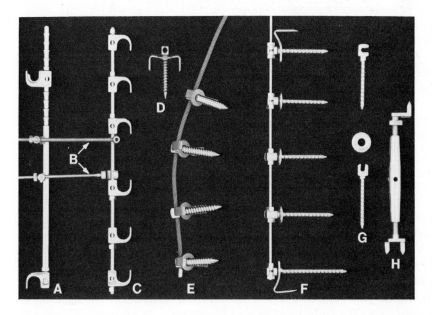

Figure 13 Surgical implants used in the correction of spinal deformities. *A*, Harrington distraction rod; *B*, transverse loading rods; *C*, Harrington compression apparatus with six hooks; *D*, Dwyer screw and staple; *E*, Dwyer screws on cable; *F*, Zielke screws and threaded rod; *G*, Zielke screws and washer; *H*, Pinto distractor (this is not an implant).

the hooks facing each other and tightening appropriately placed nuts, a compressive force is applied. A short compression rod can be combined with a transverse loading system of Cotrel (*B* in Fig. 13) or Armstrong [132, 133].

The biomechanics of instrumentation [134] involves first the bony laminae around which the hooks are placed. Waugh [135] showed that the thoracic laminae fail with a distractive force of 370 N. To reduce this tendency in some cases, especially with bone that is soft, the forces are spread over a larger area by the use of methyl methacrylate, commonly referred to as "bone cement" [136, 137]. In clinical practice we have found it unusual for the hook to cut out of the laminae; more often the problem is dislocation of the upper hook from the lamina, due to inadequate bending of the rod to follow a kyphosis.

Waugh [135] used strain gauges fixed to an outrigger that was attached to the hooks, in some cases prior to insertion of the distraction rod. During correction the axial distractive force was 200 to 300 N, but at times it rose as high as 680 N. The forces decreased significantly over the next few minutes—a demonstration of relaxation. Nachemson and Elfstrom [127, 138] repeated the experiments by using a rod incorporating telemetry. Their findings confirmed the figures of Waugh, with forces of 200 to 400 N being found. The force fell rapidly in the first 60 min and then over the next few days, reaching a plateau at 10 days in which the value was 33 to 38 percent of the initial force. Schultz and Hirsch [139, 140] mathematically analyzed the correction of a scoliotic curve. Their findings confirm the principles of curve correction stated earlier. Initially a small distractive force gave a large degree of correction; then larger forces were necessary for small amounts of correction—conversion of a short-radius curve to a long-radius curve. This shows that attempts to improve the anchoring system are not worthwhile, and that excessive distractive forces do not give greater correction.

Are there any ways to increase correction? Nordwall [141] found that intervertebral disk wedging correlates strongly with the outcome of correction in idiopathic scoliosis. Schultz and Hirsch [139, 140], from a mechanical viewpoint, found the disk to be the main restraint for correction and proposed that disk removal will give better correction with larger or more rigid curves. Waugh [135] found that cutting the posterior ligaments did not affect the distractive force and thus did not increase correction. The addition of a compressive system should theoretically increase correction. Waugh [135] found that this did not reduce the force on the distraction system, although Hall and Gillespie [142] found that only in curves under 50° was better correction obtained with the compression system. Theoretically, the use of a transverse force should increase correction (Fig. 9) for all degrees of curvature, but especially with long-radius curves. In clinical experience the compression rod and transverse force have not been found to significantly increase correction. Generally they increase the stability of the instrumentation so that no loss or minimal loss of correction occurs during the time the fusion is becoming solid [143]. The use of disk excision is discussed in the next subsection.

The recently introduced technique of Luque [144] is interesting. In this procedure a rod is contoured to the spine, the contouring being slightly less than maximum preoperative correction. The rod is secured to each lamina by a wire passing around the lamina. Correction and fixation are obtained at each vertebral level, and thus a very stable system results. In addition, the ligamentum flavum has to be removed to pass the wire, and this ligament, as has been mentioned, is one of the main restraining ligaments of the spine.

A note is necessary regarding the site of the fusion mass. The bone chips act as a scaffold for the bone-forming cells, the site and extent of the fusion thus depending on the bone graft. Early fusion techniques involved splitting the spinous processes and placing bone in this area. Such narrow fusions had a high failure rate. Formation of a wide fusion mass from the tip of the transverse process to the tip of the transverse process gives a more rigid stable fusion [10]. In addition, extra bone should be placed on the concavity of the curve because bone force lines are formed in accordance with Wolff's law, and as there are more compressive forces on the concavity of the curve, the bone in this area will better stabilize the curve. This is important with larger curves, where the bone must span the concavity of the scoliosis to stabilize the curve (Fig. 14).

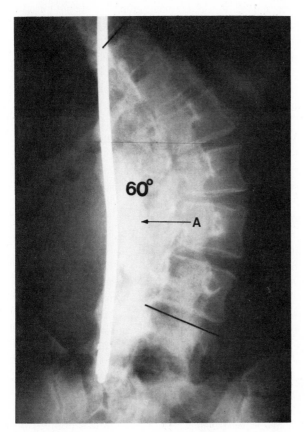

Figure 14 Radiograph of a lumbar curve showing the fusion mass *A* spanning the concavity of the curve.

Anterior approach The importance of the anterior structures is well shown in the experimental work of Rolander [16]. He fixed all the posterior elements except the pedicles with bone cement and found that significant motion occurred at the interspace with physiological loading. This shows that there is significant motion due to the elastic properties of bone with a solid and adequate posterior fusion. An interbody fusion would eliminate this motion and provide marked rigidity. In situations where the posterior fusion is expected to be of poor quality, or where there is a high incidence of failures of the posterior technique (pseudarthrosis), anterior fusion is indicated. This can be a simple fusion or can be supplemented by instrumentation.

It is possible to add instrumentation to an anterior fusion with the technique of Dwyer et al. [145] or Zielke. The initial stage is anterior exposure of the spine and complete disk removal in the area of the scoliosis. Screws with either staples (Dwyer) or washers (Zielke) are placed through the vertebral body to engage both cortices of the body, the screw entering the body on the convexity of the curve. A braided cable is passed through the screw heads in the Dwyer technique while a threaded rod and nuts are used in the Zielke procedure (Fig. 13). Compressive forces are applied to correct the curve, the nuts maintaining correction in the Zielke procedure. With the Dwyer cable, the screwheads are crimped onto the cable. The principle is thus compression on the convexity of the curve with small increments of correction being obtained at each disk space. Micheli and Hall [146] modified the Dwyer instrumentation by using a solid rod. Dunn [147, 148] has devised an anterior stabilization device consisting of a heavy threaded rod with screws and connectors for use with instability with trauma or after anterior bone excision.

The manner in which the screw is inserted will determine the correcting force (Fig. 15). A screw inserted across the vertebral body will correct pure scoliosis as in *A*. With insertion from anterior to posterior, the correcting force will create kyphosis, and thus this direction is ideal for correcting lordosis (*B*). An angle between these directions, as in *C*, will correct lordoscoliosis. If there is a significant rotatory prominence, a screw entering anterior to *A* will have a derotatory vector.

As with the Harrington procedure, the critical area is the interface between the instrumentation and bone. Dunn and Bolstad [149] evaluated this fixation *in vitro*, testing toggle strength and the force necessary to extract the screw. The screw alone had the least fixation, followed by the screw and staple, screw and methyl methacrylate, and finally the combination of screw, staple, and methyl methacrylate. Each step progressively increases the area of contact between the instrumentation and the bone. In clinical practice, screw-and-staple fixation is sufficient as long as the bone is not weakened and the opposite cortex of the vertebra is engaged by the screw tip.

There is only one study on the measured forces with Dwyer instrumentation. Shapiro et al. [150] performed experiments *in vitro* and *in vivo* in dogs. The compressive forces at one level have been reported to be 450 N. This does not accurately reflect the actual load placed on the cable. Once the screw is crimped on

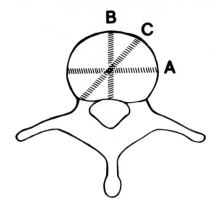

Figure 15 Direction of Dwyer screw insertion. A screw inserted transversely across the vertebral body in direction *A* corrects pure scoliosis. When inserted from anterior to posterior in direction *B*, the screw corrects lordosis. A screw inserted between these two directions, as in direction *C* will correct lordoscoliosis.

the cable, the tension in that portion of the cable falls rapidly. When dogs with tension gauges implanted on the cable were stressed in the first few weeks after surgery, the cable tension increased markedly. This increase was not seen 8 to 12 mo later, the bodies then being solidly fused.

The biomechanical forces were assessed by White and Panjabi [92] (Fig. 16). The corrective bending moment at each disk space is the tension on the cable F multiplied by the perpendicular distance L of this force from the instantaneous axis of rotation (LAR) of that motion segment; that is, $M = F \times L$. The distance L is very small, and thus large forces are necessary to produce a significant corrective moment.

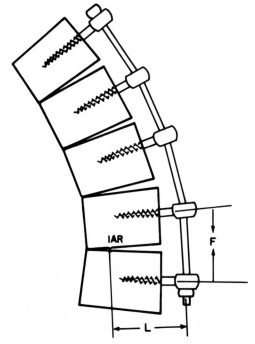

Figure 16 Biomechanical principle of Dwyer instrumentation. Compressive forces are applied on the convexity of the curve. The corrective bending moment at each disk space equals the tension F in the cable multiplied by the distance L from the force to the axis of rotation (IAR). As L is very small, large forces are necessary to produce a significant corrective moment. *(From White and Panjabi [92].)*

In general, anterior instrumentation is used clinically to obtain correction, to achieve anterior fusion, and to increase the rigidity of the spine while fusion is occurring. The ideal curves have proved to be lumbar or thoracolumbar curves in patients with neuromuscular disease, e.g., spina bifida, poliomyelitis, and cerebral palsy. Anterior instrumentation is not used above T9 because of the proximity of the heart and great vessels to the metal and the narrowness of the interspaces, which prevent much correction. This technique is also occasionally used in adults with idiopathic scoliosis [151]. It has been found that the anterior fusion and instrumentation alone are rarely sufficient to stabilize the spine but must be combined with a posterior fusion and Harrington instrumentation.

5 KYPHOSIS

Kyphosis, by definition, is a posterior angulation of the spine. The normal thoracic kyphosis is taken to be between $20°$ and $40°$ as measured by the Cobb method. Posterior angulation in the thoracic area above $45°$ is abnormal, as is any kyphosis in the cervical and lumbar areas—areas that are normally lordotic [23].

Normal spinal balance is maintained by bony, ligamentous and muscular forces. This balance is more delicate than in the frontal plane, as the spine in the sagittal plane is eccentrically placed, and an especially delicate balance exists at the apex of the thoracic kyphosis (Fig. 17a). There is a normal flexion bending moment due to the weight of the head and thorax plus the powerful abdominal muscles that flex the spine. These are counteracted by the spine extensors, which, as they lie very close to the axis of motion, are inefficient. The extension moment is increased by the hydraulic effect of the intrathoracic and intraabdominal pressures, these being maintained by the muscular action of the abdominal and intercostal muscles.

5.1 Classification

Problems of kyphosis can be classified etiologically, as follows:

1. Postural
2. Scheuermann's disease
3. Congenital
    a. Failure of formation
    b. Failure of segmentation
4. Neuromuscular
5. Myelomeningocoele
6. Posttraumatic
7. Inflammatory
8. Postsurgical
9. Postirradiation

10. Metabolic
11. Skeletal dysplasias
12. Collagen disease
13. Tumor
14. Neurofibromatosis
15. Inflammatory

Kyphosis may also be classified biomechanically:

1. Failure in tension (posteriorly)
    a. Ligamentous (trauma)
    b. Bony (postlaminectomy)
    c. Muscular (muscle paralysis)
2. Failure in compression (anteriorly)
    a. Bone weakness (osteoporosis, tumor, metabolic, Scheuermann's)
    b. Bone deformity (congenital, postirradiation, Scheuermann's, trauma)
    c. Bone loss (infection, trauma)
3. Unclassified (postural)

The biomechanical classification is more applicable to kyphosis than to scoliosis, as sagittal-plane deformities are biomechanically easier to explain. The sagittal-plane deformity often occurs alone, but in some cases is combined with a frontal-plane deformity, giving kyphoscoliosis. In severe cases of scoliosis, especially those of neuromuscular origin, the severe rotation of the spine gives the clinical appearance of a posterior angulation of the apical vertebrae. This is not true kyphosis, but a "rotatory kyphosis" or a "kyphosis scoliosis" as described by Stagnara [152].

Two important differences exist between scoliosis and kyphosis. In pure kyphosis the deformity remains in the sagittal plane, with no rotation being present. Once kyphosis is abnormal, the angulation increases, progression being far more common than with scoliosis. Clinically, thoracic scoliosis, when severe, results in thoracic cage distortion, abnormal breathing mechanics, and eventually lung and heart failure [36, 37]. Thoracic kyphosis, on the other hand, does not result in breathing problems unless very severe. The spinal cord is stretched and compressed in kyphosis, and this can result in paralysis [153].

5.2 Biomechanics

The biomechanics of kyphosis and its production is shown in Fig. 17. There is a normal flexion moment on the spine, as shown in Fig. 17*a*. Muscular forces and the righting reflex counteract this tendency. This righting reflex is well shown in the balance between kyphosis and lordosis in that an increased thoracic kyphosis will result in an increase in the lumbar and cervical lordosis to maintain the upright position with the head positioned over the pelvis.

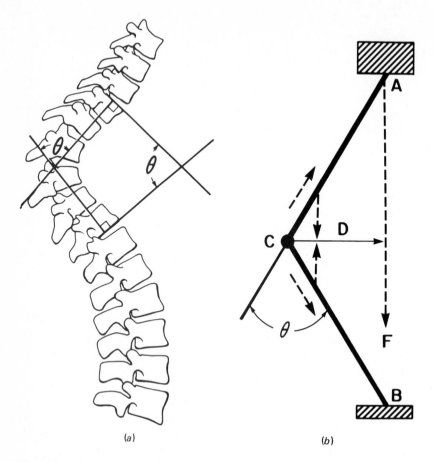

(a)   (b)

Figure 17 Biomechanics of kyphosis. (*a*) Spine with kyphosis showing normal flexion moment of thoracic spine, which is counteracted by muscular forces and the righting reflex. (*b*) Simplified model with two solid limbs *AC* and *CB* connected by a torsional spring at *C*. The flexion force due to the weight of the head and trunk acts at *A*. At the apex of the deformity *C*, the anterior structures resist compressive forces, while the posterior structures resist traction forces. The flexion bending moment equals the product of the force *F* and the perpendicular distance *D* of this force from apex of the deformity.

Kyphosis can occur in any area of the spine, but is more easily understood biomechanically if the most vulnerable area—the thoracic spine—is considered. The kyphosis is represented mechanically as in Fig. 17*b*. Two solid links *AC* and *BC* are connected by a torsional spring *C*. The normal flexion force *F* due to the weight on the head and trunk acts at point *A*. It will be seen that when the system is in balance, in the area of *C*, the apex of the deformity, the anterior structures resist compressive forces, while the posterior structures resist traction forces. In the growing child the kyphosis will be perpetuated as growth obeys the Heuter-Volkmann law [25, 26]. Compression of the anterior growth plate will result in growth retardation in this area and, eventually, a wedged vertebra.

The causes of kyphosis as shown above can now be appreciated. Failures of the spine posteriorly in its ability to resist traction forces include loss of supporting structures surgically (laminectomy) or due to trauma disrupting the posterior ligaments. Muscle paralysis also decreases the resistance to traction forces. Failure to resist compression can be due to bone loss or weakening (tumor, infection, trauma, metabolic) or due to a growth disturbance (congenital, irradiation, developmental, and Scheuermann's disease). The only unclassified failure is postural kyphosis, which may be due to a combination of muscle imbalance and an immature righting reflex.

In Fig. 17b it is seen that the flexion bending moment M equals the product of the force F and the perpendicular distance D of this force from the apex of the deformity; that is, $M = F \times D$. An increase in F will result in increasing deformity, as will an increase in D. The latter is the more important, as the flexion moment will increase as the curve increases, resulting in a progressive deformity. For example, the normal bending moment at T8 has been calculated to be 105 kg·cm; with an increased kyphosis with a 4-cm increase in D, the moment is 155 kg·cm. An additional factor in curve progression is anterior growth retardation, as discussed above.

5.3 Treatment

Before a discussion of treatment, it must be appreciated that, although increased sagittal-plane deformity can theoretically occur in any area of the spine, the most common sites by far are the thoracic and thoracolumbar areas. As with scoliosis, the shape of the curve can vary. Stagnara et al. [154] have divided the curves into "regular" (long radius) and "angular" (short radius). In addition, the angular kyphosis may vary in flexibility, being reducible or irreducible.

Kyphosis treatment is similar in some ways to scoliotic treatment, and differs in others. The role of axial and transverse forces follows the same principles as in scoliosis, and force curves similar to those shown in Fig. 9 apply. In kyphotic deformities the anterior structures resist correction, and, in addition, as anterior support is necessary for stabilization, the anterior approach to the spine is routine in kyphosis treatment.

Exercises [23] Exercises play a role in the postural deformity and in early, flexible Scheuermann's disease. This disease of unknown cause presents with back pain and kyphosis with radiological changes of vertebral wedging and bone end-plate irregularity. This kyphosis shows a high propensity to progress. The exercises given are those to strengthen the thoracic extensors and abdominal flexors.

Spinal orthoses [107] Spinal orthoses are used for Scheuermann's disease and occasionally for severe postural kyphosis. The main orthosis is the Milwaukee brace, the same basic design as for scoliosis, with pads attached to the posterior uprights to exert pressure in the area of the kyphosis (Fig. 18a). The pelvic section is fabricated to control lumbar lordosis, and the neck ring is slightly lower posteriorly than in scoliosis.

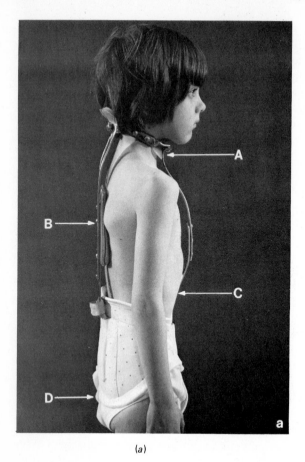

(a)

Figure 18 Milwaukee-brace treatment of kyphosis. (*a*) Lateral view of patient in Milwaukee brace, the force points being the same as in part *b* .

Biomechanically, the three-point principle is operative (Fig. 18*b*). The pelvic section is more stable in the sagittal plane than the frontal plane. The kyphosis pads exert force at the apex *B* of the curve, with the abdominal apron *C* of the pelvic girdle anteriorly and the lower edge *D* of this girdle posteriorly being the other two force points. There is a tendency for the upper arm of the kyphosis to incline into flexion. This is counteracted by the normal righting reflex, which is stimulated by the throat mold (force point *A*), causing spine extension.

If an underarm brace (TLSO) is used with a sternal pad for midthoracic kyphosis, it proves to be ineffective (Fig. 18*c*). The force due to the sternal pad *A*1 is too close to the apex of the deformity to be efficient. In addition, the kyphosis can increase by bending over this pad. If, however, the apex is lower, for example in the thoracolumbar area, this underarm brace is more effective, as the three-point system is more balanced.

Surgical procedures To correct and stabilize kyphosis, a pure sagittal-plane deformity, three possible forces can be applied. These are axial distraction, a transverse force, and compression on the convexity of the curvature, the forces being used alone or in combination. The surgical approaches in kyphosis are posterior and anterior. As with scoliosis, the objectives of the surgical procedure are correction of the deformity and fusion of the spine in this corrected position. The site of the fusion mass is important biomechanically, i.e., anterior, posterior, or combined.

In Fig. 19 a solid posterior fusion is compared to a solid anterior fusion. After a posterior fusion (Fig. 19a), the force F on the kyphosis lies anterior to the fusion, and thus a bending moment is still present. This results in the fusion being under tension. The fusion will fail in tension following Wolff's law [24], and a progressive deformity will result due to the pseudarthrosis at the point of failure—the apex of the curve. In addition, in a case of a posterior fusion, the tight anterior structures (intervertebral disk and anterior longitudinal ligament) cannot be released; thus with some correction the fusion is under tension.

An anterior fusion consists of removal of the intervertebral disks in the area of proposed fusion and cutting of the anterior longitudinal ligament. The placement of the fusion bone will depend on the type of kyphosis present. In a "regular" kyphosis and reducible angular kyphosis, bone is placed in the disk spaces and, in addition, a trough can be cut into the vertebral bodies and a rib placed in this trough to provide stability for correction. In Fig. 19b this fusion mass is

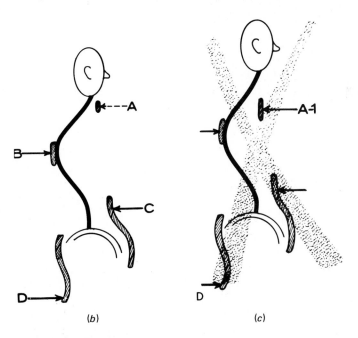

(b)   (c)

Figure 18 *(Cont.)* *(b)* Three-point system for correction of kyphosis. The kyphosis pads *B* exert pressure over the kyphosis. The abdominal apron *C* exerts counterpressure, while the throat mold *A* induces an upright stance with the patient's righting reflex. The posterior aspect *D* of the pelvic girdle helps stabilize the brace. *(c)* If a sternal pad *A*1 is used, an effective corrective system is impossible with thoracic kyphosis. *(Parts b and c from Moe et al. [23].)*

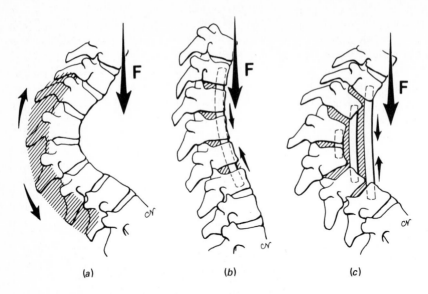

Figure 19 (*a*) With a posterior fusion for kyphosis, the flexion force *F* lies anterior to the fusion, with a bending moment being present. This results in the fusion being under tension. (*b*) "Regular" kyphosis with inlay graft, showing the fusion mass lying near the line of action of the flexion force *F*. The fusion is under compression. (*c*) With an "angular" kyphosis, antierior struts of bone span the curve. The resulting anterior fusion lies close to the flexion force *F* and is under compression.

demonstrated as lying near the line of force of the bending moment. This fusion is under compression. When the kyphosis is more "angular" and irreducible, struts of bone are placed anteriorly, spanning the concavity of the curve (Fig. 19*c*). These struts of rib or fibula are placed in cavities in the vertebral bodies, and the spaces between the struts and the disk spaces are also filled with bone. This bone is important, as the struts are remote from their blood supply and become avascular and fracture. With the additional bone a continuous bony plate is formed, which allows early revascularization to take place. The fusion mass thus lies in the concavity of the curve, close to the line of force and under compression. The biomechanical importance of an anterior fusion with kyphosis has been discussed by White et al. [155]. In addition, the clinical experience and role of anterior fusion have been presented in many papers [156 to 160]. The closer the anterior strut is located to the line of compressive forces, the more effective it is in supporting the kyphosis. Often the limiting factors in the placement of this strut are the anatomical structures in the concavity of the curve.

As has been discussed earlier, for the greatest rigidity and stability of the spine, an anterior and posterior fusion is optimal. With a kyphotic deformity this gives a thick anteroposterior fusion mass to resist the bending moments. The posterior fusion must thus be as thick as possible. The question now arises as to the length of the posterior fusion. Even with an anterior fusion of sufficient thickness (and length), it has been found that if the posterior fusion is of the same vertebrae, the spine buckles over the fused area, increasing the deformity. A posterior fusion extending into the lordotic areas adjacent to the kyphosis is necessary for optimal stability. The line of force then passes through the posterior fusion above the kyphosis, then through the anterior fusion, and then through the posterior fusion below the kyphosis (Fig. 20a). This is seen clinically when the bone lying in this force line becomes more dense, showing changes in accordance with Wolff's law (Fig. 20b).

The types of forces and instrumentation used for correction of kyphosis can now be discussed. For an axial force to be effective it must be applied at the ends of a curve—at A and B in Fig. 17b. Longitudinal traction alone, as with scoliosis, is

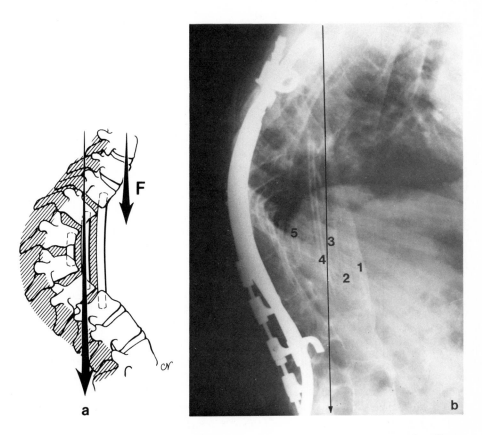

Figure 20 (a) Anterior fusion combined with a posterior fusion extending into the adjacent lordotic curves. The line of force passes through the posterior fusion above the kyphosis, then through the anterior fusion and the posterior fusion below the kyphosis. (b) Radiograph of a combined fusion for kyphosis. A solid anterior fusion spans the concavity of the kyphosis, and five struts are seen. The line of force passing through the fusion mass is shown.

more effective for an angular, short-radius deformity. In kyphosis there is tethering on the concavity of the curve, and thus preoperative longitudinal traction will not affect the rigid apex of the curve, but rather straighten the ends of the kyphosis and place the spinal cord under traction [153]. Once these tight structures have been released, traction is more effective. This can be applied at the time of the anterior fusion by forceful manual distraction of the spine combined with a transverse force on the curve (see below) while the bone strut is being inserted. A distraction instrumentation has been designed by Pinto et al. [161] (Fig. 13). This comes in four sizes and uses the turnbuckle principle. It can be used at the time of anterior fusion to correct the kyphosis while the bone strut is inserted. Once inserted, the strut maintains an axial distractive force. The distracting device is then removed, as it is not an implant. In the time between the anterior and posterior surgeries, traction is used in conjunction with a transverse force to gain correction.

A Harrington distraction rod can be used with some kyphoses to gain correction [155]. The principle is shown in Fig. 21. With distraction, tensile forces F are generated. Additional forces are generated at the sites of contact of the rod and the spine. At the sites of hook insertion, forces F_1 will tend to pull the hooks out of the bone. At the apex of the curve, force T acts to correct the kyphosis. Although this theoretical three-point system should be effective, in practice it is not. The limiting factors are F_1 and T. Except for flexible or mild kyphoses, the rod has to be contoured for the deformity, being made slightly straighter than the spine. On insertion, this will generate forces F_1 and T, but as the corrective force becomes larger, so does the force to pull out the hooks. In addition, when a rod is contoured, distraction of the rod results in buckling, and in that case the tensile

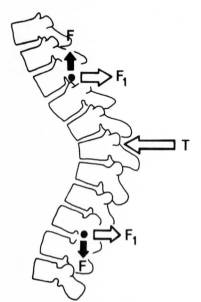

Figure 21 Harrington distraction rod used for kyphosis generates the forces shown. Distractive forces F are generated at sites of hook insertion. At these sites, forces F_1 will tend to pull the hooks out of the bone. These forces are counteracted by the force T generated by the rod at the apex of the kyphosis. This system is only effective for a mild or flexible kyphosis. *(From White et al. [155].)*

forces become smaller. A distraction rod is thus useful only for mild or flexible kypho-sis. It is used in the cases where kyphosis is associated with scoliosis, being contoured for the kyphosis and inserted to stabilize the spine rather than gain correction.

The second corrective force used for kyphosis is a transverse force. This can be applied during the anterior fusion in combination with distraction. The anesthetist applies longitudinal traction to the head while direct pressure is applied over the apex of the deformity. While these corrective forces are being applied, a strut is inserted into prepared notches in the vertebral bodies to maintain the correction. A transverse force is used when traction is used as mentioned earlier. The force is applied by placing the spine on an extension frame, or by placing rolls under the kyphosis. When used for a mild, flexible kyphosis, a Harrington distraction rod applies a transverse force for correction.

The third force that can be used to correct kyphosis is compression applied posteriorly, on the convexity of the curve. This can be applied by using Gruca-Weiss springs or Harrington distraction rods. With pure kyphosis, double instrumentation is used, one on each side of the spine. When the kyphosis is associated with scoliosis, a Harrington distraction rod is used on the concavity to correct the scoliosis, and a compression system on the convexity to correct the kyphosis.

Gruca-Weiss springs consist of heavy springs with hooks on both ends. The hooks are inserted around the transverse process or under the lamina at the upper and lower ends of the curve. Gruca [162] first introduced these springs in 1956 for the correction of scoliosis; they were placed on the convex side of the curve to create a moment for correction of the rotation in the frontal plane. They were largely unsuccessful in this. In 1975 Weiss [163] reintroduced the springs for correction of kyphosis, especially after trauma. The springs, when under tension, exert a considerable compression force, but with significant or rigid kyphosis the amount of correction obtained is minimal [164]. In addition, the stability obtained with springs is minimal [164, 165].

The Harrington compression system applies compression to the spine, the forces acting at the points of insertion of the hooks (Fig. 13). The hooks are applied around the transverse processes in the thoracic spine and under the laminae in the lower thoracic and lumbar areas. Multiple areas of correction are obtained by using multiple hooks, one at each vertebral level, with no hooks inserted at the apical 1 to 3 levels. As mentioned, with a pure sagittal deformity a compression system is inserted on each side of the spine. When analyzed mechanically by Panjabi and White [166], this system was found to provide little corrective force. They only used two hooks for fixation of the rod, and stated that, owing to the flexible nature of the rod, no corrective transverse force is large but there is minimal correction. When the system is used with multiple hooks, the effect is different. With compression at each segment, it achieves its result in the same way as the Dwyer instrumentation. With tightening of the nuts on the rod, compressive forces are generated at each level on the convexity of the curve. With progressive tightening of all the nuts and hooks of the system, progressive correction results.

The stability of these three systems has been tested by Stauffer and Neil [164] in cadaver spines. The disruptive moment applied to the instrumented spine was a combination of flexion and axial rotatory moment. The Harrington compression rod supplied the maximum stability, followed by the Harrington distraction rod, and least of all the springs. Similar studies of Meyer et al. [165] confirmed these findings.

6 TRAUMA

An appreciation of the mechanics and kinematics of the normal spine is necessary for a discussion of the changes that occur with injury. The ligaments impart intrinsic stability to the spine and are able to absorb some suddenly applied forces. The anterior longitudinal ligament is twice as strong as the posterior longitudinal ligament. The coordinate system is shown in Fig. 3, and, as mentioned, there is a normal range of motion of rotation around the three axes (Fig. 4). Translational or shear motions are normally not present in the spine. Coupling of spine motions is important, and an appreciation of the different stiffnesses of areas of the vertebral column is necessary in understanding spine injuries. Great variations exist in each individual with respect to bone and ligament strength, range of motion at each spinal segment, and the stiffness and flexibility of different areas of the spine.

When a force is applied to the spine, the muscles and ligaments absorb the initial force; once their capacity is reached, failure occurs, with a spinal injury resulting. The most common mechanisms of injury are automobile accidents, diving accidents, and falls from a height. Flexion, extension, and compression injuries predominate, the most common sites being the thoracolumbar area followed by the cervical spine. At the thoracolumbar area the orientation of the facet joints changes from thoracic to lumbar, and because of this there is an abrupt change in the stiffness of the spine.

The integrity of the spine and thus its stability, as mentioned, depend on the ligamentous supports of the motion segment. Roaf [8] has shown that the ligaments are most vulnerable to shear and rotatory forces, but can fail when stretched beyond their mechanical limit. The experiments of White et al. [167 to 169] on sectioning of ligaments demonstrated their role in clinical spine stability in the cervical and thoracic spine. The sectioning was done from anterior to posterior and then posterior to anterior, with testing of the stability of the motion segment after each ligament was sectioned. The anterior ligaments stabilize the spine in extension, while the posterior ligaments stabilize the spine in flexion. With sectioning there were small increments of change followed by a sudden disruption and loss of stability. Once the facets were removed in the cervical spine, there was less angular and more horizontal displacement with a flexion moment [170]. In the thoracic spine, when the ligaments were sectioned from posterior to anterior, failure occurred after cutting of the rib articulations. In sectioning in the opposite direction, failure occurred after cutting of the posterior longitudinal ligament [10, 171, 172].

The maximum disruptive force is applied to the spine at the moment of impact, and at this time the displacement is maximum [173 to 177]. When first seen clinically, the spine is in a less displaced, partially reduced position. The forces acting at the moment of impact vary in their magnitude, rate, and site of application. It must be appreciated that the resultant moment on the spine depends on the position of the vertebrae at the time of impact. This was well shown by the monkey experiments of Gosch et al. [178], in which an axial force on the cervical spine produced different injuries depending on the position of the head and neck at the moment of impact. When an axial compressive force is applied in the line of the instantaneous axis of rotation, a compression moment results. When applied anterior to the axis, a flexion moment results; and when applied posterior, the moment is one of extension. The injuries are discussed below in terms of a single-axis displacement. It must be understood that this rarely occurs clinically, the displacement normally occurring around more than one axis and producing a complex motion.

In discussing spinal injuries, two aspects are important—spinal-cord involvement and stability. The spinal cord suffers maximum injury at the moment of impact. In addition, the spinal canal may be distorted owing to the bony displacement, and bone or disk fragments in the canal may be pressing on the neural tissue. This can result in no neurological deficit, or a complete lesion with no neurological function below the site of injury, or some function may be retained (incomplete lesion). As discussed, the stability of the spinal column can be divided into anterior and posterior stabilizing columns, a loss of integrity of both columns resulting in instability [179]. Clinically, instability can occur in the acute stage with bone and ligament damage, or later when healing has occurred [180]. The healing power of ligaments is poor, and thus once bony healing has occurred, the ligamentous disruption can cause chronic instability. This is aided by the fact that a large number of spinal injuries result in kyphosis, and with posterior ligament disruption, a progressive deformity results.

One of the first descriptions of spinal injuries was that of Holdsworth [181] in 1963, with emphasis placed on the mechanism of injury and the resultant lesions found. The moments produced at the time of injury as a result of impact are flexion, extension, compression, distraction, rotation, and shear. These rarely occur alone, most injuries being due to a combination of moments. By careful analysis of the history, accompanying injuries, and high-quality x-rays, the exact mechanism of spinal injury can be determined [182].

6.1 Spinal Injuries

Compression An axial compressive force applied directly in the line of the spine leads to compression of the disk and vertebral body. The disk is less compressible than the bone, and blood is initially squeezed out of the vertebral body, the bone acting as a shock absorber [183]. The disk remains intact and bulges into the bony vertebral end plates with subsequent failure of the bone, fracture of the end plate, and compression of the cancellous bone. This results in a bursting injury of the vertebral body with concomitant loss of height. Bone is forced in all directions, especially posteriorly into the spinal canal, with pressure on the spinal cord. Neurological damage is thus common with this injury. Owing to the type of bony injury, this lesion is stable.

Distraction Distraction or tension injuries are unusual. The injury, a horizontal splitting of the spine, occurs through bone, soft tissue, or a combination of these. Pure distraction or distraction combined with flexion occurs in the thoracolumbar area. This was described by Chance [184] and Rennie and Mitchell [185] and is referred to as the "seat belt injury." The lap seat belt holds the pelvis while the trunk moves forward into flexion and distraction on impact. This force disrupts both stabilizing columns with variable damage to the spinal cord.

Flexion When a flexion moment is applied, the vertebral bodies approximate and the spinous processes distract, with the posterior ligaments being placed under tension. The ligaments withstand the longitudinal stress in the line of their fibers very well, and the failure occurs anteriorly, with anterior compression of the vertebral body causing a wedge compression fracture. Kaufer [186, 187] has calculated that the compressive forces on the vertebral body are equal to four times the tensile forces on the spinous process or supraspinous ligaments. With extreme flexion there can be failure posteriorly either with avulsion of bone or through the supraspinous ligament. This injury shows acute stability, and spinal-cord damage is rare. The flexion moment can be associated with rotation (see below) or compression, the flexion-rotation injury being the most common type of spinal injury.

Extension Extension injuries occur almost exclusively in the cervical spine. With a flexion force the spine is protected from extreme flexion as the chin hits the sternum. With extension the protection is absent, and extreme extension is possible. The anterior longitudinal ligament is placed under stress, and approximation of the spinous processes occurs. Failure occurs posteriorly with fracture of the facets or neural arch, and occasionally the anterior longitudinal ligament avulses a small fragment of vertebral body. In addition, the anterior neck structures are placed under tension with possible muscle or esophageal tears, as is seen in the clinical syndrome of "whiplash" [188, 189]. With extreme extension, the upper cervical spine is placed under a shear moment, with possible resultant bone (odontoid) or ligament (transverse ligament of axis) failure.

Rotation Pure axial rotatory injuries are rare, rotation usually being combined with flexion. Roaf [8] has shown that the ligaments fail in rotation, and Gosch [178] demonstrated that for dislocation, flexion or extension of the spine must be combined with rotation. Evans [190] showed that when rotation and flexion forces are combined, the posterior ligaments fail first, and when rotation and extension moments are combined, the anterior ligaments fail first.

In the cervical spine, axial rotation produces facet subluxation or dislocation. As mentioned, flexion-compression injuries are the most common. These forces cause disruption posteriorly, either through ligaments or bone, with subsequent disruption anteriorly, the exact injury depending on the proportion of flexion and rotatory forces present. With a large rotatory force in the thoracolumbar area, a shear fracture of the vertebral body occurs—the "slice fracture" of Holdsworth. This group of injuries shows the most acute instability and, due to the extreme displacement, the highest incidence of spinal-cord and nerve-root injury.

Lateral bending A lateral bending force results in failure of the lateral mass in the cervical spine and of the vertebral body in the lumbar spine. This is analogous to an anterior wedge fracture due to pure flexion and is also a stable injury, rarely associated with a neurological deficit.

Translation Translation or shear forces may occur in the anteroposterior or lateral planes. A large force is necessary to cause this injury, as both structural columns of the spine have to be damaged for this displacement to occur. These lesions are very unstable, with spinal-cord damage being common.

6.2 Treatment

Spinal injuries, as shown, involve a combination of a bony injury and injury to the spinal cord and nerves. The latter is the more important, but in the long run both aspects must be addressed as they are interdependent. In the initial assessment the bony lesion is either stable or unstable. The neurological evaluation will show no loss or loss that is partial or complete [191].

The spinal-cord damage occurs either due to gross malalignment of the spinal canal, or due to bone or disk fragments encroaching on the canal with no malalignment being present. The cord injury occurs at the moment of impact, but further cord injury must be prevented. All pressure on the cord due to canal malalignment or bone fragments must be removed [192]. Surgical unroofing via a laminectomy has proved to be ineffective and may lead to later instability [180, 193 to 197]. It has been well shown that reduction of the fracture with realignment of the spine and spinal canal will "decompress" the spinal cord [194, 198 to 200]. This method of postural reduction was first popularized by Guttmann [201, 202] and reviewed by Frankel et al. [203]. In the cervical area, skull traction achieves the same result [204]. This method is very costly; the hospitalization is prolonged, as rehabilitation cannot be started till the fracture has healed. Careful and constant nursing care is necessary for regular turning and skin care. In addition, late instability problems still occur if the ligaments do not heal. This method is not effective for burst fractures in which bone fragments encroach on the spinal canal.

Neurological improvement occurs with fracture reduction, which decompresses the cord. There is a higher rate of neurologic recovery in patients with reduced fractures than in those with nonreduced fractures. In addition, further cord damage is prevented [198]. Incomplete neurological lesions are improved in this manner, and some recover completely [193, 203].

What, then, is the role of surgical stabilization in spinal injuries? Stabilization has been shown to allow rapid rehabilitation with decreased hospital stay, fewer complications, and less nursing care [71, 130, 131, 174, 179, 187, 194, 197, 199, 205 to 209.

The specific injuries that require stabilization depend on the spine injury, the spinal-cord damage, and the philosophy of the specific surgeon. In general, acutely unstable injuries should be stabilized. In the cervical spine, stabilization is generally external via a halo cast, with surgery used when indicated to remove bone impinging on the spinal cord. In the thoracolumbar area, operative stabilization is used. The large majority of injuries are accompanied by some kyphosis, as the disrupting forces are flexion and rotation. The basic principles are those discussed under the treatment of a flexible kyphosis and shown in Figs. 20 and 21. The instrumentation available for this stabilization are the Harrington compression and distraction rods, Gruca-Weiss springs [163, 210], and Meurig-Williams plates. The latter, attached to the spinous processes, are completely ineffective in stabilizing the spine. The work of Stauffer and Neil [164] and Meyer et al. [165] has shown that the Harrington compression rod provides the maximum stability, followed in effectiveness by the distaction rod and then the Gruca-Weiss springs. With a fracture there is some shortening of the spine, and the Harrington distraction rod has proved to be the most practical for stabilization and restoring the alignment of the spine.

The Harrington distraction rods are inserted at least two levels above and two levels below the site of injury. With a three-point correcting principle, the rods restore the anterior longitudinal ligament to its normal length. The ligament acts as a hinge allowing proper realignment to take place. In cases where severe instability is present with disruption of the anterior longitudinal ligament, a circumferential wire is placed around the spinous processes above and below the site of injury to prevent excessive distraction.

Biomechanically, the distraction rod exerts forces as shown in Fig. 22b. The axial distractive force F results in a tension force F_2 in the anterior longitudinal ligament. At the site of hook insertion, a force F_1 tending to dislodge the hook is present. To counteract this force, the rod exerts a transverse force T at the site of injury to stabilize the spine. The transverse forces F_1, T, and F_2 thus act on the three-point principle. In cases where bone still encroaches on the spinal canal with pressure on the spinal cord, it is possible to remove half a lamina and the pedicle and facet area, visualize the canal, and remove this bone or disk [174, 211]. A fusion is performed at the same time, usually along the transverse processes, to give eventual bony stabilization.

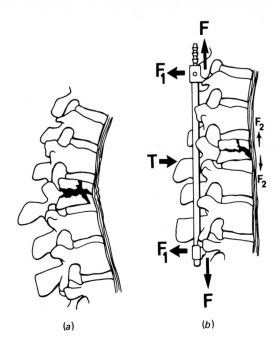

Figure 22 Treatment of a spine fracture with Harrington distraction rods. (*a*) Flexion-rotation injury with bony disruption, instability, kyphosis, and bone encroachment on the spinal canal. (*b*) Use of the Harrington distraction rod exerts an axial distractive force F at the sites of hook insertion, and places the anterior longitudinal ligament under a tension force F_2. At the sites of hook insertion, forces F_1 tend to dislocate the hook, and the rod exerts a transverse force T at the apex of the kyphosis. The forces F_1, T, and F_2 act on the three-point principle to stabilize the kyphosis. With restoration of the vertebral height and correction of the kyphosis, the bone encroachment on the spinal canal is reduced.

Some cases of trauma require surgery after the acute stage. These are usually cases where instability is present and leads to a progressive kyphosis [180]. This instability can be due to anterior bony loss at the time of injury, or loss of posterior stability due to ligamentous damage or a laminectomy. The principles of treatment and the anterior and posterior approach are the same as discussed above under the treatment of kyphosis. In addition, many of these cases have bone impinging on the spinal cord at the apex of the kyphosis, with neurological loss. This bone is removed at the time of the anterior fusion, with decompression of the spinal cord.

REFERENCES

1. D. Lucas and B. Bresler, Stability of Ligamentous Spine, *Biomechanics Lab. Rept. 40*, University of California, San Francisco, 1961.
2. J. M. Morris, Biomechanics of the Spine, (in press).
3. O. Messerer, "Uber Elasticitat und Festigkeit der menschlichen Knocken," Cottaschen, Stuttgart, 1880.
4. O. Perry, Fracture of the Vertebral End-Plate in the Lumbar Spine, *Acta Orthop. Scand. Suppl.*, vol. 25, 1957.
5. G. H. Bell, O. Dunbar, J. S. Beck, and A. Gibb, Variation in Strength of Vertebrae with Age and Their Relation to Osteoporosis, *Calcif. Tissue Res.*, vol. 1, p. 75, 1967.
6. I. R. Harris and MacNab, I. Structural Changes in the Lumbar Intervertebral Discs. Their Relationship to Low Back Pain and Sciatica, *J. Bone Jt. Surg.*, vol. 36B, p. 304, 1954.

7. A. L. Nachemson and J. Evans, Some Mechanical Properties of the Third Lumbar Inter-Laminar Ligament, *J. Biomech.,* vol. 1, p. 211, 1968.
8. R. Roaf, A Study of the Mechanics of Spinal Injuries, *J. Bone Jt. Surg.,* vol. 42B, p. 810, 1960.
9. A. A. White, Kinematics of the Normal Spine as Related to Scoliosis, *J. Biomech.,* vol. 4, p. 405, 1971.
10. A. A. White and M. M. Panjabi, "Clinical Biomechanics of the Spine," Lippincott, Philadelphia, 1978.
11. A. A White and M. M. Panjabi, Kinematics of the Human Spine, *Spine,* vol. 3, p. 16, 1978.
12. E. Agostini, G. Mognoni, G. Torri, and G. Miserocki, Forces Deforming the Rib Cage, *Respir. Physiol.,* vol. 2, p. 105, 1966.
13. E. Lysell, Motion in the Cervical Spine, *Acta Orthop. Scand. Suppl.* vol. 123, 1969.
14. M. M. Panjabi, R. A. Brand, and A. A. White, Mechanical Properties of the Human Thoracic Spine: as Shown by Three-Dimensional Load-Displacement Curves, *J. Bone Jt. Surg.,* vol. 58A, p. 642, 1976.
15. C. Hirsch and A. Nachemson, A New Observation on the Mechanical Behavior of Lumbar Discs, *Acta Orthop. Scand.,* vol 23, p. 254, 1954.
16. S. D. Rolander, Motion of the Lumbar Spine with Special Reference to the Stabilizing Effect of Posterior Fusion, *Acta. Orthop. Scand. Suppl.,* vol. 90, 1966.
17. M. H. Berkson, A. Nachemson, and A. B. Schultz, Mechanical Properties of Human Lumbar Spine Motion Segments. Part II: Responses in Compression and Shear; Influence of Gross Morphology, *J. Biomech. Eng.* (in press).
18. H. S. Lin, U. K. Liu, and K. H. Adams, Mechanical Response of the Lumbar Intervertebral Joint under Physiological Loading, *J. Bone Jt. Surg.,* vol. 60A, p. 41, 1978.
19. K. Y. Liu, G. Ray, and C. Hirsch, The Resistance of the Lumbar Spine to Direct Shear, *Orthop. Clin. N. Am.,* vol. 6, p. 33, 1975.
20. K. Markolf, Deformation of the Thoracolumbar Intervertebral Joint in Response to External Loads: A Biomechanical Study Using Autopsy Material, *J. Bone Jt. Surg.,* vol. 54A, p. 511, 1972.
21. A. B. Schultz, D. N. Warwick, M. H. Berkson, and A. L. Nachemson, Mechanical Properties of Human Lumbar Spine Motion Segments. Part I: Responses in Flexion, Extension, Lateral Bending and Torsion, *J. Biomech. Eng.* (in press).
22. A. L. Nachemson, A. B. Schultz, and M. H. Berkson, Mechanical Properties of Human Lumbar Spine Motion Segments, *Spine,* vol. 4, p. 1, 1979.
23. J. H. Moe, R. B. Winter, D. S. Bradford, and J. E. Lonstein, Scoliosis and Other Spinal Deformities, Saunders, Philadelphia, 1978.
24. J. Wolff, Über die innere Architecture der Knochen und ihre Bedeutung für die Frage von Knochenwachstum, *Virchows Arch. A,* vol. 50, p. 589, 1870.
25. C. Heuter, Anatomische Studien an den Extremitaten Gelenken neugeborener und erwachsener. *Virchows Arch. A,* vol. 25, p. 575, 1862.
26. R. Volkmann, Chirurgische Erfahrungen ueber Knochenverbiegungen und Knochenwachstum, *Arch. Pathol. Anat.,* vol. 24, p. 512, 1862.
27. A. R. Shands and H. B. Eisberg, The Incidence of Scoliosis in the State of Delaware, *J. Bone Jt. Surg.,* vol. 37A, pp. 1243–1248, 1955.
28. W. J. Kane and J. H. Moe, A Scoliosis-Prevalence Survey in Minnesota, *Clin. Orthop.,* vol. 69, pp. 216–218, 1970.
29. J. E. Lonstein, Screening for Spine Deformities in Minnesota Schools, *Clin. Orthop.,* vol. 126, p. 33, 1977.
30. E. J. Rogala, D. S. Drummond, and J. Gurr, Scoliosis: Incidence and Natural History. A Prospective Epidemiological Study, *J. Bone Jt. Surg.,* vol. 60A, p. 173, 1978.

31. I. V. Ponseti, V. Pedrini, R. Wynne-Davies, and G. Duval-Beaupere, Pathogenesis of Scoliosis, *Clin. Orthop.*, vol. 120, p. 268, 1976.
32. H. R. Cowell, J. N. Hall, and G. D. MacEwen, Genetic Aspects of Idiopathic Scoliosis, *Clin. Orthop.*, vol. 86, pp. 121-131, 1972.
33. E. Riseborough and R. Wynne-Davies, A Genetic Survey of Idiopathic Scoliosis in Boston, Massachusetts, *J. Bone Jt. Surg.*, vol. 55A, pp. 974-982, 1973.
34. R. Wynne-Davies, Familial Idiopathic Scoliosis, A Family Survey, *J. Bone Jt. Surg.*, vol. 50B, pp. 24-30, 1968.
35. D. Collis and I. Ponseti, Long-term follow-up of Patients with Idiopathic Scoliosis Not Treated Surgically, *J. Bone Jt. Surg.*, vol. 51A, pp. 425-445, 1969.
36. A. L. Nachemson, A Long-Term Follow-up Study on Non-Treated Scoliosis, *Acta Orthop. Scand.*,, vol. 39, pp. 466-476, 1968.
37. U. Nilsonne and K. Lundgren, Long Term Prognosis in Idiopathic Scoliosis, *Acta Orthop. Scand.*, vol. 39, p. 456, 1968.
38. R. Wynne-Davies, Genetic and Other Factors in the Aetiology of Scoliosis, unpublished thesis, University of Edinburgh, 1973.
39. A. L. Nachemson, Terapeutiská Framsteg inom Skoliosomrodet, *Lakartidningen*, vol. 73, pp. 953-961, 1976.
40. G. D. MacEwen, Experimental Scoliosis, in P. A. Zorab (ed.), "Proceedings of a Second Symposium on Scoliosis. Causation," Livingstone, Edinburgh, 1968.
41. A. L. Nachemson and T. Sahlstrand, Etiologic Factors in Adolescent Idiopathic Scoliosis, *Spine*, vol. 2, p. 176, 1977.
42. A. Langenskiold, A Summary of 16 Years Experimental Research on the Pathogenesis of Scoliosis, in P. Zorab (ed.), "Scoliosis and Muscle," chap. 19, pp. 163-171, Heinemann, London, 1974.
43. A. Langenskiold and J. E. Michelsson, The Pathogensis of Experimental Progressive Scoliosis, *Acta Orthop. Scand. Suppl.*, vol. 59, pp. 1-26, 1962.
44. J. Michelsson, The Development of Spinal Deformity in Experimental Scoliosis, *Acta Orthop. Scand. Suppl.*, vol. 81, 1965.
45. R. Roaf, The Late Results of Unilateral Growth Arrest of the Spine for Scoliosis, *Acta Orthop. Scand.*, vol. 33, p. 393, 1958.
46. S. Wilner, Factors Contributing to Structural Scoliosis, Studentlitteratur, University of Lund, 1972.
47. S. Willner, A Study of Height, Weight, and Menarche in Girls with Idiopathic Structural Scoliosis, *Acta Orthop. Scand.*, vol. 46, pp. 71-83, 1975.
48. A. Nordwall and S. Willner, A Study of Skeletal Age and Height in Girls with Idiopathic Scoliosis, *Clin Orthop.*, vol. 110, pp. 6-10, 1975.
49. E. Agostini, P. Scalella, and D. Fabris, Indagini sull 'escrezione di idrossipolina totale in pazienti affeti dia scoliosis, *Clin. Ortop.*, vol. 25, p. 205, 1974.
50. T. Y. Balaba, Some Biochemical Aspects of Scoliosis and Their Pathogenetic Significance, *Reconstr. Surg. Traumatol.*, vol. 13, pp. 191-209, 1972.
51. P. F. Benson, Hydroxyproline Excretion in Idiopathic, Congenital and Paralytic Scoliosis, *Arch. Dis. Child.*, vol. 47, p. 476, 1972.
52. M. J. O. Francis, M. C. Sanderson, and R. Smith, Skin Collagen in Idiopathic Adolescent Scoliosis and Marfans, *Clin. Sci. Mol. Med.*, vol. 51, p. 467, 1976.
53. P. A. Zorab, Normal Creatinine and Hydroxyproline Excretion in Young Persons, *Lancet*, vol. 2, pp. 1164-1165, 1969.
54. P. A. Zorab, Urinary Total Hydroxyproline Excretion in Normal Scoliosis Children, pp 112-116 in "Scoliosis and Growth," Churchill Livingstone, Edinburgh, 1971.
55. P. A. Zorab, S. Clark, Y. Cotrel, and A. Harrison, Bone Collagen Turnover in Idiopathic Scoliosis Estimated from Total Hydrozyproline Excretion, *Arch. Dis. Child.*, vol. 46, p. 828, 1971.

56. M. W. Fidler and R. L. Jowett, Muscle Imbalance in the Aetiology of Scoliosis, *J. Bone Jt. Surg.*, vol. 58B, pp. 200-201, 1976.
57. M. W. Fidler, R. L. Jowett, and J. D. G. Troup, Histochemical Study of the Function of Miltifidus on Scoliosis, in "Scoliosis and Muscle," chap. 22, pp. 184-192, Heinemann, London, 1974.
58. S. Hoppenfeld, Histochemical Findings in Paraspinal Muscles of Patients with Idiopathic Scoliosis in "Scoliosis and Muscle," chap. 12, pp. 113-114, Heinemann, London, 1974.
59. G. S. G. Spencer, Muscle and Enzyme Staining in Scoliosis, in "Scoliosis and Muscle," chap. 11, pp. 103-112, Heinemann, London, 1974.
60. P. Tsairis, A Histochemical Study of Paraspinal Muscles in Idiopathic Scoliosis, in "Scoliosis and Muscle," chap. 13, pp. 115-120, Heinemann, London, 1974.
61. R. Yarom, G. C. Robin, and R. Gorodetsky, X-Ray Fluorescence of Muscles in Scoliosis, *Spine*, vol. 3, p. 142, 1978.
62. R. Yarom and G. C. Robin, Studies of Spine and Peripheral Muscles from Patients with Scoliosis, *Spine*, vol. 4, p. 12, 1979.
63. N. K. Chin and A. C. Yau, Nerve Endings in Back Muscles of Patients with Genetic Scoliosis, *Orthop. Trans.*, vol. 2, p. 266, 1978.
64. J. B. Redford, T. R. Butterworth, and E. L. Clements, Use of Electromyography as a Prognostic Aid in the Management of Idiopathic Scoliosis, *Arch. Phys. Med. Rehabil.*, vol. 50, pp. 433-438, 1969.
65. Y. C. Wong, A. C. M. C. Yau, W. D. Low, N. K. Chin, and F. P. Lisowki, Ultrastructural Changes of Back Muscles of Idiopathic Scoliosis, *Spine*, vol. 2, p. 251, 1977.
66. K. Yamada and H. Yamamoto, Neuro-Muscular and Neuro-Humoral Approaches to the Etio Pathology of Idiopathic Scoliosis, presented at Japanese Scoliosis Society and Scoliosis Research Society Meeting, Kyoto, Japan, October, 1977.
67. K. Yamada, H. Yamamoto, T. Ikata, Y. Nakagawa, I. Kinoshita, A. Tezuka, and T. Tamura, A Neurological Approach to the Etiology and Treatment of Scoliosis, *J. Bone Jt. Surg.*, vol. 53A, p. 197, 1971.
68. Y. Yamauchi, H. Asaka, and E. Sakata, Scoliosis and Abnormal Occular Movement, presented at Scoliosis Research Society meeting, Hong Kong, October, 1977.
69. T. Sahlstrand, R. Örthengren, and A. Nachemson, Postural Equilibrium in Adolescent Idiopathic Scoliosis, *Acta. Orthop. Scand.*, vol. 49, p. 354, 1978.
70. R. Herman, J. Stuyck, H. Yamamoto, D. MacEwen, R. Maulucci, and B. Herr, Vestibular Functioning in Idiopathic Scoliosis, presented at the Annual Meeting of the Orthopedic Research Society, San Francisco, February, 1979.
71. P. R. Harrington, Instrumentation in Spine Instability Other than Scoliosis, *S. Afr. J. Surg.*, vol. 5, p. 7, 1969.
72. J. H. Moe and D. N. Kettleson, Analysis of Curve Pattern and Preliminary Results of Milwaukee Brace Treatment in 169 Patients, *J. Bone Jt. Surg.*, vol. 52A, p. 1509, 1970.
73. J. R. Cobb, Outline for the Study of Scoliosis, *Am Acad. Orthop. Surg. Lect.*, vol. 5, p. 261, 1948.
74. T. Thulbourne and R. Gillespie, The Rib Hump in Idiopathic Scoliosis, *J. Bone Jt. Surg.*, vol. 58B, p. 64, 1976.
75. C. J. Levine, N. J. Spielholz, and G. L. Engler, EMG Activity of Paravertebral Muscles in Progressive Idiopathic Scoliosis, paper presented at Annual Meeting, Scoliosis Research Society, Boston, September, 1978.
76. R. Waters and J. Morris, An in Vitro Study of Normal and Scoliotic Interspinous Ligaments, *J. Biomech.*, vol. 6, p. 343, 1973.
77. A. Nordwall, Mechanical Properties of Tendinous Structures on Patients with Idiopathic Scoliosis, *J. Bone Jt. Surg.*, vol. 56A, p. 443, 1974.
78. A. A. White, Analysis of the Mechanics of the Thoracic Spine in Man, *Acta Orthop. Scand. Suppl.*, vol. 127, 1969.

79. A. Arkin, The Mechanics of the Structural Changes on Scoliosis, *J. Bone Jt. Surg.*, vol. 31A, pp. 180–188, 1949.
80. E. Carey, Scoliosis—Etiology, Pathogenesis and Prevention of Experiment Rotary Lateral Curvature of the Spine, *J. Am. Med. Assoc.*, vol. 98, pp. 103–110, 1932.
81. O. Lindahl and E. Raeder, Mechanical Analysis of Forces Involved in Idiopathic Scoliosis, *Acta Orthop. Scand.*, vol. 32, p. 27, 1962.
82. R. Roaf, Rotative Movements of the Spine with Special Reference to Scoliosis, *J. Bone Jt. Surg.*, vol. 40B, pp. 312–332, 1958.
83. R. Roaf, The Basic Anatomy of Scoliosis, *J. Bone Jt. Surg.*, vol. 48B, p. 786, 1966.
84. E. Sommerville, Rotational Lordosis: The Development of the Single Curve, *J. Bone Jt. Surg.*, vol. 34B, pp. 421–427, 1952.
85. S. P. Rogers, Mechanics of Scoliosis, *Arch. Surg.*, vol. 26, p. 962, 1933.
86. T. Belytschko, T. Andriacchi, A. Schultz, and J. Galante, Analog Studies of Forces in Human Spine, *Comput. Tech. J. Biomech.*, vol. 6, p. 361, 1973.
87. M. M. Panjabi and A. A. White, A Mathematical Approach for Three Dimensional Analysis of the Mechanics of the Spine, *J. Biomech.*, vol. 4, p. 3, 1971.
88. A. B. Schultz, H. Larocca, J. Galante, and T. P. Andriacchi, A Study of Geometrical Relationships in Scoliosis Spines, *J. Biomech.*, vol. 5, p. 409, 1972.
89. S. Swank, J. E. Lonstein, J. H. Moe, R. B. Winter, and D. S. Bradford, Surgical Treatment of Adult Scoliosis, paper presented at Annual Meeting, Scoliosis Research Society, Boston, September, 1978.
90. A. B. Schultz and J. Galante, A Mathematical Model for the Study of Mechanics of Human Vertebral Column, *J. Biomech.*, vol. 3, pp. 405–416, 1970.
91. M. Vercauteren, Etiological and Pathological Approach to Idiopathic Scoliosis, *Acta Orthop. Belg.*, vol. 38, pp. 429–445, 1972.
92. A. A. White and M. M. Panjabi, Clinical Biomechanics of Scoliosis, *Clin. Orthop.*, vol. 118, p. 100, 1976.
93. R. A. Dickson and K. D. Leatherman, Cotrel Traction, Exercises, Casting in Treatment of Idiopathic Scoliosis, *Acta Orthop. Scand.*, vol. 49, p. 46, 1978.
94. Y. Cotrel, Traction in the Treatment of Vertebral Deformity, *J. Bone Jt. Surg.*, vol. 57B, p. 260, 1975.
95. R. N. Hensinger and G. D. MacEwen, Evaluation of the Cotrel Dynamic Spine Traction in the Treatment of Scoliosis, *Orthop. Rev.*, vol. 3, p. 27, 1974.
96. R. L. DeWald, Halo and Halo Hoop in Scoliosis Management, in Hugo A. Keim (ed.), "Third Annual Post-Graduate Course of the Management and Care of the Scoliosis Patient," New York Orthopedic Hospital, Columbia Presbyterian Medical Center, December, 1971.
97. R. L. DeWald, T. M. Mulcahy, and A. B. Schultz, Force Measurement Studies with the Halo-Hoop Apparatus in Scoliosis, *Orthop. Rev.*, vol. 2, no. 12, pp. 17–31, 1973.
98. R. L. DeWald and R. D. Ray, Skeletal Traction for the Treatment of Severe Scoliosis, *J. Bone Jt. Surg.*, vol. 52A, p. 233, 1970.
99. L. M. Letts, G. Palakar, and W. P. Bobechko, Operative Skeletal Traction in Scoliosis, *J. Bone Jt. Surg.*, vol. 57A, p. 616, 1975.
100. W. C. Pinto, Role of Traction in Preoperative Correction of Scoliosis, paper presented at Annual Meeting, Scoliosis Research Society, San Francisco, September, 1974.
101. P. L. Ramsey, J. Wickersham, H. Kingsbury, and D. Lou, Mechanical Analysis of Cotrel Traction in Idiopathic Scoliosis, *J. Bone Jt. Surg.*, vol. 58A, p. 157, 1976.
102. A. L. Nachemson and A. Nordwall, Effectiveness of the Operative Cotrel Traction for Correction of Idiopathic Scoliosis, *J. Bone Jt. Surg.*, vol. 59A, p. 504, 1977.
103. J. L. Cummine, J. E. Lonstein, J. H. Moe, R. B. Winter, and D. S. Bradford, Reconstructive Surgery for Scoliosis in the Adult, *J. Bone Jt. Surg.*, vol. 61A, p. 1151, 1979.
104. J. P. O'Brien, The Halo-Pelvic Apparatus, *Acta Orthop. Scand. suppl.*, vol. 163, 1975.

105. J. M. Carlson, Basic Mechanics of Orthotic Treatment of Pediatric Spine Deformity (submitted for publication).
106. R. L. Waters and J. M. Morris, Effects of the Spinal Support on the Electrical Activity of Muscles of the Trunk, *J. Bone Jt. Surg.*, vol. 52A, p. 51, 1970.
107. R. B. Winter and J. M. Carlson, Modern Orthotics for Spinal Deformities, *Clin. Orthop.*, vol. 126, p. 5, 1977.
108. W. P. Blount, A. C. Schmidt, D. D. Keever, and E. T. Leonard, The Milwaukee Brace in the Operative Treatment of Scoliosis, *J. Bone Jt. Surg.*, vol. 40A, p. 511, 1958.
109. W. P. Blount and J. H. Moe, "The Milwaukee Brace," Williams and Wilkins, Baltimore, 1973.
110. R. Cockrell and J. Risser, Plastic Body Jacket in the Treatment of Scoliosis, exhibit at Annual Meeting, American Academy of Orthopedic Surgery, Las Vegas, 1973.
111. J. Murphy, The Lexan Jacket in the Conservative Treatment of Scoliosis, a Comparison of Results Obtained with the Milwaukee Brace, *J. Bone Jt. Surg.*, vol. 57A, p. 136, 1975.
112. H. L. Shufflebarger and R. P. Keiser, Milwaukee Brace Treatment of Idiopathic Scoliosis: A Review of One Hundred and Twenty-Three Completed Cases, *Clin. Orthop.*, vol 118, p. 19, 1976.
113. W. P. Blount and D. Mellencamp, Long Term Results of Idiopathic Scoliosis Treated with the Milwaukee Brace, *Clin. Orthop.*, vol. 126, p. 47, 1977.
114. W. Carr, J. H. Moe, R. B. Winter, J. E. Lonstein, and D. S. Bradford, Long Term Follow-up of Patients Treated with the Milwaukee Brace, *Orthop. Trans.*, vol. 2, p. 279, 1978.
115. T. P. Andriacchi, A. B. Schultz, T. B. Belytschko, and R. L. DeWald, Milwaukee Brace Correction of Idiopathic Scoliosis, *J. Bone Jt. Surg.*, vol. 58A, p. 806, 1976.
116. A. L. Nachemson and J. M. Morris, In Vivo Measurements of Intra-Discal Pressure, *J. Bone Jt. Surg.*, vol. 46A, p. 1077, 1964.
117. M. Lindh, The Effect of Sagittal Curve Changes on Brace Correction of Idiopathic Scoliosis (submitted for publication).
118. G. V. B. Cochran and T. R. Waugh, The External Forces in Correction of Idiopathic Scoliosis, *Proc. Scoliosis Res. Soc., J. Bone Jt. Surg.*, vol. 51A, p. 201, 1969.
119. J. Galante, A. Schultz, R. L. DeWald, and R. D. Ray, Forces Acting in the Milwaukee Brace of Patients Undergoing Treatment for Idiopathic Scoliosis, *J. Bone Jt. Surg.*, vol. 52A, p. 498, 1970.
120. T. Mulcahy, J. Galante, R. DeWald, A. Schultz, and J. C. Hunter, A Follow-up Study of Forces Acting on the Milwaukee Brace on Patients Undergoing Treatment for Idiopathic Scoliosis, *Clin. Orthop.*, vol. 93, p. 53, 1973.
121. A. B. Schultz and J. O. Galante, Measurement of Forces Exerted in the Correction of Idiopathic Scoliosis Using Three-Component Dynamometers, *Exp. Mech.*, vol. 9, p. 419, 1969.
122. R. G. Alexander, The Effects on Tooth Position and Maxillofacial Vertical Growth During Treatment of Scoliosis with the Milwaukee Brace, *Am. J. Orthod.*, vol. 52, p. 161, 1966.
123. P. B. Caldwell, An Evaluation of the Modified Milwaukee Brace, M. S. D. thesis, University of Baylor Dental College, 1972.
124. C. C. Howard, A Preliminary Report of Infraocclusion of the Molars and Premolars Produced by Orthopaedic Treatment of Scoliosis, *Int. J. Orthod.*, vol. 12, p. 434, 1926.
125. W. R. Logan, The Effect of the Milwaukee Brace on the Developing Dentition, *Dent. Pract.*, vol. 12, p. 447, 1962.
126. R. O. Northway, R. G. Alexander, and M. L. Riolo, A Cephalometric Evaluation of the Old Milwaukee Brace and the Modified Milwaukee Brace in Relation to the Normal Growing Child, *Am. J. Orthod.*, vol. 65, p. 341, 1974.
127. A. L. Nachemson and G. Elfstrom, Intravital Wireless Telemetry of Axial Forces in Harrington Distraction Rods in Patients with Idiopathic Scoliosis, *J. Bone Jt. Surg.*, vol. 53A, p. 445, 1971.

128. T. Andriacchi, A. Schultz, T. Belytschko, and R. DeWald, Milwaukee Brace Correction of Idiopathic Scoliosis; a Biomechanical Analysis, *J. Bone Jt. Surg.*, vol. 57A, p. 582, 1975.

129. J. Moe and R. Gustilo, Treatment of Scoliosis: Results in 196 Patients Treated by Cast Correction and Fusion, *J. Bone Jt. Surg.*, vol. 46A, pp. 293–312, 1964.

130. P. R. Harrington, Technical Details in Relation to the Successful Use of Instrumentation in Scoliosis, *Orthop. Clin. No. Am.*, vol. 3, p. 49, 1972.

131. P. R. Harrington and J. H. Dickson, The Development and Further Prospects of Internal Fixation of the Spine, *Isr. J. Med. Sci.*, vol. 9, pp. 773–778, 1973.

132. G. W. D. Armstrong and S. H. G. Connock, A Transverse Loading System Applied to a Modified Harrington Instrumentation, *Clin. Orthop.*, vol. 108, pp. 70–75, 1975.

133. S. H. G. Connock and G. W. D. Armstrong, A Transverse Loading System Applied to a Modified Harrington Instrumentation, *J. Bone Jt. Surg.*, vol. 53A, p. 194, 1971.

134. G. Shen, L. Gilbertson, W. D. Erwin, J. H. Dickson, and P. R. Harrington, Biomechanical Aspects of Harrington Instrumentation, paper presented at the Annual Meeting, Scoliosis Research Society, Boston, September, 1978.

135. T. R. Waugh, Intravital Measurements during Instrument Correction of Idiopathic Scoliosis, *Acta Orthop. Scand. Suppl.*, vol. 93, pp. 1–87, 1966.

136. E. D. Dawson and L. Herron, Use of Methyl methacrylate in Spinal Instrumentation, *Orthop. Trans.*, vol. 2, p. 271, 1978.

137. T. R. Waugh, Biomechanical Basis for Utilization of Methyl methacrylate Treatment of Scoliosis, *J. Bone Jt. Surg.*, vol. 53A, p. 194, 1971.

138. G. Elfstrom and A. Nachemson, Telemetry Recordings of Forces in Harrington Distraction Rod–A Method for Increasing Safety in the Operative Treatment of the Scoliosis Patient, *Clin. Orthop.*, vol. 93, p. 158, 1973.

139. A. B. Schultz and C. Hirsch, Mechanical Analysis of Harrington Rod Correction of Idiopathic Scoliosis, *J. Bone Jt. Surg.*, vol. 55A, pp. 983–992, 1973.

140. A. B. Schultz and C. Hirsch, Mechanical Analysis Techniques for Improved Correction of Idiopathic Scoliosis, *Clin. Orthop.*, vol. 100, p. 66, 1974.

141. A. Nordwall, Studies in Idiopathic Scoliosis Relevant to Etiology, Conservative and Operative Reaction to Treatment, *Acta Orthop. Scand. Suppl.*, vol. 150, pp. 1–78, 1973.

142. J. E. Hall and R. Gillespie, Idiopathic Scoliosis Treatment by Harrington Rod and Spine Fusion, *J. Bone Jt. Surg.*, vol. 53A, p. 198, 1971.

143. J. L. Briard, personal communication, 1979.

144. E. R. Luque and A. Cardoso, Segmental Correction of Scoliosis with Rigid Internal Fixation, *Orthop. Trans.*, vol. 1, p. 136, 1977.

145. A. Dwyer, N. Newton, and A. Sherwood, An Anterior Approach to Scoliosis. A Preliminary Report, *Clin. Orthop.*, vol. 62, p. 192, 1969.

146. L. Micheli and J. E. Hall, Use of Modified Dwyer Instrumentation in Anterior Stabilization of the Spine, *Orthop. Trans.*, vol. 2, p. 270, 1978.

147. H. K. Dunn, Internal Fixation of the Spine, New Inplant, paper presented at Annual Meeting, Scoliosis Research Society, Boston, September, 1978.

148. H. K. Dunn, New Instrumentation for Anterior Spine Stabilization, *Orthop. Trans.*, vol. 2, p. 248, 1978.

149. H. K. Dunn and K. E. Bolstad, Fixation of Dwyer in Scoliosis, paper presented at the Annual Meeting, Scoliosis Research Society, San Francisco, September, 1974.

150. F. D. Shapiro, A. P. Dwyer, and D. Rowell, Telemetric Monitoring of Cable Tensions following Dwyer Spinal Instrumentation in Dogs, *Spine*, vol. 3, p. 213, 1978.

151. R. B. Winter, Combined Dwyer and Harrington Instrumentation and Fusion in the Treatment of Selected Patients with Painful Idiopathic Scoliosis, *Spine*, vol. 3, p. 135, 1978.

152. P. Stagnara, presidential address, presented at Annual Meeting, Scoliosis Research Society, Boston, September, 1978.

153. J. E. Lonstein, J. H. Moe, R. B. Winter, S. Chou, and W. Pinto, Cord Compression due to Spinal Deformity, *Spine*, vol. 5, p. 331, 1980.

154. P. Stagnara, J. Gounod, A. Campo-Paysaa, C. Vauzelle, R. Fauchet, D. Maxoyer, B. Biot, C. Poncet, J. C. DeMauroy, and B. Villard, Arthodeses trans-thoraciques dans le traitement des cyphoses et des cyphoscoliosis, *Int. Orthop.*, vol. 1, pp. 199-214, 1977.

155. A. A. White, M. M. Panjabi, and C. L. Thomas, The Clinical Biomechanics of Kyphotic Deformities, *Clin. Orthop.*, vol. 128, p. 8, 1977.

156. K. B. Ahmed, D. S. Bradford, J. H. Moe, R. B. Winter, and J. E. Lonstein, Anterior Spine Surgery in the Treatment of Kyphotic Spine Deformity, *Orthop. Trans.*, vol. 1, p. 135, 1977.

157. D. S. Bradford, J. H. Moe, F. J. Montalvo, and R. B. Winter, Scheuermann's Kyphosis. Results of Surgical Treatment by Posterior Spine Arthrodesis in Twenty-Two Patients, *J. Bone Jt. Surg.*, vol. 57A, p. 439, 1975.

158. H. S. Y. Fang, G. B. Ong, and A. R. Hodgson, Anterior Spinal Fusion. The Operative Approaches, *Clin. Orthop.*, vol. 35, p. 16, 1964.

159. R. B. Winter, J. H. Moe, and J. F. Wang, Congenital Kyphosis. Its Natural History and Treatment as Observed in a Study of One Hundred Thirty Patients, *J. Bone Jt. Surg.*, vol. 55A, p. 223, 1973.

160. R. B. Winter and J. E. Hall, Kyphosis in Childhood and Adolescence, *Spine*, vol. 3, p. 285, 1978.

161. W. C. Pinto, O. Avanzi, and R. B. Winter, An Anterior Distractor for the Intraoperative Correction of Angular Kyphosis, *Spine*, vol. 3, p. 309, 1978.

162. A. Gruca, Protocol of the 41st Congress of Indian Orthopedics and Trauma, Bologna, 1956.

163. M. Weiss, Dynamic Spine Allopasty after Fracture and Spinal Cord Injury, *Clin. Orthop.*, vol. 112, p. 150, 1975.

164. E. S. Stauffer and J. L. Neil, Biomechanical Analysis of Structural Stability of Internal Fixation in Fractures of the Thoracolumbar Spine, *Clin. Orthop.*, vol. 112, p. 159, 1975.

165. P. R. Meyer, M. Pinzur, E. Lautenschlasger, and W. R. Dobozi, Measurement of Internal Fixation Device Support–Thoracic Lumbar Spine, scientific exhibit at American Academy of Orthopedic Surgery, Las Vegas, 1977.

166. M. M. Panjabi and A. A. White, Biomechanical Analysis of Gruca-Weiss and Harrington Instrumentation on the Treatment of Kyphosis (to be published).

167. A. A. White, R. M. Johnson, M. M. Panjabi, and W. O. Southwick, Biomechanical Analysis of Clinical Stability in the Cervical Spine, *Clin. Orthop.*, vol. 109, p. 85, 1975.

168. A. A. White, M. M. Panjabi, S. Saha, and W. O. Southwick, Biomechanics of the Axially Loaded Cervical Spine: Development of a Safe Clinical Test for Ruptured Cervical Ligaments, *J. Bone Jt. Surg.*, vol. 57A, p. 582, 1975.

169. A. A. White, W. O. Southwick, and M. M. Panjabi, Clinical Instability on the Lower Cervical Spine, *Spine*, vol. 1, p. 15, 1976.

170. M. M. Panjabi, A. A. White, and R. M. Johnson, Cervical Spine Mechanics as a Function of Transection of Components, *J. Biomech.*, vol. 8, p. 327, 1975.

171. A. A. White and C. Hirsch, The Significance of the Vertebral Posterior Elements in the Mechanics of the Thoracic Spine, *Clin. Orthop.*, vol. 81, p. 2, 1971.

172. A. A. White, M. M. Panjabi, and J. N. Hausfeld, A Systematic Approach to the Problem of Clinical Stability in the Thoracic Spine, paper presented at Annual Meeting, Scoliosis Research Society, Boston, September, 1978.

173. G. M. Bedbrook, Use and Disuse of Surgery in Lumbo-Dorsal Fractures, *J. West. Pac. Orthop. Assoc.*, vol. 6, pp. 5-26, 1969.

174. J. R. Flesch, L. L. Leider, D. L. Erickson, S. N. Chou, and D. S. Bradford, Harrington Instrumentation and Spine Fusion for Thoracic and Lumbar Spine Fractures, *J. Bone Jt. Surg.*, vol. 59A, p. 143, 1977.

175. L. Guttmann, Surgical Aspects of the Treatment of Traumatic Paraplegia, *J. Bone Jt. Surg.*, vol. 31B, p. 339, 1949.

176. L. Guttmann, Initial Treatment of Traumantic Paraplegia, *Proc. R. Soc. Med.*, vol. 47, pp. 1103-1109, 1954.

177. L. Guttmann, Spinal Deformities in Traumatic Paraplegia and Tetraplegia Following Surgical Procedure, *Paraplegia*, vol. 7, pp. 38-58, 1969.

178. H. H. Gosch, E. Gooding, and R. C. Schneider, An Experimental Study of Cervical Spine and Cord Injuries, *J. Trauma*, vol. 12, p. 570, 1972.

179. R. P. Kelly and T. E. Whitesides, Jr., Treatment of Lumbodorsal Fracture Dislocations, *Ann. Surg.*, vol. 167, pp. 705-717, 1968.

180. B. Malcolm, D. S. Bradford, R. B. Winter, and S. Chou, Late Post-Traumatic Kyphotic Deformity of the Spine, paper presented at Annual Meeting, Scoliosis Research Soceity, Boston, Septermber, 1978.

181. F. W. Holdsworth, Fractures, Dislocations and Fracture Dislocations of the Spine, *J. Bone Jt. Surg.*, vol. 45B, p. 6, 1963.

182. H. B. Griffith, J. R. W. Cleave, and R. G. Taylor, Changing Patterns of Fracture in the Dorsal and Lumbar Spine, *Br. Med. J.*, vol. 1, p. 891, 1966.

183. H. F. Farfan, J. W. Cossette, H. G. Robertson, R. V. Wells, and H. Kraus, The Effects of Torsion on the Lumbar Intervertebral Joints; the Role of Torsion in the Production of Disc Regeneration, *J. Bone Jt. Surg.*, vol. 52A, p. 468, 1970.

184. G. O. Chance, Note on a Type of Flexion Fracture of the Spine, *Br. J. Radiol.*, vol. 21, p. 452, 1948.

185. W. Rennie and N. Mitchell, Flexion Distraction Fractures of the Thoracolumbar Spine, *J. Bone Jt. Surg.*, vol. 55A, pp. 386-390, 1973.

186. H. Kaufer, The Thoracolumbar Spine, in A. C. Rockwood, Jr., and D. P. Green (eds.), "Fractures," Lippincott, Philadelphia, 1972.

187. H. Kaufer and J. T. Hayes, Lumbar Fracture-Dislocation: A Study of 21 Cases, *J. Bone Jt. Surg.*, vol. 48A, pp. 712-730, 1966.

188. N. Gotten, Survey of 100 Cases of Whiplash Injuries after Settlement of Litigation, *J. Am. Med. Assoc.*, vol. 162, p. 865, 1956.

189. I. MacNab, Acceleration Injuries of the Cervical Spine, *J. Bone Jt. Surg.*, vol. 46A, p. 1797, 1964.

190. D. K. Evans, Fractures and Dislocation of the Spine, in R. Furlong (ed.), "Clinical Surgery," vol. 12, Butterworth, Washington, D.C., 1966.

191. R. Braakman and L. Penning, Mechanisms of Injury to the Cervical Cord, *Int. J. Paraplegia*, vol. 10, p. 314, 1973.

192. T. E. Whitesides and S. G. A. Shah, On the Management of Unstable Fractures of the Thoracolumbar Spine; Rationale for Use of Anterior Decompression and Fusion and Posterior Stabilization, *Spine*, vol. 1, p. 99, 1976.

193. H. H. Bohlman, Traumatic Fractures of the Upper Thoracic Spine with Paraplegia, *J. Bone Jt. Surg.*, vol. 56A, p. 1299, 1974.

194. J. H. Dickson, P. R. Harrington, and W. D. Erwin, Harrington Instrumentation in the Fractured Unstable Thoracic and Lumbar Spine, *Tex. Med.*, vol. 69, p. 91, 1973.

195. T. H. Morgan, G. W. Wharton, and G. N. Austin, The Results of Laminectomy on Patients with Incomplete Spinal Cord Injuries, *J. Bone Jt. Surg.*, vol. 52A, p. 822, 1970.

196. H. V Pelosof and P. R. Harrington, Progressive Quadriplegia in a Paraplegia Patient, *Arch. Phys. Med. Rehabil.*, vol. 54, pp. 530-532, 1973.

197. J. B. Roberts and P. H. Curtiss, Stability of the Thoracic and Lumbar Spine in Traumatic Paraplegia following Fracture or Fracture-Dislocation, *J. Bone Jt. Surg.*, vol. 52A, pp. 1115-1130, 1970.

198. D. S. Bradford and R. C. Thompson, Fractures and Dislocation of the Spine, Indications for Surgical Intervention, *Minn. Med.*, vol. 58, p. 711, 1976.

199. J. H. Dickson, P. R. Harrington, and W. D. Erwin, Reduction and Stabilization of the Severely Fractured Spine Using Harrington Instrumentation, paper presented at Annual Meeting, Scoliosis Research Society, Ottawa, September, 1976.

200. J. Lewis and B. McKibben, The Treatment of Unstable Fracture-Dislocations of the Thoraco-Lumbar Spine Accompanied by Paraplegia, *J. Bone Jt. Surg.*, vol. 56B, p. 603, 1974.

201. L. Guttmann, "Initial Treatment of Traumatic Paraplegia and Tetraplegia Spinal Injuries," Morrison and Gibb, London, 1963.

202. L. Guttmann, Management of the Spinal Fractures, in "Spinal Cord Injuries, Comprehensive Management and Research," Blackwell, Oxford, 1973.

203. H. L. Frankel, D. O. Hancock, G. Hyslop, J. Melzak, L. S. Michaelis, G. H. Ungar, J. D. S. Vernon, and J. J. Walsh, The Value of Postural Reduction in the Initial Management of Closed Injuries of the Spine with Paraplegia and Tetraplegia, *Paraplegia*, vol. 7, p. 179, 1969.

204. R. Bailey, Fractures and Dislocations of the Cervical Spine: Orthopedic and Neuro-Surgical Aspects, *Postgrad. Med.*, vol. 35, p. 588, 1964.

205. J. Bohler, Operative Treatment of Fractures of the Dorsal and Lumbar Spine, *J. Trauma*, vol. 10, p. 1119, 1970.

206. L. Bohler, "The Treatment of Fractures," 5th ed., vol. 1, Grune and Stratton, New York, 1956.

207. D. S. Bradford, The Role of Internal Fixation and Spine Fusion in Thoracic and Lumbar Spine Fractures, in S. N. Chou and E. L. Seljeskog (eds.), "Spinal Deformities and Neurological Dysfunction," Raven, New York, 1977.

208. D. S. Bradford, B. A. Akbarnia, R. B. Winter, and E. L. Seljeskog, Surgical Stabilization of Fracture and Fracture Dislocation of the Spine, *Spine*, vol. 2, p. 185, 1977.

209. A. A. Katznelson, Stabilization of the Spine in Traumatic Paraplegia, *Paraplegia*, vol. 6, pp. 33–37, 1969.

210. M. Weiss, Parallel Springs Used to Control Fractures of the Spine, *Int. Orthop.*, vol. 1, p. 275, 1978.

211. D. L. Erickson, L. L. Leider, and W. E. Brown, One-Stage Decompression Stabilization for Thoracolumbar Fracture, *Spine*, vol. 2, p. 53, 1977.

212. R. T. Woodburne, "Essentials of Human Anatomy," Oxford, New York, 1978.

213. T. P. Andriacchi, A. B. Schultz, T. B. Belytschko, and O. J. Galante, A Model for Studies of Mechanical Interactions between the Human Spine and Rib Cage, *J. Biomech.*, vol. 7, p. 497, 1974.

214. F. R. Convery, M. A. Minteer, R. W. Smith, and S. M. Emerson, Fracture Dislocation of the Dorsal-Lumbar Spine, *Spine*, vol. 3, p. 160, 1978.

215. M. Hohl, Soft-Tissue Injuries of the Neck in Automobile Accidents. Factors Influencing Prognosis, *J. Bone Jt. Surg.*, vol. 56A, p. 1675, 1974.

216. M. M. Panjabi, Three-Dimensional Mathematical Model of the Human Spine Structure, *J. Biomech.*, vol. 6, p. 671, 1973.

217. M. M. Panjabi, W. Hooper, A. A. White, and J. K. Kristaps, Posterior Spine Stabilization with Methyl methacrylate, *Spine*, vol. 2, p. 241, 1977.

218. A. B. Schultz, A Biomechanical View of Scoliosis, *Spine*, vol. 1, p. 162, 1976.

219. K. Zielke and B. Pellin, Electronic Pressure Gauge for Harrington Instrumentation, *Z. Orthop.*, vol. 2, pp. 229–232, 1973.

ELEVEN

A BIOMECHANICAL BASIS
FOR TREATMENT OF INJURIES
OF THE DORSOLUMBAR SPINE

Rae R. Jacobs
Dhanjoo N. Ghista

Compression usually causes fracture of the vertebral body, which can be reduced by distraction; being cancellous, the bone heals rapidly. Tension usually dislocates the posterior joints by rupturing the ligamentous complex. If the anterior bone is sufficiently intact to resist compressive loads, a compression system is suitable; otherwise, distraction rods contoured to resist bending are necessary. Spinal fusion is required because ligamentous healing is not sufficiently strong.

Flexion injuries result in combinations of varying degrees of disruption of the posterior ligamentous complex and fracture of the vertebral bodies. Rotational injury usually fractures the facet joints. Both the $\frac{1}{4}$-in distraction rods and the $\frac{3}{16}$-in compression system adequately control rotational instability. Fusion is necessary as these comminuted fractures destroy the facet joints. Only through an understanding of mechanics can a rational stabilization technique be developed.

The quantitative biomechanical approach to dorsolumbar injury presented in this chapter (1) analyzes the forces applied to the spine—especially those exerted on the structures that have failed, (2) classifies the types of injuries, and (3) provides the basis for injury reduction modalities and stabilization modes and devices by computation of the stresses and forces in the spinal structures at the injury site as well as in the injury reduction-stabilization devices.

1 INTRODUCTION

Although nonoperative treatment of dorsolumbar spine injuries has been the standard around the world, surgery offers two major advantages. The first is decompression of the neurologic structures with possible greater neurologic recovery in partial lesions. The historical approach has been to perform a laminectomy. In this procedure bone posterior to the neurologic structures is removed, but frequently the offending lesion is an anterior bone fragment from a vertebral body fracture. In addition, because of flexion angulation, the neurologic structures are stretched over the anterior deformity. Partial stability is afforded by the stretched posterior structures. Thus, laminectomy would, by removal of this stabilizing factor, cause spinal instability. It is more appropriate to obtain neurologic decompression by reduction of the fracture dislocation. Fair alignment of angular deformity can easily be obtained by closed methods, but open reduction allows anatomical correction of both angular and translational deformity. Also, any remaining fragments of bone or disk material in the canal can be removed through a posterolateral approach. The instrumentation used for reduction of the injury should also provide sufficient stability for immediate ambulation—the second advantage of surgical management.

2 BIOMECHANICAL APPROACH

Only by a mechanical analysis of the forces applied to the spine can one determine what structures have been injured and how their functions should be replaced by spinal instrumentation (Table 1). An axial-distraction-type injury results in facet capsule disruption. Axial compressive loading of the spine results in vertebral body fracture. Flexion injury results in a bending force being applied to the spine, with compressive loading anteriorly and tensile loading posteriorly. The result is a combination of varying degrees of vertebral body fracture and facet capsule disruption. Rotational forces lead to disruption of the facet complex including both fracture and ligamentous disruption. Most injuries involve a combination of forces. A careful history and examination usually suggest the type of force applied to the spine and the resultant structural injury. A patient in an automobile with the seat belt applied is likely to have a distraction type of injury, whereas a person who falls from a height, landing in the sitting position or on the feet, is more likely to have

Table 1 Mechanics of spinal injury

Applied force	Resulting failure
Axial distraction	Facet capsule disruption
Axial compression	Body fracture
Flexion	Facet capsule disruption ± body fracture
Rotation	Facet fracture

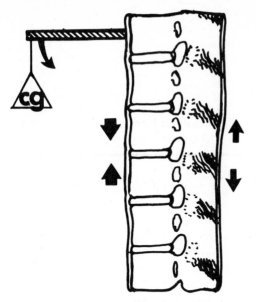

Figure 1 The center of gravity is located anterior to the spine and therefore imposes a flexion load. This results in compression of the vertebral bodies, which are anterior, and tension in the ligamentous complex, which is posterior. This basic principle is essential to understanding the nature of an injury and the selection of a stabilization technique.

an axial-compression-type injury. A person thrown from an automobile and landing on the shoulder, where there is usually an abrasion, most commonly has a combination flexion-rotation injury causing vertebral body fracture with facet fracture and capsular disruption. The extent of fracture can be determined by radiographs and tomograms. Posterior ligamentous injury may be apparent if there is widening between the spinous processes posteriorly, but a more consistent indication is the presence of pain, tenderness, swelling, and a gap between the spinous processes in the area of injury observable on physical examination. Frequently the deformity present on initial recumbent radiographs is far less than that at the time of injury, owing to spontaneous reduction. Extension injuries of the dorsolumbar spine are quite rare and will not be considered.

Roaf [1], in 1960, demonstrated that all spinal injuries can be reproduced by applying various combinations of forces to the spine, such as compression, flexion, rotation, and extension. Compressive forces are chiefly absorbed by the vertebral body, resulting in fracture. Rotational injury is the most common cause of posterior ligamentous disruption. Kelly and Whitesides [2] point out that the anterior column structures of the spine, the vertebral bodies, are under compressive loads; and the posterior structures, the ligamentous complex, are under tensile loads (Fig. 1). An understanding of this concept is basic to internal fixation of the spine. Only by analyzing the injury to determine if either or both of these structures is incompetent can a suitable form of internal fixation be selected.

We have divided our cases into four biomechanical types. Distraction injuries are those in which the bony elements have a single plane fracture, or there is only ligamentous disruption resulting in a dislocation. The flexion-distraction injury described by Grantham et al. [3] is a typical example resulting from seat-belt

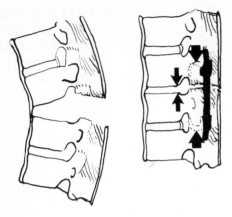

Figure 2 The simplest type of injury to understand mechanically is the flexion-distraction dislocation injury, which results in posterior ligamentous disruption and a single-plane fracture through the vertebral body or rupture through the disk space anteriorly. The anterior structures are sufficiently intact to withstand compressive loads, and therefore only the posterior structures need to be replaced. This is appropriately done with a Harrington compression apparatus for acute stabilization and bone grafting across the same area for permanent stability.

injuries. These injuries are amenable to a posterior compression fixation device that replaces the absent posterior ligamentous structures while the anterior bony elements withstand the compressive loads (Fig. 2).

Patients with anterior crushing of the vertebral body and total paraplegia are also amenable to posterior compression-type fixation because it is not necessary to reconstruct the normal anatomy if the neurologic structures are destroyed. In the paraplegic patient, the advantage of immobilizing only two or three spinal segments with a rigid compression system outweighs the theoretical advantage of anatomical reduction by the long Harrington distraction rods, which immobilize five to seven segments and are frequently less stable (Fig. 3). A compression system utilizes the tension band principle with bone carrying the anterior compressive stress and the implant carrying the posterior tensile stress, similar to a plate applied to the lateral aspect of the femur.

In burst fractures the entire vertebral body is disrupted and unable to withstand any compressive loads. There is also a fracture that may best be considered a potential burst fracture in which the entire vertebral body is involved, although there may not be displacement into the spinal canal. Widening of the pedicles indicates this type of fracture but is not always present. The Harrington distraction

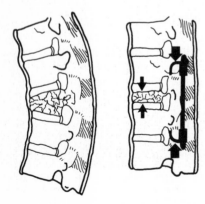

Figure 3 A fracture of the vertebral body with total paraplegia can be treated first by a posterior compression system correcting the angular deformity but not restoring vertebral height. The advantage is immobilization of only one or two segments of the spine instead of four to six as would be the result when using distraction rods; spinal mobility is important for the paraplegic patient.

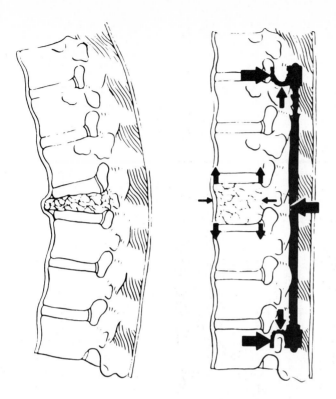

Figure 4 A burst fracture is one in which there is maximal compressive load and minimal flexion component resulting in complete fracturing of the entire vertebral body, usually with widening of the pedicles, but the posterior ligamentous complex remains intact. This injury is best treated by reestablishing vertebral body height using a Harrington distraction rod posteriorly. This rod, applied posterior to the structure that is to be distracted, must function as a three-point fixation device; therefore, it must have contact with the lamina at the area of injury. The ligamentous structures surrounding the bony fragments pull them into position when they are tensed to their anatomical length. The forces exerted by the rod on the spine are shown in the figure. Note the anteriorly directed force exerted by the rod on the vertebral column to resist flexion bending. Compared to the compression injury, there is a posterior displacement of the neutral axis (of a section through the crushed body) to almost coincide with the lamina edges. Thus, under flexion, these points are not displaced. However, under the action of the torso weight these points are displaced toward each other. Thus rod hooks would need to be placed to prevent this relative displacement. The required orientation of the rod hooks, to prevent this relative displacement of the points toward each other, calls for a distraction rod, as shown on the right.

rod lengthens the spine, thereby restoring vertebral body height and also supporting the weight of the upper half of the body (Fig. 4). The center of gravity of the body above the injury site and the ligaments connecting the two injured segments of the spine, being anterior to the laminae in the hooks, contribute to a flexion bending moment on the spine. Thus maintaining the patient in extension will both decrease the bending force and keep the laminae well-seated in the hooks.

The last category of injury is the fracture-dislocation combining both an anterior bony fracture and a posterior ligamentous injury (Fig. 5). In this case the vertebral body cannot withstand compressive loads; nor can the posterior structures withstand the tensile component of bending. These injuries must also be treated with a distracting beam-column to restore normal anatomy. The forces applied to the spine are totally resisted by the rod acting as a laterally loaded beam-column. As Stauffer and Nell [4] emphasized, an understanding of the principle of three-point fixation is essential to the proper use of the Harrington distraction rod in fracture treatment. In this injury, the rod functions as a beam-column, loaded by end-compressive forces and end-flexion moments (not shown in Fig. 5) caused by the eccentrically applied weight of the torso above the level of injury. Additionally, the spine exerts lateral bending forces on the rod; reciprocally the rod hooks pull posteriorly on the

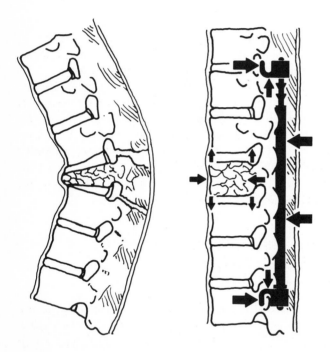

Figure 5 The fracture-dislocation group includes all those injuries in which there are both posterior ligamentous disruption and anterior vertebral body fracture. Thus there is no component of the spine able to withstand the stresses that must be transferred across the area of injury. Harrington distraction rods are also indicated in this injury. The rods must be applied in such a way as to obtain four-point bending, with the hooks at either end of the rod pulling the spine posteriorly, and the laminae on either side of the area of injury being pushed anteriorly by the central portion of the rod. The rod must be contoured to the desired normal shape of the spine in the area of injury. In the lumbar spine this requires the use of rods with a square end inferiorly, and similar type hooks with lordotic contouring of the rod. The square-ended rod is essential to prevent the rod from spinning around posteriorly and resulting in a kyphotic contour. Failure to contour the rods properly may result in distraction of the posterior portion of the spine without elevation of the vertebral body anteriorly, producing a flexion deformity rather than correcting it. This is very dangerous, as it stretches the neurologic structures, resulting in further neurologic damage.

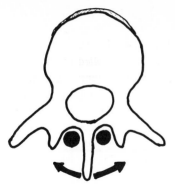

Figure 6 Rotational instability results from ligamentous injury and/or fracture in the area of the facet joints. Distraction rods produce rotational stability by impingement of the rod against articular processes and the spinous processes in the area of injury, and by the hooks superiorly and inferiorly. Using the $\frac{3}{16}$-in threaded rod as a compression device with superior and inferior hooks being placed over the laminae with a minimum of one intact lamina between the hook sites will result in a similar type of impingement on attempted rotation. The $\frac{1}{8}$-in compression rod with multiple hooks above and below is more difficult to apply and offers less resistance to rotational instability.

spine and the rod pushes anteriorly on the laminae immediately above and below the injury. To achieve reduction, the rods must be contoured to the curvature of that area of the normal spine. Failure to recognize this essential feature of the technique results in inadequate reduction, instability, and neurologic damage.

Rotational instability may be a component of any of the previously described injuries if the facet joints are fractured or if there is significant translational deformity of the anterior structures. Fracture dislocations nearly always are rotationally unstable. Rotational stability can be provided by a posterior beam lying between the spinous processes medially and the facet processes laterally, extending over several vertebral levels (Fig. 6). Both ends of the rod are attached to the spine by the hooks. Rotation associated with posterior lateral motion is prevented by the impingement of the rod on the adjacent structures.

3 BIOMECHANICAL ANALYSES OF REDUCTION AND FIXATION OF THE FOUR MAJOR CATEGORIES OF SPINAL INJURIES

In this section we present the biomechanical analyses of the Harrington rod distraction and compression systems to provide reduction and fixation of the above mentioned categories of spinal injuries. In all the analyses and equations in this section, for the purpose of quantitatively illustrating the biomechanical basis of fracture-fixation mode (without loss of generality) we assume that the injury is sustained at the L1 level and that the anatomical and anthropometric values correspond to that of a 150-lb (69-kg) man, of 5-ft 10-in (1.78-m) height.

At the site of injury a transverse section of the spine is subjected to (1) normal compressive stresses caused by the total weight of the body segment ΣW_i above the level of injury, as well as (2) flexion bending stresses caused by the flexion moment M_w due to the eccentricities x_i of these segmental weights W_i with respect to the neutral axis of the transverse spinal section (Fig. 7). Forward bending dramatically increases the bending load by increasing the lever arm x_i while correspondingly reducing the compressive force.

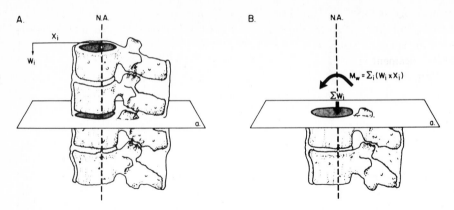

Figure 7 Loading situation on the spinal column. *A*. W_i is the weight of a body segment acting anteriorly eccentric by x_i with respect to the neutral axis of the spinal cross section *a-a* normal to its longitudinal axis *s*. *B*. The effect of the segmental body weights about the section *a-a* is a direct compression force W_i and a flexion bending moment M_w ($=\Sigma W_i x_i$).

In the normal spine the compressive stresses resulting from the flexion moment are resisted primarily by the vertebral body (and the intervertebral disk), while the resulting tensile stresses are resisted primarily by the facet joint capsules and also by the ligmentum flavum, the interspinous ligament, and the supraspinous ligament. However, in the event of ligamentous disruption (as in the case of distraction injury, Fig. 2) or vertebral body crushing (as in the case of burst fractures, Fig. 4), the spine undergoes a drastic flexion curvature under the action of the flexion bending moment induced by the eccentrically located body segment weight vector (Fig. 7), which can cause further damage to the neurological structures while also critically straining the ligamentous structures.

The Harrington rod (compression or distraction) system is designed to reduce the stress on the neurological structures and maintain the spine in as near normal form as possible. The analysis provided here will serve to biomechanically (1) illustrate this role of the Harrington rod system, (2) justify the use of the appropriate compression or distraction system, (3) determine the order of magnitude of the forces and stresses that can be induced in the implanted Harrington devices, and (4) develop guidelines for the safe prescription of the forces in the Harrington rods so as not to impair the structural integrity of the spinal structures such as the laminae, the vertebral body, and the ligaments; the guidelines depend on the nature of injury and the corresponding Harrington rod system employed to reduce it.

The analytical simulation of fractured spinal injury and correction procedure here employs very basic mechanics-of-materials formulations and should be regarded as only an initial attempt at invoking biomechanical rationale to this complex problem.

3.1 The Distraction-Dislocation Injury

As can be observed in the schematic illustration of Fig. 2, the ligamentous structures are ruptured. Consequently, under the influence of the flexion bending moment M_w induced by the body segment weights (whose lines of action are eccentric with respect to the neutral axis of the spinal cross section), as shown in Fig. 7, the spine becomes unstable (see Figs. 2 and 8) because of the inability of the posterior ligamentous structures to sustain the induced tensile stresses.

Thus the role of the Harrington rod compression system is to serve as a tension member of the now composite "spine-rod" beam structure. Now, with the Harrington compression rods in place (Figs. 2 and 8), a transverse cross section of this hybrid spine-rod beam at the dislocation site (Fig. 8) is subjected to (1) a pure compressive force ΣW_i acting at the neutral axis, and (2) a bending moment M_w caused by the eccentricities of W_i around the neutral axis. The compressive force ΣW_i induces compressive stresses in the vertebral body as well as in the rods. On the other hand, in resisting the moment M_w the compression is borne by the vertebral body while the two Harrington rods sustain the tension; an analogy may be made to bending a reinforced concrete beam where the concrete bears the compressive stress and the steel reinforcement rods bear the tensile stress.

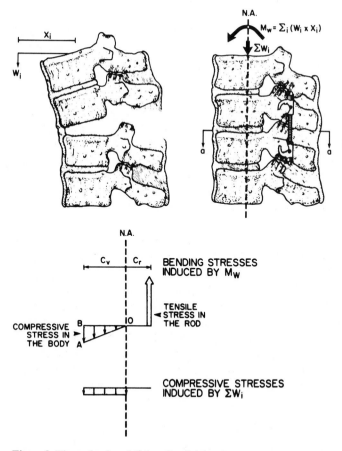

Figure 8 Biomechanics of dislocation injury.

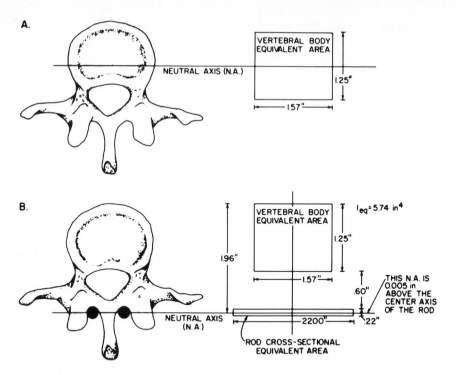

Figure 9 Equivalent bending moment resisting sections of the injured spinal segment (involving posterior ligamentous disruption) and the rod-reinforced spinal segment. Note the posterior shift of the neutral axis in the case of the reinforced section.

The higher modulus of the rods has the effect of shifting the neutral axis posteriorly (Fig. 9) and (as illustrated in the qualitative normal bending stress distribution diagram of Fig. 8) thereby reducing the value of the maximum compressive stress on the anterior edge of the vertebral body ($\sigma_{v,c}^m$ in Fig. 8) caused by the greater moment arm (OB) with respect to the neutral axis. In the absence of the rods and even if, for example, some ligamentous structures were intact, the neutral axis would shift anteriorly, thereby reducing the value of OB in Fig. 8 and concomitantly requiring a higher value of the maximum compressive stress $\sigma_{v,c}^m$ in order to provide the requisite bending resistance to M_w.

The normal bending stresses in the vertebral body and in the rods caused by M_w are obtained by sequentially carrying out the following steps.

(1) The neutral axis of the hybrid spine-rod cross section (Fig. 9b) is determined by computing the effective areas of the vertebral body and the rods, where (as shown in Fig. 9b) the lateral dimension of the rod is multiplied by the ratio of its Young's modulus to the Young's modulus of the vertebral body in compression. It is noted that (based on Fig. 9a and b) the effect of the rods is to shift the neutral axis considerably posteriorly.

(2) The moment of inertia of the hybrid spine-rod equivalent section (I_{eq}) is computed; and for the representatively dimensioned cross section (Fig. 9) the moment of inertia is 5.74 in^4.

(3) The maximum compressive stress at the anterior edge of the vertebral body is

$$\sigma_{v,c} = \frac{M_w}{I_{eq}} C_v \tag{1}$$

where $C_v = C_{v,eq}^a$ (the distance from the neutral axis to the anterior edge) $= 1.96$ in, and M_w is the sum of the moments of the segmental weights W_i above the level of the injury with respect to the neutral axis; according to Fig. 7, M_w (for L1 level of injury) varies from 32 in·lb (3.6 N m), in the case of the subject holding the back straight, to an extreme of 400 in·lb (45 N m) in the case of the subject bending forward with the back horizontal at $90°$ to the vertical. Thus from Eq. (1) the value of the maximum compressive stress in the vertebral body is given by

$$\sigma_{v,c} = \frac{M_w}{I_{eq}} C_{v,eq}^a = \frac{(400)(1.96)}{5.74} = 136 \text{ lb/in}^2 \qquad (0.94 \text{ MPa}) \tag{2}$$

which, together with $\Sigma W_i / A_{sp}$ ($\simeq 25$ psi or 0.16 MPa), is considerably less than the allowable value of 700 lb/in^2 (4.85 MPa).

(4) The average tensile stress in the rod is given by

$$\sigma_{r,t} = \frac{M_w}{I_{eq}} C_{r,eq} \frac{E_r}{E_v} \tag{3}$$

where $C_{r,eq}$ is the distance of the rod from the neutral axis of the equivalent section, and E_r / E_v is the ratio of the Young's moduli of the rod and the vertebral body. On substituting the respective values, we get

$$\sigma_{r,t} = \left(\frac{400}{5.74}\right) (0.005) \left(\frac{30 \times 10^6}{6 \times 10^3}\right) = 1742 \text{ lb/in}^2 \qquad (12.1 \text{ MPa}) \tag{4}$$

The unstrained rod is assumed to be of length equal to the distance between the intended attachment points of the rods to the laminae when the spine, adjusted by distraction to its near-normal anatomical length, is unstrained by M_w (in the absence of ΣW_i, or in its unloaded configuration); thus, the spine is stressed only when the moment M_w due to body segment weights (ΣW_i above the injured section) acts on the spine. Hence, from a design viewpoint we demand that the allowable tensile stress in the rod material $\sigma_{r,t}$ be at least twice the value of the induced tensile bending stress given by Eqs. (3) or (4), so that we need to have

$$\sigma_{r,t} \left(= \frac{M}{I_{eq}} C_{r,eq} \frac{E_r}{E_v} \right) \leqslant \frac{\sigma_{r,t}^*}{2} \tag{5}$$

Now since $\sigma_{r,t}$ was computed to be 1742 lb/in^2 (12.1 MPa), and $\sigma_{r,t}^* = 30 \times 10^3$ lb/in^2 (206 MPa), the criterion of Eq. (5) is easily satisfied.

In addition, we must ensure that the force exerted by the rod hook ($=\sigma_{r,t} \times$ rod area A_r) on the lamina does not induce a compressive force over the lamina edge, that exceeds the allowable bearing force of the lamina $P_{l,c}^*$ by a safety-factor of two, so that

$$\sigma_{r,t} A_r \leqslant \frac{P_{l,c}^*}{2} \tag{6}$$

where A_r is the cross-sectional area of the rod, and $\sigma_{r,t}$ is given by Eq. (5). For a representative rod diameter of $\frac{1}{8}$ in, where $A_r = .049$ in^2 (0.32 cm^2), and $\sigma_{r,t} = 1742$ lb/in^2 (12.1 MPa), the compressive force on the lamina equals 75 lb (332 N), which is less than the allowable compression fracture force of the lamina (about 200 lb) by a safety-factor of two.

3.2 Anterior Crushing of the Vertebral Body with Total Paraplegia

In the injury illustrated in Fig. 3, a posterior portion of the vertebral body is intact, while its anterior segment has reduced compression bearing capacity. Also, because the posterior ligaments are ruptured, a posterior compression device is inserted in order to substitute the tension-strain resisting function of the ruptured ligaments, with the intact posterior vertebral body serving as the compression member.

The main difference between this type of injury and the previously discussed distraction-dislocation injury is that in this case the compression bearing area of the vertebral body is reduced, which results in a greater compressive stress in the vertebral body and greater tensile stress in the compression rod. For analysis purposes, i.e., in order to compute the values of these stresses, we can assume a reduced total contact area (i.e., moment of inertia) of the vertebral body and reduced compression-failure stress limit; or we can assume a reduced value of Young's modulus and compression strength for the anterior crushed position of the vertebral body; or even more conservatively, we can assume that the anteriorly crushed portion should not be permitted to bear any compression and that the intact segment should bear all of the compression load.

We will adopt the last mentioned approach, which results in a reduced value of I_{eq} as well as altered values of $C_{v,eq}^a$ and $C_{r,eq}$ in Eqs. (2) and (4). Hence we ascertain that the compressive stresses sustained by the intact portion of the vertebral body and by the lamina do not exceed their allowable limits, for example, for an assumed 50 percent anterior crushing of the vertebral body.

For the purpose of analysis we assume that the effective moment resisting portion of the vertebral body is only the remaining intact posterior 50 percent portion of the vertebral body. Thus for a 90° bending, the maximum compressive stress at the anterior edge of the intact vertebral body is given by

$$\sigma_{v,c} = \frac{M_w}{I_{eq}} C_{v,eq}^a = \left(\frac{400}{3.094}\right)(1.3305) = 172 \text{ lb/in}^2 \qquad (1.189 \text{ MPa}) \qquad (7)$$

which, together with $\Sigma W_i / A_{sp}$ ($\simeq 50$ psi or 0.32 MPa), is considerably less than the allowable value of 700 lb/in^2 (4.85 MPa), thereby ensuring the structural integrity of the remnant intact vertebral body.

The average tensile stress in the rod $\sigma_{r,t}$ is given (as in Eq. (3)) by

$$\sigma_{r,t} = \frac{M_w}{I_{eq}} C_{r,eq} \frac{E_r}{E_v} = \left(\frac{400}{3.094}\right)(0.012)\left(\frac{30 \times 10^6}{6 \times 10^3}\right) = 7741 \text{ lb/in}^2 \qquad (53.8 \text{ MPa})$$
$$(8)$$

The force P exerted by the rod on the lamina is then given by

$$P = \sigma_{r,t} A_r = 7751 \text{ lb/in}^2 \times 0.049 \text{ in}^2 = 379 \text{ lb} \qquad (1678 \text{ N}) \qquad (9)$$

It is seen that this value for M_w caused by $90°$ forward bending considerably exceeds the allowable fracture force of the lamina of 200 lb. As a result, immediately after surgery and until the crushed anterior segment of the vertebral body increases its compressive strength by healing, the paraplegic patient has to be restricted to at most $30°$ forward bending, for which $M_w = 200$ in·lb and the compressive force on the lamina is $P = \sigma_{r,t} A_r = 140$ lb, which is then less than the allowable value of 200 lb. In addition, the concomitant use of appropriate bracing provides compensatory extension moment in order to reduce the value of M_w and hence reduce the crushing force on the lamina edge, thereby further stabilizing the spine. As the crushed amount of vertebral body increases, the compression resisting segment of the hybrid spine-rod cross section decreases, so that in the limiting case the rod no longer serves its role as a tension member to resist M_w in conjunction with the intact portion of the vertebral body serving as the complementary compression member. Therefore, in the case of almost complete crushing of the vertebral body (which corresponds to spinal injury category 4 of fracture-dislocation), the use of a Harrington distraction rod is recommended; this case will be discussed later.

3.3 Burst and Wedge Fractures of the Vertebral Body

In this type of injury, the vertebral body is completely crushed (Fig. 4) and is incapable of withstanding any compressive stress from the combined external loading of a compressive load W_i at the neutral axis along with a flexion moment $M_w \ (= \Sigma_i W_i x_i)$. The role of the Harrington fracture-stabilizing system is to prevent the already crushed vertebral body from sustaining any compressive stress under the action of ΣW_i and M_w. The wedge-compression fracture may be a more extreme example of this injury, but only when the posterior ligamentous structures are intact. Because the crushed vertebral body cannot provide any compression bearing area, the rods must sustain all of the compression due to both ΣW_i and M_w.

Now with the vertebral body totally crushed and incapable of resisting M_w, the neutral axis of the transverse spinal cross section moves posteriorly to the crushed body and may be assumed to lie close to the edges of the lamina. Thus under the action of the flexion moment, since the longitudinal segment of the spine through the neutral axis does not undergo strain, the lamina edges that the rod hooks are to be attached to have negligible relative displacement. However, under the ΣW_i the lamina edges will be displaced toward each other. Thus the net strain along the longitudinal edge of the lamina (or in the spinal longitudinal section through the neutral axis) is compressive (Fig. 4).

To prevent this compressive strain, in turn stabilizing the spine, and hence to prevent further compressive stress in the vertebral body, distraction rods must be implanted (as shown in Fig. 4) in order to stabilize the fractured spine after the normal spinal anatomy has been restored by surgery. The rods are implanted with the upper rod hooks passing under the lamina edges and the lower rod hooks over the lamina edges in a configuration that bears the compression caused by the attachment points displacing toward each other.

Because the crushed vertebral body is incapable of bearing compression, the distraction rods bear ΣW_i completely, while the rods and the spinous ligaments together constitute the flexion moment resisting unit (wherein the rods and the ligaments respectively function as compression and tension members).

It may be reasonably assumed that the rod carries the full compression load ΣW_i so that the distraction force in each rod is on the order of 25 lb (111 N). The M_w moment-resisting spinal cross section consists of equivalent cross sections of the rod and ligaments. Since the cross section of the ligaments is relatively negligible, it can be assumed that the rod also totally sustains the bending moment M_w. It is important that the implanted rod firmly abut against the lamina to provide rigidity to the spine and to enable the spine and the rod to deform and function as one unit under the action of the lateral forces exerted by the rod and the spine's laminae on each other (Fig. 4). Hence, if the rod is contoured to abut against the lamina, these lateral forces offer resistance to the spine to develop a destabilizing curvature in the sagittal plane; in fact, this spinal curvature or lateroposterior deflection is limited to that of the relatively stiffer rod.

To contain the spinal deformation so as to ensure the spine's fracture fixation, the rod has to be properly contoured. Further, we need to check that the compressive load ΣW_i does not exceed its buckling load value by a safety-factor of two. Then the maximum lateroposterior deflection of the spine will be limited to that sustained by the rod functioning as a beam-column under the axial load ΣW_i and end-moments M_w. We now evaluate the buckling load as well as the central or mid-span maximum lateral deflection of the rod. For the buckling load of each rod of moment of inertia I_r (based on its diameter d_r) and length l_r to be greater than its axial load $\Sigma W_i/2$ by a safety-factor of two, we need to have

$$\frac{\pi^2 E_r I_r}{l_r^2} \geqslant 2 \ \frac{\Sigma W_i}{2}$$

where E_r, I_r, l_r are the values of the rod's Young's modulus, moment of inertia, and length, respectively. For representative values of $E_r = 30 \times 10^6$ lb/in², $I_r = 1.92 \times 10^{-4}$ in⁴, and $l_r = 5.5$ in, the value of the buckling load is 1877 lb (8.35 kN), which is an order of magnitude times the body weight above the injury level, and certainly much greater than ΣW_i. Thus, there is no danger of the rod buckling.

Let us now compute the center-span (lateral) deflection of the rod (in the sagittal plane), in the role of an equivalent beam-column under the action of axial force $\Sigma W_i/2$ and the end-bending moments $M_w/2$. The associated formula for the center-span deflection (from Timoshenko [5]) is:

$$\delta_c = \frac{M_w l_r^2}{16 E_r I_r} \frac{2(1 - \cos u)}{u^2 \cos u} \tag{10}$$

where
$$u = \frac{k l_r}{2} = \frac{l_r}{2} \left(\frac{\Sigma W_i/2}{E_r I_r} \right)^{1/2} \tag{11}$$

By substituting the earlier mentioned values of E_r, l_r, I_r, we obtain the value of δ_c as 0.25 mm, which alleviates the danger of the fragmented body herniating against the spinal cord.

Finally, we can confirm that the compressive force carried by each rod, equal to P (25 lb), is much less than the compressive fracture strength of the lamina, i.e., the value of $[P/(P_{l,c}^*/2)]$ is very small.

We now analyze why when the vertebral body is only partially crushed in what may be termed a wedge type fracture of the vertebral body, the distraction rod should not be used, but instead the compression rod is needed for fracture fixation. Although this type of injury is not generally predominant, the analysis offers a solution for the more plausible case of near-complete crushing of the body. For example, if there is an intact, posteriorly located segment of the vertebral body, then the neutral axis of the spinal cross section shifts more anteriorly (relative to its location in the case of burst injury) and lies within the area of the intact portion of the vertebral body. Thus, under the combined action of the flexion moment M_w and body segment weight ΣW_i, the portion of the vertebral body anterior to the neutral axis undergoes a compression strain, while the portion of the spinal transverse cross-section posterior to the neutral axis undergoes a tensile strain.

In that situation, the lamina edges of transverse spinal cross sections on either side of the injured body (around which the rod hooks are placed) are displaced away from each other. Thus the stabilizing rod hooks have to be placed in a mode that limits this relative displacement. This implies that the rod's upper hook should be over the lamina edge while the lower hook should be under it (i.e., a compression rod is to be employed), so that when the rod's attachment sites get displaced away from each other, the rod is put in tension while limiting this displacement; concomitantly, the spine is subjected to compression.

Thus, as illustrated in Fig. 3, bilateral compression rods are recommended to provide fracture fixation and stabilization of the injured spine. The original, unstrained length of the rod is selected to be equal to the curved distance (along the edges of the laminae) between the intended points of attachment of the rod hooks, when the spine is unstrained by the flexion bending moment induced by the segmental body weight ΣW_i. When, under the influence of the flexion bending moment (M_w, Fig. 7), the spine develops a flexion curvature, the compressive rod system exerts a compressive force P posteriorly eccentric to the neutral axis of the spine segment's transverse cross section; thereby the rod is intended to exert an extension bending moment to counter the flexion bending moment M_w.

Our initial task is to analyze the hybrid spine-rod beam structure and to determine the magnitude of the compression force P exerted by each rod at its points of attachment to the laminae. Thereafter, constraint equations ensure the structural integrity of the rods, laminae, vertebral body, and the supra-spinous ligaments; i.e., they ensure that the allowable failure stresses of these components are not exceeded. We will also determine the percent limiting amount of body fracture that can be stabilized by compression rods (without the stress in the vertebral body exceeding its allowable limit with a safety-factor of two), beyond which the use of distraction rods becomes necessary.

Because the ligamentous structures are intact in the case of incomplete wedge crushing of the vertebral body, as opposed to their being ruptured as in the case of distraction-dislocation and compression of injuries previously discussed, the spinal column is stable on its own, relative even to the case of burst injury discussed earlier. The attachment of the rods in response to the external loading ΣW_i and the associated flexion moment M_w (Fig. 7) induces compressive forces on the spine at the points of attachment to the lamina. These compressive forces cannot be determined by static analysis alone; rather, compatibility of strain between the spine and the rods must be invoked to determine the magnitude of the forces.

For this purpose, we substitute the effect of the rods on the spine by compressive forces equal in magnitude but opposite in sense to those actually induced on the rods. We now invoke the compatibility criterion that under the action of the external loading (namely, the compressive force ΣW_i at the neutral axis and the flexion bending moment M_w) and the indeterminate forces P exerted by the rods on the spine, the longitudinal strain in the spine along the line of location of the rod's longitudinal axis between the points of the attachment of the rods equals the longitudinal strain in the rod.

The total longitudinal strain in the spine ϵ_{sp} is made up of the following components:

$$\epsilon_{sp}(1) = -\frac{\Sigma W_i}{A_{sp}E_{sp}} \tag{12}$$

under the action of the flexion moment M_w, where (1) I_{sp} = effective moment of inertia of the spinal cross section, consisting of the intact vertebral body and the ligaments; and (2) C_r = distance from the neutral axis of the spinal cross section of the line of location of the rod axis.

$$\epsilon_{sp}(2) = \frac{M_w}{I_{sp}E_{sp}} C_r \tag{13}$$

under the action of the flexion moment M_w, where (1) I_{sp} = moment of inertia of the spinal cross section, which incorporates the contributions of the intact vertebral body and the ligaments; and (2) C_r = distance from the neutral axis of the spinal cross section to the line of location of the rod axis.

$$\epsilon_{sp}(3) = -\frac{2P}{A_{sp}E_{sp}} \tag{14}$$

due to the rod-induced compressive forces $2P$, and

$$\epsilon_{sp}(4) = -\frac{2PC_r}{I_{sp}E_{sp}} C_r \tag{15}$$

due to the extension bending moment $2PC_r$.

By equating the total longitudinal strain in the spine along the line of location of the rod's axis to the strain sustained by the rod (equal to P/A_rE_r, where A_r = cross-sectional area and E_r = Young's modulus of the rod), we obtain [from Eqs. (12)–(15)] the following compatibility equation:

$$\left| -\frac{\Sigma W_i}{A_{sp}E_{sp}} + \frac{M_w - 2PC_r}{E_{sp}I_{sp}} C_r - \frac{2P}{A_{sp}E_{sp}} \right| = \frac{P}{A_rE_r} \tag{16}$$

For the same dimensional cross section, as considered in the case of dislocation injury, let us evaluate the above equation and compute the value of P for the case of an L1 level of injury sustained by a 150-lb man, for a number of cases with increasing amounts of fracture. For these cases the values of the quantities employed in Eq. (16) are listed in Table 2 along with the computed values of P.

Our computations show that with increasing amounts of fracture of the vertebral body, the value of the tensile strain in the spine along the longitudinal axis of the lamina (or along the axis of the rod), represented in Eq. (16) by the term

$$\epsilon_{sp}(1) + \epsilon_{sp}(2) = \frac{M_w}{E_{sp}I_{sp}} C_r - \frac{\Sigma W_i}{A_{sp}E_{sp}} \tag{17}$$

keeps increasing from a value of 3.37×10^{-2} at one-fifth vertebral body fracture to 0.215 at four-fifths vertebral body fracture. Hence, the value of P (applied by the compression rod as a compressive force on the spine) needed to maintain reduction of the injury deformation also increases from 12.8 lb (57 N) to 17.3 lb (77 N). Since in this state of vertebral body fracture the points of attachment of the rod (under the combined action of M_w and ΣW_i) must displace away from each other, the hooks must counter it by passing over instead of under the attachment point at the top end of the rod and under it at the bottom end.

However, with further fracture, the value of the compression bearing vertebral body area A_{sp} tends to zero, so that the value of the compressive strain component, $\Sigma W_i/A_{sp} E_{sp}$ in Eq. (17), becomes very large; on the other hand, the values of both C_r and I_{sp}, in the term $(M_w/E_{sp}I_{sp}) C_r$ remain finite. Thus with near-complete fracture of the vertebral body, the total strain in the spine along the longitudinal edge of the lamina (i.e., along the axis of the rod), as given by Eq. (17), switches from tensile to compressive. At this transition stage when, as shown in Fig. 10, the force in the compression rod becomes zero, it can no longer serve its intended purpose without its hooks slipping out of place, and distraction rods become necessary.

Another factor also works against using compression rods for near-complete fracture of the vertebral body; this is the value of the compressive stress in the remnant intact vertebral body segment. As a result of decreasing compression bearing cross section A_{sp}, the value of the compressive stress at the anterior edge of the vertebral body (at C_v^a from the neutral axis) due to ΣW_i, P, and M_w, namely

$$\sigma_v^a(1) = \frac{\Sigma W_i + 2P}{A_{sp}} + \frac{M_w}{I_{sp}} C_v^a \tag{18}$$

becomes very high. The compensatory tensile stress at the anterior edge of the vertebral body due to the extension moment exerted by the rod, namely

$$\sigma_v^a(2) = \frac{2PC_r}{I_{sp}} C_v^a \tag{19}$$

is then just not adequate to maintain the value of the net compressive stress $[\sigma_v^a(1) - \sigma_v^a(2)]$ from encroaching the limiting value of vertebral body failure (σ_v^*), i.e., for

Table 2 Values of quantities in compatibility equation, Eq. (16), and computed values of P for an L1 injury[a]

Fraction of vertebral body crushed	ΣW_i (lb)	M_w (in·lb)	E_{sp} (lb/in²)	A_{sp} (in²)	I_{sp} (in⁴)	C_r (in)	A_r (in²)	E_r (lb/in²)	P (lb)	$\sigma_{r,t}$ (=P/A_r)	$\dfrac{\sigma_{r,t}}{\sigma^*_{r,t}/2}$	$\dfrac{P}{P^*_{l,c}/2}$	C_s (in)	$\sigma_{s,t}$ (lb/in²)	$\dfrac{\sigma_{s,t}}{\sigma^*_{s,t}/2}$	C^a_v (in)	σ^a_v (lb/in²)	$\dfrac{\sigma^a_v}{\sigma^*_v/2}$
$\frac{1}{5}$	47.4	32.2	6000	1.57	0.165	1.19	0.098	30×10^6	10.9	112	0.0075	0.099	2.19	4.15	0.036	0.52	63.8	0.182
$\frac{2}{5}$	47.4	32.2	6000	1.18	0.083	1.07	0.098	30×10^6	12.8	131	0.0087	0.116	2.07	6.0	0.053	0.40	85.0	0.242
$\frac{3}{5}$	47.4	32.2	6000	0.98	0.057	1.01	0.098	30×10^6	13.8	141	0.0094	0.125	2.01	7.62	0.067	0.32	100.8	0.288
$\frac{4}{5}$	47.4	32.2	6000	0.78	0.038	0.98	0.098	30×10^6	15.1	154	0.0103	0.137	1.93	10.45	0.092	0.28	130.0	0.371
1	47.4	32.2	6000	0.39	0.018	0.79	0.093	30×10^6	17.3	177	0.0118	0.158	1.79	24.2	0.212	0.18	259.0	0.740

[a] $\sigma^*_{r,t} = 30 \times 10^3$ lb/in² (206 MPa); $P^*_{l,c} = 220$ lb (979N); $\sigma^*_{s,t} = 228$ lb/in² (1.57 MPa); $\sigma^*_v = 700$ lb/in² (4.83 MPa).

452

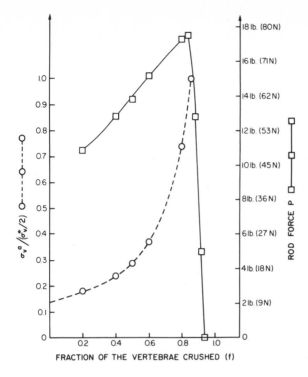

Figure 10 Variations of (1) the ratio of maximum compressive stress induced in the vertebral body to half its allowable value $[\sigma_v^a/(\sigma_v^*/2)]$, and (2) the force in the compression rod P with the fraction of vertebral body crushed.

$$\sigma_v^a = \sigma_v^a(1) - \sigma_v^a(2) \leqslant \frac{\sigma_v^*}{2} \qquad (20)$$

thereby indicating the inadequacy of the compression rod device for such a large fracture involvement. In the above equation, as the percent of fracture increases, the value of A_{sp} decreases; hence the value of the term $(\Sigma W_i + 2P)/A_{sp}$ increases, thereby suggesting a limiting value of the percent of fracture at which the value of $\sigma_v^a/(\sigma_v^*/2)$ exceeds unity. The last column in Table 2 lists the computed values of $\sigma_v^a/(\sigma_v^*/2)$ for increasing amount of fracture. Figure 10 also shows a plot of $\sigma_v^a/(\sigma_v^*/2)$ vs. the fracture fraction f for the compression rod device. Note that for $f = .85$, the compression rod yields a compressive stress in the vertebral body that exceeds $\sigma_v^*/2$, thereby necessitating the employment of distraction rods instead of compression rods.

It is worthwhile noting from the graphs in Fig. 10 that whereas for a fracture involvement greater than 85 percent the compressive stress in the vertebral body exceeds its allowable safe limit (thereby contraindicating use of the compression rod), yet until the fracture involvement reaches 94 percent there does not exist a compressive strain between the rod attachment points to permit a tension rod to remain in place. Therefore a possible solution for an almost complete fracture involvement is to use a new hook design (illustrated in Fig. 11c), which could enable the rod to function in both compression and distraction modes.

Finally, let us check that in the compression mode of fixation, the structural integrities of the laminae and the posterior ligaments are also maintained. Table 2

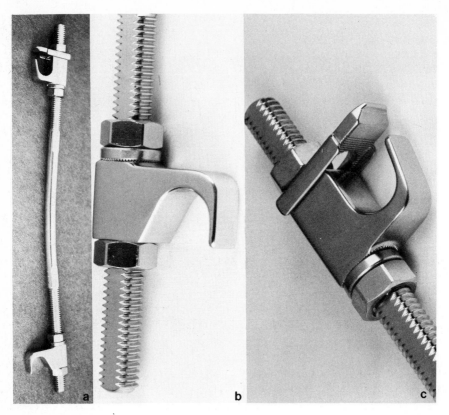

Figure 11 Spinal fixation is more rigid and stronger with this 8-mm rod. (*a*) The hooks are fixed to the rod by nuts and grooved washers keyed to the rod, preventing rotation; (*b*) the upper hook has two components; (*c*) the top locks the lamina in the hook. Patent pending.

presents the values of the ratio of the force in the rod to the force required to fracture the lamina by a safety-factor of two, namely $P/(P_{l,c}^*/2)$, which confirms the structural integrity of the lamina. Then the condition for the tensile stress $\sigma_{s,t}$ in the supraspinous ligaments not exceeding the allowable tensile stress in the ligament by a safety-factor of two is:

$$\sigma_{s,t} = \left[\frac{(M_w - 2PC_r)}{I_{sp}}\ C_s\right]\frac{E_l}{E_v} \leqslant \frac{\sigma_{s,t}^*}{2} \tag{21}$$

where (1) A_{sp} is the bearing area of the intact vertebral body cross section, (2) I_{sp} is the effective moment of inertia of the spine (i.e., the intact body and ligaments) cross section, (3) C_r and C_s are the distances from the center of the rod and the supraspinous ligaments to the neutral axis of the spine (intact body and ligaments) cross section. The computed quantities involved in the evaluation of Eq. (21) for various extents of fracture are provided in the columns of Table 2. The values of the ratio $\sigma_{s,t}/(\sigma_{s,t}^*/2)$ in Table 2 show that the stresses incurred by the supraspinous ligaments are well below their allowable limits.

3.4 Fracture-Dislocation Injury

This injury combines the severities of distraction-dislocation injuries and burst and wedge fractures of the vertebral body. Not only is the crushed vertebral body incapable of sustaining compressible stress without the fragments impinging against the cord, but also the ruptured posterior interspinous ligaments cannot sustain tensile stress. As a result, under the action of the external body segment weight ΣW_i and the resulting bending moment M_w, this spinal segment develops a significant and unstable flexion curvature. This flexion curvature is a result of the crushing of the spine's fractured and fragmented vertebral body and the con-comitant inability of the interspinous ligaments to provide resistance to the flexion bending, which endangers the cord being impinged by the fragments of the crushed vertebral body.

In order to stabilize this injury, the spine must be kept distracted while it is under the action of the external loading ΣW_i and M_w. This procedure alleviates the compressive stress on the spine, and in so doing, retracts the crushed body fragments away from the cord in an attempt to restore the normal anatomy. Thus the distraction-rod fixation mode could be adopted as in the case of burst type injury.

The analysis presented earlier for the fractured spinal fixation mode for burst fractures, by means of distraction rods acting as beam-columns, can then apply for this case also, although in this case the severity of the injury is compounded by the rupture of the supraspinous ligaments. As shown in the case of burst injury, the distraction rod functioning as a beam-column, with compression forces and bending moments applied at its ends, is stable in the upright position, but becomes more precarious as the patient leans forward. Therefore it is relevant to check if the lamina can slide out of the hook at different levels of imposed end moments and compressive loads associated with varying degrees of bending.

Assuming that the line joining the tip of the hook and the lamina edge makes an angle of $45°$ with the horizontal, we need to check if the levels of the axial force ($\Sigma W_i/2$, along the axis of the rod) and the end moment (due to the eccentricity of $\Sigma W_i/2$ with respect to the rod) on the rod, associated with varying degrees of bending (denoted by the angle α of the back of the rod axis with respect to the horizontal), will cause the angles of rotation θ (with respect to the vertical) at the ends of the rod to exceed $45°$ (thus causing the hooks to slip out). Therefore we need to ensure that the value of θ, given by the following expression from [5], is less than $45°$ (or $\pi/4$ radians):

$$\theta = \frac{\Sigma(W_i/2)(x_i \sin\alpha + h_i \cos\alpha)l_r}{2E_r I_r}\left(\frac{\tan u}{u}\right) = \frac{\pi}{4} \tag{22}$$

where

$$u = \frac{kl_r}{2} = \frac{l_r}{2}\left[\frac{\Sigma(W_i/2)\sin\alpha}{E_r I_r}\right]^{1/2} \tag{23}$$

and E_r, l_r, and I_r are the Young's modulus, length, and moment of inertia of the rod; x_i is the eccentricity of a body segment weight W_i with respect to the rod axis; and h_i is the height of a body segment above the level of the hook.

Based on Eqs. (22) and (23), it is found that for α (the angle of the bend) varying from $0°$ to $90°$, the value of the end rotation of the rod θ remains an order of magnitude less than $\pi/4$. Thus there is no danger of disengagement or slipping of the hooks. Again, a safeguard against this possibility would be to employ the hook design shown in Fig. 11c. The above mentioned beam-column role of the rods with the new hook design in totally carrying both ΣW_i and M_w is one possibility of the fraction-fixation mode. An alternative method, although surgically more involved, is a compression rod or spring acting as a tension member in conjunction with either a vertebral body graft or prosthetic plug acting as a compression member. Accordingly, a prosthetic plug could be designed to have the linear stiffness and strength characteristics of the natural vertebral body, for example, equal to 550 lb/in^2 (3.79 MPa) and 800 lb/in^2 (5.5 MPa), respectively; the tension-resisting spring could have the linear stiffness characteristics, equal to 100 lb/in^2 (0.69 MPa).

4 CLINICAL EXPERIENCE

In our series of dorsolumbar spine injuries there were 3 distraction injuries, 9 compression injuries, 32 burst fractures, and 62 fracture dislocations. As expected, there was little neurologic deficit in the first two categories of injury, but 50 percent of the burst fractures and two-thirds of the fracture dislocations had major neurologic involvement (Table 3).

Early neurologic decompression and spinal stabilization were evaluated in this study of 106 fractures of the dorsolumbar spine in 100 patients. Thirty-two patients were treated with varying periods of recumbency followed by external immobilization. Thirteen were treated with Meurig-Williams spinous-process plates. Harrington rods were used in the remaining 55 cases. The injuries were similarly distributed throughout the thoracolumbar spine for all three treatment methods (Table 4). The 58 fractures associated with "paraplegia" are those in which there was no useful motor function below the level of the lesion. The 48 ambulatory injuries were those associated with at least some useful motor function below the lesion. The proportion of paraplegic cases was nearly the same in all treatment groups.

All cases included in this study were considered to be "unstable." Our understanding of this term is somewhat different from that proposed by Holdsworth [6]. First, any injury of the dorsolumbar spine sufficiently severe to be associated with a neurologic deficit is assumed to be mechanically unsound for early ambulatory treatment without internal fixation. Second, injuries that may result in

Table 3 Distribution of injuries by type

	Distraction	Compression	Burst	Fracture dislocation
Paraplegic	1	0	17	40
Ambulatory	2	9	15	22
Total	3	9	32	62

Table 4 Distribution of injuries through the thoracolumbar spine[a]

Site	Recumbent	Meurig-Williams plates	Harrington rods
		Treatment	
T1			
T2			
	x		
T3			
	x		x
T4			
	x		xo
T5			x
T6			o
			x
T7	x		
	xo		
T8			xo
T9	x		x
	xx		o
T10			
	xxx	x	xo
			o
T11			
T12	o	o	xo
	xo		xxxo
L1	xxoo	xxxxx	xxxxxxoo
	xoo		xxxxxxxxooo
L2	xx	xxo	xo
	oo		xxo
	o		oooo
L3	xoo	o	ooooo
	x	o	
L4			xoo
	oo	o	o
L5	o		xo

[a] x = paraplegic (58); o = ambulatory (48); total injuries = 106.

neurologic damage are also considered unstable. A vertebral body fracture where the fragments might become displaced into the canal with early ambulatory treatment should be stablized to prevent neurologic injury. If there is evidence of posterior ligamentous disruption on physical examination or on x-ray, this is also an indication of instability because neurologic damage may result from increasing flexion deformity. Rotational instability can likewise lead to neurologic damage, but in most cases of rotational injury neurologic deficit is apparent initially.

The third indication of instability is an injury that may lead to "chronic instability." Although there may not be any neurologic damage initially, nor any likely to occur in the immediate postinjury period, it may develop later, owing to progressive deformity. The so-called stable compression fracture is frequently in this category, and, as pointed out by Nash et al. [7], may develop neurologic deficit. In addition, any vertebral body compression fracture involving a loss of anterior vertebral height of over 50 percent has a high likelihood of late mechanical instability. Back pain may develop at the site of the injury or inferior to the resulting gibbus, owing to a compensatory lordosis. Soreff [8] reviewed 147 compression fractures over 8 yr postinjury, and found objective physical and radiologic abnormalities correlated with symptoms and disability. Injuries in the thoracolumbar, and especially the lumbar, spine lead to greater disability than in the thoracic area. In addition, neurologic deficit may result from late progressive deformity. All these problems can be avoided by correction of the deformity and stabilization at the time of injury. Late treatment of these problems is far more difficult.

Harrington instrumentation was developed for correction of scoliotic deformities but has also been found useful in spinal injury. A 47-yr-old diabetic was involved in a collision when she lost consciousness secondary to a hypoglycemic episode. She sustained a burst fracture of L3 with loss of plantar flexion and dorsal flexion of the ankles, and some weakness of the quadriceps bilaterally (Fig. 12).

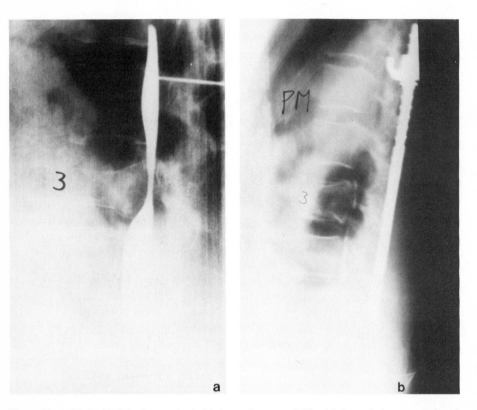

Figure 12 A 47-yr-old diabetic sustained this burst fracture of L3 with loss of plantar and dorsal flexion of the ankles and some weakness of the quadriceps bilaterally. The fracture was reduced with Harrington rods, and because of posterior ligamentous disruption, a fusion was performed across the area of injury.

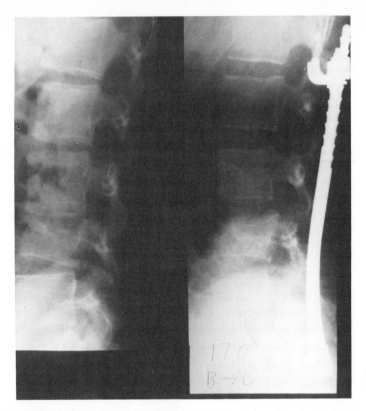

Figure 13 A 17-yr-old male sustained this burst fracture of L4 associated with slight sacral sparing. An open reduction and internal fixation with distraction rods were performed with the inferior hooks on the sacral alae. Note that the rods are contoured both anteriorly into the normal lordotic curve and toward the midline so as to apply anterior pressure on the lamina of L4.

Within 24 h, an open reduction with bilateral Harrington distraction rods was performed from L1 to L5. Because of posterior ligamentous disruption across the area of injury, a fusion was performed from L2 to L4. The patient was ambulated in a Jewett brace 2 weeks postsurgery. By 6 weeks the neurologic deficit had cleared. One year following surgery the rods were removed, and the fusion found to be solid. Three months later flexion films demonstrated maintenance of the reduction and an increase in flexibility of the spine.

A 17-yr-old male was involved in an automobile accident, resulting in paraplegia with slight sacral sparing due to a burst fracture of L4 (Fig. 13). Open reduction and internal fixation with distraction rods were performed without laminectomy or fusion. Note that the rods are contoured to the normal lumbar lordosis, providing contact with the lamina adjacent to the area of fracture. With lower-lumbar fractures, the lower hook must rest on the sacral ala, as the S1 lamina does not have sufficient strength to withstand the high stresses. In addition, square-ended rods that insert into square holes in the inferior hooks are necessary to maintain the rods in the proper position when they are contoured in this manner.

5 RESULTS OF CLINICAL STUDIES

The first reason for considering surgical treatment was neurologic decompression. Neurologic improvement was evaluated by assigning the numbers 1 through 5 to the Frankel classes A through E, respectively. The observed increase, that is, the observed minus the initial value, was divided by the maximum improvement possible, that is, 5 minus the initial value. This gives a percent recovery. For a Frankel B that improved to a D, the percent recovery would be $(4 - 2)/(5 - 2) = 66.7$ percent. As the E-group could not improve and none of the A-group cases did improve, only the B, C, and D or partial-lesion cases were considered. In no case did the neurologic function decrease. Laminectomy appeared to have no beneficial effect (Table 5). Neurologic improvement with rods was somewhat better, rather than worse, when compared with recumbent treatment (53 percent compared to 44 percent). The group treated with plates was probably too small to be considered.

The anatomical results were measured on AP and lateral x-rays. Less than 10 percent displacement and 15° of angulation in both views was considered anatomical. Over 50 percent displacement or 45° of angulation in either view was considered unsatisfactory. All other cases were considered satisfactory. In the recumbent group 82 percent of the cases were satisfactory and 14 percent unsatisfactory, with only one case anatomical (Table 6). With the use of spinous process plates the anatomical results were worse, probably due to the destablizing effect of surgery and the relatively poor fixation obtained. In contrast, open reduction and internal fixation with Harrington rods resulted in two-thirds of the cases being anatomically reduced in both the paraplegic and ambulatory groups.

The effect of treatment on rehabilitation was evaluated by studying the number of weeks required for paraplegic patients to be up in wheelchairs performing independent transfers, and for ambulatory candidates to be walking (Table 7). The use of Meurig-Williams plates had no effect on the rehabilitation of paraplegic patients, but there was some slight decrease in the time required in the ambulatory group. In contrast, Harrington-rod treatment allowed wheelchair use in half the time in paraplegic patients. Even greater improvement occurred in the ambulatory patients—walking in 2.5 weeks compared with 7.1 weeks. Thus, the overall rehabilitation time was cut from 9 weeks to 4 weeks.

The complication rate of 18 percent in the recumbent group was reduced to 7

Table 5 Percent recovery via Frankel classification

	Treatment			
	Recumbent	Meurig-Williams plates	Harrington rods	Total
Laminectomy	43%	0%	53%	50%
No laminectomy	46%	57%	53%	51%
Both	44%	50%	53%	51%

Table 6 Radiographic evaluation of fracture reduction

| | Percent | | |
| | Recumbent | Meurig-Williams plates | Harrington rods |
Result			
Unsatisfactory	$\frac{5}{34} = 14\%$	$\frac{5}{13} = 38\%$	$\frac{1}{51} = 2\%$
Satisfactory	$\frac{28}{34} = 82\%$	$\frac{8}{13} = 61\%$	$\frac{16}{51} = 31\%$
Anatomical	$\frac{1}{34} = 2\%$	$\frac{0}{13} = 0\%$	$\frac{34}{51} = 67\%$

percent in the 55 patients treated with Harrington rods. Two patients sustained pulmonary emboli; therefore, we now use prophylactic anticoagulation. In an early case treated with a sacral bar, persistent drainage developed but was resolved with implant removal. One case of hook dislodgement occurred with the use of the S1 foramina for a lower hook site. Also, the patient was inadvertently allowed to use an overhead trapeze, producing high flexion loads.

There is currently some controversy concerning the appropriate type of Harrington rod. In cases where the anterior bony column is intact such that compressive loads can be resisted, and where there is posterior ligamentous damage, compression rods appear to be a more satisfactory fixation device because they replace the injured posterior ligaments. They are also appropriately used in paraplegic patients for correcting angulation without reestablishing vertebral body height. In our series we selected compression fixation in nine cases (Table 8). As indicated by the proportion of only satisfactory reductions, this type of equipment was frequently used in paraplegic patients for correction of angulation. In using a compression rod posteriorly, it is imperative that the bone column be sufficiently intact anteriorly to support the compressive component of the eccentrically applied forces. Tomograms are frequently necessary to prove this. If the anterior column is not intact, both angulation and displacement of fragments into the canal can occur.

A question arises regarding the length of the rods and the indication for fusion. Should the rods be placed from two levels above to two levels below the area of injury with a fusion equal to the length of the rods, as recommended by Dickson et al. [9], or three levels above to three levels below with no fusion, as recommended by Peterson and Armstrong [10]? In our series, using the former method, anatomical

Table 7 Effect of treatment on rehabilitation time

| | Rehabilitation time (weeks) | | |
| | Recumbent | Meurig-Williams plates | Harrington rods |
Patients			
Paraplegic	10.5 ± 0.9	10.0 ± 0.5	5.3 ± 0.6
Ambulatory	7.1 ± 1.3	5.4 ± 2.4	2.5 ± 0.3
Total	9.1 ± 0.8	8.2 ± 0.8	4.0 ± 0.4

Table 8 Results for compression and distraction rods[a]

	Compression rods	Distraction rods	
		Fusion (2 + 2)	Short fusion or none (3 + 3)
Result			
Unsatisfactory	$\frac{0}{9}$	$\frac{0}{20}$	$\frac{0}{29}$
Satisfactory	$\frac{4}{9} = 44\%$	$\frac{6}{20} = 30\%$	$\frac{5}{29} = 17\%$
Anatomical	$\frac{5}{9} = 56\%$	$\frac{14}{20} = 70\%$	$\frac{24}{29} = 82\%$

[a]One case was unreduced.

reduction was achieved in only 70 percent of the 20 cases. By using the latter approach, with fusion confined to the area of injury in fracture dislocation, or no fusion at all in burst fracture, anatomic reduction was achieved in 82 percent of the cases (Table 8).

This apparent better control of the spinal segments has a mechanical explanation. For the fixation device to function by resisting bending, rather than simply by distraction, accurate contouring of the rod to the normal shape of the spine in the area of injury is required. The use of a straight rod in the normally kyphotic upper thoracic spine will result in overcorrection or, more likely, fracture of the lamina. In the lordotic lumbar spine the rod must be curved anteriorly into the concavity. With proper contouring the midportion of the rod exerts an anterior force on the lamina adjacent to the injury. If the vertebra subjected to this anterior force is adjacent to the one with the hook, a mere 4-mm gap between the rod and the lamina will result in $10°$ of angulation (Fig. 14). It is frequently impossible to contour the rod properly over the short distance between two adjacent vertebrae to obtain an accurate reduction. In contrast, with the "three above and three below" method, the rod can easily be contoured to obtain proper contact with the lamina. The lamina-rod error required to produce a $10°$ error in reduction is then nearly 1 cm. The lamina contact with the smooth portion of the rod, rather than the ratchet area, decreases the error; accordingly, the ratchet portion of the rod below the top hook should be as short as possible. This is because the bending moment increases linearly from the top hook to the point of contact of the rod with the lamina, and the solid portion of the rod is nearly three times stronger than the notched area.

There is another mechanical reason for using a longer internal fixation device. The rods act as a beam subjected to three-point bending stress by the superior and inferior hooks being attached to the spine and the central portion of the rod impinging on the two laminae adjacent to the area of instability. If the hook is placed into one vertebra and the rod impinges on the lamina of the immediately adjacent vertebra, as in the "two above and two below" technique, the lever-arm length to resist the bending movement is 3 cm (Fig. 15). In the "three above and three below" approach, the lever arm increases to 6 cm, resulting in a 50 percent decrease in the force applied to the bone by the fixation device. Absolute

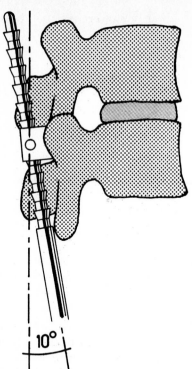

Figure 14 The better control of the spinal segment on either side of the injury with the "three above and three below" technique, as compared with the "two above and two below" method, has a mechanical basis. When the rod is in contact with the lamina two vertebrae away from the hook, a 4-mm gap may exist between the rod and the lamina of the vertebra adjacent to the hook owing to either the notches on the rod or minimal lordosis. With the "two above and two below" method, flexion would occur until the rod impinged on the lamina, resulting in 10° of angulation.

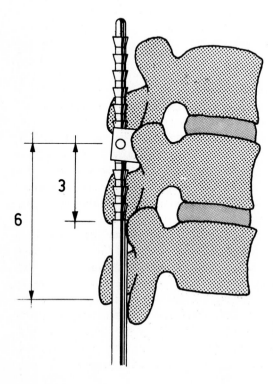

Figure 15 Use of the longer fixation technique increases the lever arm from 3 cm for two vertebrae to 6 cm for three vertebrae, thus decreasing the force applied to the bone by 50 percent. Greater bending movements can therefore be resisted with less likelihood of fracture and hook dislodgement.

463

Table 9 Levels fused

	Fused to rods	Short fusion or none	
Number of cases	20	16	13
Average number of levels fused	4.80 ± 0.29	1.41 ± 0.30	

anatomical reduction is imperative, particularly in using the distraction rod with posterior ligamentous insufficiency. Residual flexion deformity results in the force direction at the hook tending to disengage the lamina from the hook. The anterior lip of the hook must never tilt anteriorly with respect to an axial line through the vertebra.

We are also interested in maintaining spinal flexibility. When fusion was carried out over the length of the rods, the average number of levels fused was 4.8. In contrast, in the short-fusion approach the number was 1.4 levels (Table 9). The result is a more normally flexible spine. This latter technique requires a second procedure to remove the rods which is performed after a minimum of a year. In all cases thus far we have found the fusions to be solid; and flexion films following the removal of the rods have demonstrated maintenance of the reduction. We have had no cases of back pain related to the hook sites or the immobilization of the spine by the Harrington rods for the 1-yr period. In one case a patient failed to return for rod removal until 18 mo following injury, at which time one of the rods was broken. The patient had no symptoms referable to this.

6 EXPERIMENTAL DATA

Operative stabilization of dorsolumbar spinal injuries offers many advantages, but a rational selection of an appropriate implant requires knowledge of the rigidity and strength provided. Furthermore, some devices are appropriate only for certain types of injuries. In the case of flexion with varying amounts of axial load, the injuries are biomechanically divided into three types: posterior ligamentous disruption with dislocation but minimal body fracture, anterior vertebral body fracture with the posterior ligaments intact, and a combined injury resulting in both fracture and dislocation.

In posterior injuries, the anterior bone is able to transmit the compressive component, but the function of the ligaments must be replaced. With a vertebral body fracture, the opposite is the case. In combined injuries, the entire load must be transmitted by the implant in the initial postoperative period.

Studies [11] were undertaken on the internal fixation of dorsolumbar injuries produced on cadaver spines to provide quantitative data on the relative stability and strength provided by the various fixation systems.

6.1 Method

Using 40 fresh-frozen human cadaver spines, these injuries were produced at T11-12 and stabilized as follows:

Posterior injury: Weiss springs, Harrington distraction rods 3 + 3 (three vertebrae above to three vertebrae below the injury), Harrington transverse process compression system (two small hooks on transverse process of two vertebrae above and two below the injury), Roy-Camille plates, Harrington lamina compression system (medium hook on a single lamina above and below the injury)

Anterior injury: Bohler plate, single on the lateral vertebral bodies (two above and two below), Harrington distraction rods 2 + 2, and Harrington distraction rods 3 + 3

Combined injury: Harrington distraction rods, 3 + 3 and 2 + 2.

The spines were supported at T9 and L3 and loaded in four-point bending at T11 and L1 with a cross-head speed of 100 mm/min before and after injury, and then with stabilization. Angular deformation was measured by an electrogoniometer between T10-11 and L1-2. Each injury-implant condition was tested with each of 10 spines by loading to 25 N m bending moment six times and then taken to failure.

6.2 Results

The intact spines had a flexibility of $6.0° \pm 0.8°$ (mean $\pm$ SEM) under a 25-N m load. After posterior ligamentous injury, with a 10-N m bending moment, this increased to $25.3° \pm 3°$, and to $17.6° \pm 2.2°$ after anterior fracture. Combined injury resulted in $43.4° \pm 7.1°$ of deformity with no bending load. The results are tabulated in Table 10.

Posterior injury Weiss springs provided the least stability and allowed $19.8°$ of deformity with 40 N m, but did not fail. The poorest reduction occurred with the long Harrington distraction system. Both the Harrington compression system and the Roy-Camille plates provided good stability. The transverse process system failed at a much lower bending moment (47.3 N m compared with 86.2 and 87.6 N m; $p < 0.001$), and the lamina compression system absorbed the greatest energy (14.1 N m; $p < 0.02$).

Anterior injury The Bohler plate provided the poorest reduction and stability. The long Harrington distraction-rod technique gave greater stability than the short rod. Furthermore, at failure the load was one-third greater.

Combined injury Under these conditions, the improved stability of the long Harrington distraction technique was even more apparent ($3°$ compared with $19.9°$ under a 25-N m bending moment; $p < 0.01$). At failure, although twice as strong as the short

Table 10 Experimental results by injury

Implant	Stability (degrees)				Strength		
	0	5	10	25	Bending moment load (N m)	Deformation (degrees)	Energy (N m)
Posterior injury							
Weiss springs	−4.9 ± 2.5	−1.3 ± 2.7	1.5 ± 2.8	11.5 ± 2.9	40.0	19.8 ± 2.5	
Harrington distraction 3 + 3	4.0 ± 2.9	4.3 ± 3.1	5.1 ± 3.1		30.1 ± 3.3	10.9 ± 0.9	3.3 ± 1.0
Harrington compression (transverse	−5.4 ± 1.1	−4.7 ± 1.0	−4.0 ± 1.0	−2.4 ± 1.3	47.3 ± 7.8	6.7 ± 2.1	7.4 ± 2.6
Roy-Camille plate	−7.5 ± 0.7	−7.3 ± 0.8	−6.9 ± 0.8	−5.7 ± 1.0	86.2 ± 9.3	2.1 ± 1.4	9.5 ± 2.0
Harrington compression (lamina)	−8.4 ± 1.7	−8.0 ± 1.8	−7.4 ± 1.9	−5.8 ± 2.5	87.6 ± 17.0	6.0 ± 1.9	14.1 ± 2.8
Anterior injury							
Bohler plate	7.7 ± 2.1	12.4 ± 2.3	15.7 ± 2.4	19.1 ± 2.6	37.3 ± 4.0	23.8 ± 2.5	4.1 ± 0.7
Harrington distraction 2 + 2	−4.4 ± 1.5	1.1 ± 1.5	3.1 ± 1.9	5.3 ± 2.0	59.8 ± 10.0	17.4 ± 2.7	6.9 ± 1.7
Harrington distraction 3 + 3	−6.8 ± 1.6	−2.8 ± 1.5	−1.8 ± 1.4	0.9 ± 1.9	81.6 ± 10.0	13.2 ± 3.6	14.0 ± 3.5
Combined injury							
Harrington distraction 2 + 2	16.2 ± 3.7	18.1 ± 3.9	20.2 ± 3.8	19.9 ± 5.9	22.2 ± 2.4	23.8 ± 3.4	2.3 ± 0.4
Harrington distraction 3 + 3	0.2 ± 1.8	1.0 ± 1.6	2.1 ± 1.4	3.0 ± 1.0	44.1 ± 2.1	9.3 ± 1.9	5.7 ± 1.3

rod, the long rod falls far short of the strength obtained in using the same technique for anterior injuries along: bending load 44.1/81.6 N m, and energy 5.7/14.0 J.

6.3 Observations

In this study we assumed the absence of effective paraspinous muscle strength. Based on anthropometric calculations and *in vivo* human studies in progress, bending moments of 80 to 100 N m can be encountered under these conditions.

The Harrington rod requires a distraction force, usually of 40 kp, to keep the laminae on the hooks, which must be resisted by the anterior longitudinal ligament, the only remaining structure in fracture dislocations. This ligament failed at 64.2 ± 6.5 kp, with a range to as low as 49 kp. An experimental rod with a unique hook design has been developed, as shown in Fig. 11. Its lower hook is inserted through a small interlaminar opening, and the deformity is reduced. The upper hook is then driven into place, and a top "lid" placed above the upper lamina. Thus, a distraction force is not necessary to keep the laminae on the hooks. Furthermore, the hooks are locked onto the rod to prevent rotation. The upper-hook posterior pullout strength is 124 ± 13.2 kp, with only 12.5 kp of distraction. In contrast, the Harrington hook pulled out at 81.1 ± 11.4 kp with 40 kp of distraction. Thus, the problem of excessive distraction with ligament rupture and possible neurologic injury is avoided. In addition, the rod itself is four times stronger.

6.4 Conclusions

1. The Harrington lamina compression system provides maximal stability and strength for treatment of posterior ligamentous injuries of the dorsolumbar spine.
2. The long Harrington distraction-rod system affords similar stability and strength in vertebral body fractures.
3. In contrast, in fracture dislocations the long Harrington system provides superior stability but only moderate strength.
4. A new device under development avoids the high distraction forces of the Harrington rod while providing greater strength.

7 DISCUSSION

The historically accepted treatment for fractures of the dorsal and lumbar spine has been postural reduction and bed rest for 8 to 12 weeks until "stability" develops [12, 13]. Bedbrook [14] shortened this period to 6 to 8 weeks in paraplegic patients. Attempts at internal stabilization have been several. Kaufer and Hayes [15] reported 21 cases treated with open reduction, interspinous wiring, and plaster-cast immobilization for 4 mo with good results. Their type II and III injuries, 75 percent of the cases, involved vertebral body fractures, which biomechanically cannot be stabilized with only posterior tension wires. The plaster cast must be the major form of immobilization, but casts are hazardous in paraplegic patients and control only gross motion. The authors stressed that an advantage of their technique over Meurig-Williams plates was a shorter fusion. Lewis and McKibbin [16] reported 29 cases treated with Meurig-Williams plates. Their results were superior to postural reduction but had a high complication rate, 9 of the 27 requiring plate removal for pain associated with displacement. Roberts [16] reported similar results in a series of 28 paraplegic patients. Reporting on 25 patients with traumatic paraplegia, Roberts and Curtiss [18] presented a classification of fractures into three groups: wedge compression, compression burst, and rotational fracture-dislocation. The first and last groups rarely fused spontaneously and had a high incidence of instability.

Another device that functions as a posterior tension band is the Weiss spring [19], providing dynamic compression posteriorly. Obviously, this technique cannot restore normal vertebral anatomy if the vertebral body is fractured. In fact, posterior compression is quite likely to compress the fractured vertebral body further, displacing fragments into the canal and causing neurologic deficit. Furthermore, rotational stability is minimal. From a biomechanical viewpoint it should only be used for the same injuries as previously described for the compression apparatus—a relatively small portion of spinal injuries. None of these techniques really provides internal fixation, and they therefore have limited application.

All currently available anterior spinal instrumentation provides compression by tranverse vertebral body screws attached to a vertical cable or thin threaded rod. A system is being developed using a rod of sufficient diameter to allow distraction. A disadvantage of the anterior approach for spinal injuries is the inability to evaluate posterior ligamentous damage. If present, distraction will overdistract the spine, causing neurologic injury. Therefore, the anterior approach, although ideal for late neurologic decompression, has limited application to the correction of deformity and stabilization in acute trauma.

Reports of stabilization of fractures of the dorsolumbar spine with Harrington instrumentation have all shown a significant decrease in hospital morbidity and an improvement in reduction. Flesch et al. [20] reported on 40 cases, but stabilization was quite late: 70 days in cases with only instrumentation, 56 days when stabilization was performed subsequent to laminectomy, and 21 days when the two were combined. We do not agree with their technique of reduction by use of the scoliosis outrigger. This device applies distraction to the posterior structures without three-point fixation. The result may be overdistraction with an increase in the angular deformity and neurologic injury. Two of the four pseudarthroses developed in cases treated with a compression system. This surprising finding may be due to their use of the $\frac{1}{8}$-in rod with small hooks, which provides much less rotational stability than our technique using the $\frac{3}{16}$-in rod with the medium-size hooks.

A point we strongly endorse is posterior reduction first and removal of anterior fragments through the posterolateral approach if required, as in only three of our cases. A formal anterolateral approach is only necessary for late cases [21, 22]. Convery et al. [23] reported on 24 cases, 17 being paraplegic. Compression and distraction techniques were employed without regard for biomechanical principles. Dickson reported on 95 cases treated an average of 15.7 days postinjury. Although the outrigger was inserted first, they properly emphasize reduction by three-point fixation. Although the reductions were improved, neurologic recovery was no different than with treatment by closed methods. There were six broken rods, four with pseudarthroses, and six hook displacements. We strongly agree that operative reduction and stabilization should be performed as soon as possible. There is no evidence that anything is gained by waiting.

In our series [24] of 106 fractures in 100 patients, we noted improvement in neurologic status, reduction of the angular and translocational displacement, and improved rehabilitation time by treatment with Harrington instrumentation. In no case was there a deterioration in neurologic status. Immediate closed reduction is followed by operative reduction and stabilization within 24 h. Proper contouring of the Harrington rods is essential to obtaining an accurate reduction, but this point is not mentioned in any of the previous reports. In fact, Flesch et al. [20] describe a case requiring a lumbar osteotomy to restore the normal lordosis, but fail to describe its prevention by use of properly contoured rods.

Fountain et al. [25] recently reported on the problem of complications with Harrington-rod treatment in 52 cases: postoperative pain, progressive deformity, failure of instrumentation, infection, and alignment without reduction. We have had no problem with postoperative pain in our acute-fracture series, even with the use of long rods over unfused spinal segments with subsequent removal at 1 yr. The mechanical problems of progressive deformity and alignment without decompression suggest a failure to follow biomechanical principles. Both lateral operative radiographs and direct visualization through a partial laminectomy demonstrated reduction in all but three cases. We had only one hook dislodgement, one broken rod in a patient lost to follow-up until 18 mo postoperative, and no pseudarthroses. The longer-rod technique gives better control of the spinal segments and decreases the force on the bone at hook sites, contributing to our lack of pseudarthroses and only two instrumentation problems.

In spite of this progress in the stabilization of the acutely injured spine, there is still room for improvement. The Harrington instrumentation system was developed for correction of scoliosis by distraction. Spinal instability requires a device to resist high bending forces. (Note the high incidence of rod breakage and hook dislodgement reported by Dickson et al. [9].) We are developing a new system of spinal instrumentation to achieve this goal.

8 CONCLUSIONS

1. By analyzing the force applied to the spine, the structural failure can be predicted and an appropriate technique of stabilization selected. The Harrington instrumentation system can provide distraction or compression, or resist bending, as desired. Fractures, if reduced, will heal; but ligamentous disruption heals poorly and requires local spinal fusion (Table 11).

2. Operative reduction and stabilization of fracture-dislocations of the dorsolumbar spine can be performed with acceptable risk resulting in certainly no worse, and possibly improved, neurologic status, as well as a marked improvement in reduction and rehabilitation.

Table 11 Harrington instrumentation

		Stabilization	
Force	Structure	Immediate	Permanent
Compression	Anterior bone	Harrington rods, distraction	Fracture healing
Tension	Posterior ligaments	Harrington rods, compression or 3–4 point bending	Fusion
Rotation	Facet joints	Harrington rods, 2 or 3 level minimum	Fusion

3. A biomechanical analysis of the injury is essential for proper selection of a technique of stabilization.
4. The "rod long, fuse short" approach results in a more anatomical reduction and a shorter fusion, and thus a more normal spine at the completion of treatment.
5. The current Harrington instrumentation system provides a posterior compression system for use when the anterior bony column is intact, and the posterior ligaments injured. When the reverse is the case, the distraction rod is appropriate; but if both the anterior and posterior structures are injured, the Harrington distraction rod, even properly contoured to resist bending and avoiding over-distraction, is not optimal. A new device, shown in Fig. 11, has been developed to resolve this problem.

REFERENCES

1. R. Roaf, A Study of the Mechanics of Spinal Injuries, *J. Bone Jt. Surg.,* vol. 42B, pp. 810–823, 1960.
2. R. P. Kelly and T. E. Whitesides, Treatment of Lumbar Dorsal Fracture-Dislocations, *Ann. Surg.,* vol. 167, pp. 705–717, 1968.
3. S. A. Grantham, M. I. Malberg, and D. M. Smith, Thoracolumbar Spine Flexion-Distraction Injury, *Spine,* vol. 1, pp. 172–177, 1976.
4. E. S. Stauffer and J. L. Neil, Biomechanical Analysis of Structural Stability of Internal Fixation in Fractures of the Thoracolumbar Spine, *Clin. Orthop. Relat. Res.,* vol. 112, pp. 159–164, 1975.
5. S. Timoshenko and J. M. Gere, "Theory of Elastic Stability," McGraw-Hill, New York, 1961, pp. 12–14.
6. F. Holdsworth, Fractures, Dislocations, and Fracture-Dislocations of the Spine, *J. Bone Jt. Surg.,* vol. 52A, pp. 1534–1551, 1970.
7. C. L. Nash, Jr., L. H. Schatzinger, R. H. Brown, and J. Brodkey, The Unstable Stable Thoracic Compression Fracture, *Spine,* vol. 2, pp. 261–265, 1977.
8. J. Soreff, Assessment of the Late Results of Traumatic Compression Fractures of the Thoracolumbar Vertebral Bodies, Karolinska Hospital, Stockholm, 1977.
9. J. H. Dickson, P. R. Harrington, and W. D. Erwin, Results of Reduction and Stabilization of the Severely Fractured Thoracic and Lumbar Spine, *J. Bone Jt. Surg.,* vol. 60A, pp. 799–805.

10. E. W. Peterson and G. W. D. Armstrong, Immediate Reduction and Fixation of Major Spinal Fractures and Dislocations as an Aid to the Recovery of Function, *Am. Assoc. Neurol. Surg.*, Annual Meeting, San Francisco, Calif., 1976.

11. R. R. Jacobs, A. Nordwall, and A. Nachemson, Effect of Spinal Instrumentation on Dorso-lumbar Spinal Fracture Instability, *J. Biomech.*, vol. 13, p. 802, 1980.

12. H. C. Frankel, The Value of Postural Reduction in the Initial Management of Closed Injuries of the Spine with Paraplegia and Tetraplegia, *Paraplegia,* vol. 7, p. 179, 1969.

13. L. Guttmann, Spinal Deformities in Traumatic Paraplegics and Tetraplegics following Surgical Procedures, *Paraplegia,* vol. 7, pp. 38–49, 1969.

14. G. M. Bedbrook, Treatment of Thoracolumbar Dislocation and Fractures with Paraplegia, *Clin. Orthop. Relat. Res.,* vol. 112, p. 27, 1975.

15. H. Kaufer and J. T. Hayes, Lumbar Fracture-Dislocation, *J. Bone Jt. Surg.,* vol. 48A, p. 712, 1966.

16. J. Lewis and B. McKibbin, The Treatment of Unstable Fracture-Dislocations of the Thoracolumbar Spine Accompanied by Paraplegia, *J. Bone Jt. Surg.,* vol. 56B, p. 603, 1947.

17. P. H. Roberts, Internal Metallic Splintage in the Treatment of Traumatic Paraplegia, *Injury,* vol. 1, pp. 4–11, 1969.

18. J. B. Roberts and P. H. Curtiss, Stability of the Thoracic and Lumbar Spine in Traumatic Paraplegia following Fracture or Fracture-Dislocation, *J. Bone Jt. Surg.,* vol. 52A, p. 1115, 1970.

19. M. Weiss and Z. Bentkowski, Biomechanical Study in Dynamic Spondylodesis of the Spine, *Clin. Orthop. Relat. Res.,* vol. 103, p. 199, 1974.

20. J. R. Flesch, L. L. Leider, D. L. Erickson, et al., Harrington Instrumentation and Spine Fusion for Unstable Fractures and Fracture-Dislocation of the Thoracic and Lumbar Spine, *J. Bone Jt. Surg.,* vol. 59A, pp. 143–153, 1977.

21. T. E. Whitesides, Jr. and S. G. A. Shah, On the Management of Unstable Fractures of the Thoracolumbar Spine: Rationale for Use of Anterior Decompression and Fusion and Posterior Stabilization, *Spine,* vol. 1, pp. 99–107, 1976.

22. E. B. Riska, Anterolateral Decompression as a Treatment of Paraplegia following Vertebral Fracture in the Thoracolumbar Spine, *Int. Orthop.,* vol. 1, pp. 22–32, 1976.

23. F. R. Convery, M. A. Minteer, R. W. Smith, et al., Fracture Dislocation of the Dorsal-Lumbar Spine, *Spine,* vol. 3, pp. 160–166, 1978.

24. R. R. Jacobs, M. A. Asher, and R. K. Snider, Dorso-Lumbar Spine Fractures: A Comparative Study of Recumbent and Operative Treatment in One Hundred Patients, *Spine,* vol. 5, pp. 463–477, 1980.

25. S. S. Fountain, D. A. Nagel, and R. M. Jameson, Complications from Harrington Distraction Rod Fixation of Fracture-Dislocation of the Spine, *Proc. Soc. Int. Chir. Orthop. Traumatol.,* Kyoto, Japan, 1978.

INDEX